CARDIOPULMONARY ANATOMY & PHYSIOLOGY:
Essentials for Respiratory Care

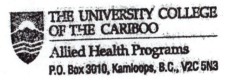

CARDIOPULMONARY ANATOMY & PHYSIOLOGY:

ESSENTIALS FOR RESPIRATORY CARE

Second edition

Terry Des Jardins, M.Ed., R.R.T.
Department of Respiratory Care
Parkland College
Champaign, Illinois

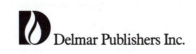 Delmar Publishers Inc.

NOTICE TO THE READER

Cover design and illustration by Precision Graphics

Delmar Staff

Executive Editor: David Gordon
Associate Editor: Adrienne C. Williams
Project Editor: Carol Micheli
Production Supervisor: Teresa Luterbach
Design Coordinator: Karen Kunz Kemp
Art Supervisor: Judi Orozco
Art Coordinator: Brian Yacur

For information, address Delmar Publishers Inc.
3 Columbia Circle, Box 15-015
Albany, New York 12212-5015

Copyright © 1993
by Delmar Publishers Inc.

printed in the United States of America
published simultaneously in Canada
by Nelson Canada,
a division of The Thomson Corporation

2 3 4 5 6 7 8 9 10 XXX 99 98 97 96 95 94 93

Library of Congress Cataloging-in-Publication Data

Des Jardins, Terry R.
  Cardiopulmonary anatomy & physiology : essentials for respiratory care / Terry Des Jardins. — 2nd ed.
    p.   cm.
  Includes index.
  ISBN 0-8273-5007-4 (textbook)
    1. Cardiopulmonary system—Physiology.   2. Cardiopulmonary system—Anatomy.   3. Respiratory therapy.   I. Title.   II. Title: Cardiopulmonary anatomy and physiology.
    [DNLM: 1. Cardiovascular System—anatomy & histology.
2. Cardiovascular System—physiology.   3. Respiratory System—anatomy & histology.   4. Respiratory System—physiology.   WF 101
D441c]
QP121.D47   1993
612.1—dc20
DNLM/DLC
for Library of Congress   92-14625
                                                                              CIP

TO JANE, JENNIFER AND MICHELLE
AND TO KEN AND ESTHER

CONTENTS

FOREWORD TO THE SECOND EDITION

When I wrote the Foreword to the first edition of Terry Des Jardins' Cardiopulmonary Anatomy and Physiology, I predicted a warm reception and continued success for that fine book. Respiratory Therapy educators agreed and this book has become a standard text in very many Respiratory Therapy Programs. Both instructors and, more importantly, students have found it informative, readable, enjoyable, and useful. No textbook can hope for more.

It is therefore with particular pleasure that I write this Foreword for the second, enlarged and improved edition of the same work. A number of minor editorial changes make it leaner and even more elegant. The three new chapters cover important areas and complement the previous edition. Several illustrations have been added and some of the illustrations from the first edition have been redrawn.

This continues to be an outstanding respiratory care text. I am very confident that the second edition will be even more popular and successful than the first one.

Terry Des Jardins has already made significant contributions to the field of respiratory care. The new edition continues to represent some of the finest educational material ever produced for this exciting and demanding health profession.

Thomas J. DeKornfeld, M.D.

PREFACE

This text is designed to provide students of respiratory care with accurate and complete information about the structure and function of the respiratory system. The book assumes no previous knowledge of respiratory anatomy or physiology. Great efforts have been made to present a comprehensive overview of the subject matter in an organized, interesting, and readable manner. The overall structure of and approach to the book is based upon both my experiences as an educator of respiratory anatomy and physiology since 1973 and on the many things I have learned from my students. In response to personal experiences and to helpful suggestions, I have employed the following pedagogic approach.

Knowledge of a *structure* is essential to the understanding of the *function* of that structure. It therefore makes little sense to present students with physiologic details without first establishing a solid foundation in anatomy. Since most college-level anatomy courses spend only a limited amount of time on the cardiopulmonary system, respiratory care educators generally had to cover this subject themselves. In regard to a suitable textbook, however, educators have usually found the cardiopulmonary section of college-level anatomy and physiology texts too introductory in nature. On the other hand, textbooks concentrating solely on the respiratory system have, historically, been too complex or esoteric.

To offset this problem, **Chapter One** provides the student with a thorough discussion of anatomic structures associated with the respiratory system. This chapter also features a large number of illustrations. The visual impact of this chapter is intended to: (1) involve the student in the learning process, (2) stimulate interest in the subject, (3) facilitate the rapid visualization of anatomic structures, and (4) help the student relate classroom knowledge to clinical experiences.

Chapters Two through **Ten** provide the major concepts and mechanisms of respiratory physiology. The discussions are comprehensive, logically organized, and, most importantly, presented at a level suitable for the average college student. When appropriate, anatomic and physiologic principles are applied to common clinical situations to enhance understanding and retention (e.g., the gas transport studies and their clinical applications to the patient's hemodynamic status). In addition, a large number of line drawings and tables appear throughout these chapters to assist in the understanding of basic principles. Chapters Two, Three, Seven, and Nine feature several unique line drawings that relate familiar visual concepts to standard graphs and nomograms. While I have found that these are often difficult for students to understand, it is important to stress that the physiology literature uses graphs and nomograms extensively to impart information.

Chapter Eleven provides the reader with the major anatomic structures and physiologic mechanisms associated with fetal and newborn gas exchange and circulation. It presents the basic cardiopulmonary foundation required to understand fetal and neonatal respiratory disorders.

Chapter Twelve presents the structure and function of the renal system. It then discusses the major cardiopulmonary problems that develop when the renal system fails.

This chapter is particularly important for respiratory care practitioners working with patients in critical care units.

Chapter Thirteen describes changes that occur in the cardiopulmonary system with age. Because the older age groups are expected to increase each year until about the year 2050, basic knowledge of this material will become increasingly important to respiratory care practitioners.

Chapter Fourteen presents the effects of exercise on the cardiopulmonary system. During heavy exercise, the components of the cardiopulmonary system may be stressed to their limits. Cardiac patients involved in exercise training after myocardial infarction, demonstrate a significant reduction in mortality and major cardiac mishaps. As our older population increases, cardiovascular rehabilitation programs will become increasingly more important to respiratory care practitioners.

Chapter Fifteen describes the effects of high altitude on the cardiopulmonary system. It provides a better understanding of chronic oxygen deprivation, which can then be applied to the treatment of chronic hypoxia caused by lung disease.

Chapter Sixteen provides an overview of high-pressure environments and their effect on the cardiopulmonary system. High-pressure environments have a profound effect on the cardiopulmonary system. The therapeutic administration of oxygen at increased ambient pressures (hyperbaric medicine) is now being used to treat a number of pathologic conditions.

At the end of each chapter there is a set of self-assessment questions designed to facilitate learning and retention. A glossary is included at the end of the text.

Finally, **Appendices** cover symbols and abbreviations, as well as units of measurement, commonly used in respiratory physiology. Also included is a nomogram that can be copied and laminated for use as a handy clinical reference tool in the interpretation of specific arterial blood gas abnormalities.

A student workbook and an instructor's guide are available from Delmar Publishers Inc. to supplement this text.

ACKNOWLEDGMENTS

A number of individuals provided important and valuable contributions in the development of the second edition of this textbook. Again, I am most thankful to Dr. Thomas DeKornfeld for his time and constructive criticism regarding the three new chapters presented in this textbook. It should also be noted that Dr. DeKornfeld spent a great deal of time in re-reading, and re-editing, the manuscript of the first edition. The numerous editorial changes provided by Dr. DeKornfeld have truly made this textbook leaner, more elegant, and student friendly.

For valuable criticism and suggestions regarding the depth, breadth, and accuracy of the manuscript and artwork for the second edition of this textbook, I extend a most sincere thank you to the following respiratory care educators: Bruce Colbert, M.S., R.R.T., University of Pittsburg at Johnstown; William A. Young, M.S., R.R.T., Amarillo College, Texas; Becky Evans, Tulsa Junior College; and Judy Bodzioney, Pima Medical Institute; The educational perspective of these individuals was very helpful.

Special mention and gratitude go to Adrianne Williams of Delmar Publishers Inc. for her help and efforts during the development of the second edition of this textbook and, importantly, in securing the clearance to redraw and improve upon a number of illustrations that were presented in the first edition. Finally, but by no means least, I extend a very special thank-you to Brian Yacur, Art/Design Coordinator, for the outstanding artwork provided by his department. The artwork illustrated in this textbook strongly facilitates the visualization—and understanding—of the material presented.

Terry Des Jardins, M.Ed., R.R.T.

CHAPTER 1

THE ANATOMY OF THE RESPIRATORY SYSTEM

OBJECTIVES

By the end of this chapter, the student should be able to:

1. List the following three major components of the upper airway:
   —Nose
   —Oral cavity
   —Pharynx
2. List the following three primary functions of the upper airway:
   —Conductor of air
   —Prevent aspiration
   —Area for speech and smell
3. List the following three primary functions of the nose:
   —Filter
   —Humidify
   —Warm
4. Identify the following structures that form the outer portion of the nose:
   —Nasal bones
   —Frontal process of the maxilla bone
   —Lateral nasal cartilage
   —Greater alar cartilage
   —Lesser alar cartilage
   —Septal cartilage
   —Fibrous fatty tissue
5. Identify the following structures that form the internal portion of the nose:
   —Nasal septum
     • Perpendicular plate of the ethmoid bone
     • Vomer
     • Septal cartilage
   —Nasal bones
   —Frontal process of maxilla bone
   —Cribriform plate of the ethmoid bone
   —Palatine process of the maxilla

—Palatine bones
—Soft palate
—Nares
—Vestibule
—Vibrissae
—Stratified squamous epithelium
—Pseudostratified ciliated columnar epithelium
—Turbinates (conchae)
  • Superior
  • Middle
  • Inferior
—Paranasal sinuses
  • Maxillary
  • Frontal
  • Ethmoid
  • Sphenoid
—Olfactory region
—Choanae

6. Identify the following structures of the oral cavity:
—Vestibule
—Hard palate
  • Palatine process of the maxilla
  • Palatine bones
—Soft palate
—Uvula
—Levator veli palatine muscle
—Palatopharyngeal muscles
—Stratified squamous epithelium
—Palatine arches
  • Palatoglossal arches
  • Palatopharyngeal arches
—Palatine tonsils

7. Identify the location and structure of the following:
—Nasopharynx
  • Pseudostratified ciliated columnar epithelium
  • Pharyngeal tonsils (adenoids)
  • Eustachian tubes
—Oropharynx
  • Lingual tonsils
  • Stratified squamous epithelium
—Laryngopharynx
  • Esophagus

(*continued*)

- Epiglottis
- Aryepiglottic folds
- Pyriform sinuses
- Stratified squamous epithelium

8. Identify the following cartilages of the larynx:
   —Epiglottis
   —Thyroid cartilage
   —Cricoid cartilage
   —Arytenoid cartilages
   —Corniculate cartilages
   —Cuneiform cartilages

9. Identify the structure and function of the following components of the interior portion of the larynx:
   —False vocal folds
   —True vocal folds
   —Vocal ligament
   —Glottis (rima glottis)
   —Epithelial lining above and below the vocal cords

10. Identify the structure and function of the following laryngeal muscles:
    —Extrinsic muscles
    - Infrahyoid group
      ○ Sternohyoid
      ○ Sternothyroid
      ○ Thyrohyoid
      ○ Omohyoid
    - Suprahyoid group
      ○ Stylohyoid
      ○ Mylohyoid
      ○ Digastric
      ○ Geniohyoid
      ○ Stylopharyngeus
    —Intrinsic muscles
    - Posterior cricoarytenoid
    - Lateral cricoarytenoid
    - Transverse arytenoid
    - Thyroarytenoid
    - Cricothyroid

11. Describe the following ventilatory functions of the larynx:
    —Primary function
    —Secondary function (Valsalva's Maneuver)

12. Describe the histology of the tracheobronchial tree, including the following components:

—Components of the epithelial lining (upper and lower airways)
- Pseudostratified ciliated columnar epithelium
- Basement membrane
- Basal cells
- Mucous blanket
  - Sol layer
  - Gel layer
- Goblet cells
- Bronchial glands (submucosal glands)
- Mucociliary transport mechanism
—Components of the lamina propria
- Blood vessels
- Lymphatic vessels
- Branches of the vagus nerve
- Smooth muscle fibers
- Peribronchial sheath
- Mast cells
  - Immunologic mechanism
—Cartilaginous layer
13. Identify the location (generation) and structure of the following *cartilaginous* airways:
—Trachea
—Carina
—Main stem bronchi
—Lobar bronchi
—Segmental bronchi
—Subsegmental bronchi
14. Identify the location (generation) and structure of the following *noncartilaginous* airways:
—Bronchioles
—Terminal bronchioles
- Canals of Lambert
- Clara cells
15. Describe how the cross-sectional area of the tracheobronchial tree changes from the trachea to the terminal bronchioles.
16. Describe the structure and function of the following components of bronchial blood supply:
—Bronchial arteries
—Azygos veins
—Hemizygous veins
—Intercostal veins

(continued)

3

17. Describe the structure and function of the following sites of gas exchange:
    —Respiratory bronchioles
    —Alveolar ducts
    —Alveolar sacs
    —Primary lobule
      • Acinus
      • Terminal respiratory unit
      • Lung parenchyma
      • Functional units
18. Discuss the structure and function of the following components of the alveolar epithelium:
    —Alveolar cell types
      • Type I cell (squamous pneumocyte)
      • Type II cell (granular pneumocyte)
    —Pulmonary surfactant
    —Pores of Kohn
    —Alveolar macrophages (Type III alveolar cells)
19. Describe the structure and function of the interstitium, including the:
    —Tight space
    —Loose space
20. Describe the structure and function of the following components of the pulmonary vascular system:
    —Arteries
      • Tunica intima
      • Tunica media
      • Tunica adventitia
    —Arterioles (Resistance vessels)
      • Endothelial layer
      • Elastic layer
      • Smooth muscle fibers
    —Capillaries
      • Single squamous epithelial layer
    —Venules and veins (Capacitance vessels)
21. Describe the structure and function of the following components of the lymphatic system:
    —Lymphatic vessels
    —Lymphatic nodes
    —Juxta-alveolar lymphatic vessels
22. Describe how the following components of the autonomic nervous system relate to the neural control of the lungs:
    —Sympathetic nervous system
      • Neural transmitters
      • Epinephrine

- Norepinephrine
- Receptors
  - Beta$_2$ receptors
  - Alpha receptors
—Parasympathetic nervous system
- Neural transmitters
  - Acetylcholine

23. Identify the effect the sympathetic and parasympathetic nervous system have on the following:
—Heart
—Bronchial smooth muscle
—Bronchial glands
—Salivary glands
—Stomach
—Intestines
—Eye

24. Identify the following structures of the lungs:
—Apex of the lungs
—Base of the lungs
—Mediastinal border
—Hilum
—Specific right lung structures
- Upper lobe
- Middle lobe
- Lower lobe
- Oblique fissure
- Horizontal fissure
Specific left lung structures
- Upper lobe
- Lower lobe
- Oblique fissure

25. Identify the following lung segments from the anterior, posterior, lateral, and medial views:
—Right lung segments
- Upper lobe
  - Apical
  - Posterior
  - Anterior
- Middle lobe
  - Lateral
  - Medial
- Lower lobe

(*continued*)

- Superior
- Medial basal
- Anterior basal
- Lateral basal
- Posterior basal

—Left lung segments
- Upper lobe
  - Upper division
    1) Apical-posterior
    2) Anterior
  - Lower division (lingular)
    1) Superior lingula
    2) Inferior lingula
- Lower lobe
  - Superior
  - Anteromedial
  - Lateral basal
  - Posterior basal

26. Identify the following components of the mediastinum:
    —Trachea
    —Heart
    —Major blood vessels
    —Nerves
    —Esophagus
    —Thymus gland
    —Lymph nodes

27. Identify the following components of the pleural membranes:
    —Parietal pleurae
    —Visceral pleurae
    —Pleural cavity

28. Identify the following components of the thorax:
    —Thoracic vertebrae
    —Sternum
      - Manubrium
      - Body
      - Xyphoid process
    —True ribs
    —False ribs
    —Floating ribs

29. Describe the structure and function of the diaphragm and include the following:
    —Hemidiaphragms
    —Central tendon
    —Phrenic nerves

—Lower thoracic nerves
30. Describe the structure and function of the following accessory muscles of inspiration:
    —Scalene muscles
    —Sternocleidomastoid muscles
    —Pectoralis major muscles
    —Trapezius muscles
    —External intercostal muscles
31. Describe the structure and function of the following accessory muscles of expiration:
    —Rectus abdominis muscles
    —External abdominis oblique muscles
    —Internal abdominus oblique muscles
    —Transversus abdominis muscles
    —Internal intercostal muscles
32. Complete the self-assessment questions at the end of this chapter.

THE UPPER AIRWAY

The upper airways consists of the **nose, oral cavity**, and **pharynx** (Figure 1–1). The primary functions of the upper airway are (1) to act as a conductor of air, (2) to prevent foreign materials from entering the tracheobronchial tree, and (3) to serve as an important area involved in speech and smell.

The Nose

The primary functions of the nose are to *filter, humidify,* and *warm* inspired air. The nose is also important as the site for the sense of smell and to generate resonance in phonation.

The outer portion of the nose is composed of bone and cartilage. The upper third of the nose (the bridge) is formed by the **nasal bones** and the **frontal process of the maxilla**. The lower two-thirds consist of the **lateral nasal cartilage**, the **greater alar cartilage**, the **lesser alar cartilages**, the **septal cartilage**, and some **fibrous fatty tissue** (Figure 1–2, page 9).

In the internal portion of the nose there is a partition, the **nasal septum**, that separates the nasal cavity into two approximately equal chambers. Posteriorly, the

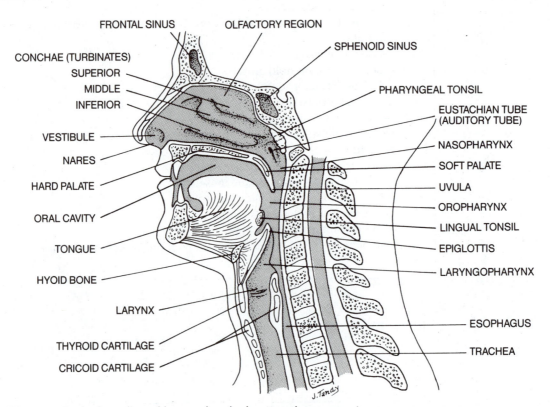

FIGURE 1–1.   Sagittal section of human head, showing the upper airway.

nasal septum is formed by the **perpendicular plate of the ethmoid bone** and the **vomer**. Anteriorly, the septum is formed by the **septal carilage**. The roof of the nasal cavity is formed by the **nasal bones**, the **frontal process of the maxilla**, and the **cribriform plate of the ethmoid bone**. The floor is formed by the **palatine process of the maxilla** and by the **palatine bones**—the same bones that form the hard palate of the roof of the mouth. The posterior section of the nasal cavity floor is formed by the superior portion of the **soft palate** of the oral cavity, which consists of a flexible mass of densely packed collagen fibers (Figure 1–3, page 10).

Air enters the nasal cavity through the two openings formed by the septal cartilage and the alae nasi, called the **nares**, or **nostrils**. Initially, the air passes through a slightly dilated area, called the **vestibule**, which contains hair follicles called **vibrissae** (see Figure 1–1). The vibrissae function as a filter and are the tracheobronchial tree's first line of defense. **Stratified squamous epithelium** (nonciliated) lines the anterior one-third of the nasal cavity (Figure 1–4A, page 11). The posterior two-thirds of the nasal cavity are lined with **pseudostratified ciliated columnar epithelium** (Figure 1–4B). The cilia propel nasal mucus toward the nasopharynx.

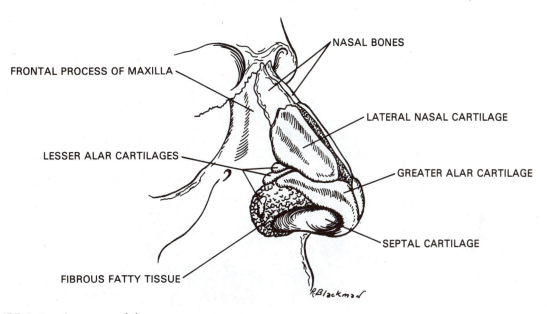

NASAL BONES

FRONTAL PROCESS OF MAXILLA

LATERAL NASAL CARTILAGE

LESSER ALAR CARTILAGES

GREATER ALAR CARTILAGE

SEPTAL CARTILAGE

FIBROUS FATTY TISSUE

RBlackman

FIGURE 1–2. Structure of the nose.

There are three bony protrusions on the lateral walls of the nasal cavity, called the **superior, middle**, and **inferior nasal turbinates**, or **conchae**. The turbinates separate inspired gas into several different airstreams. This action, in turn, increases the contact area between the inspired air and the warm, moist surface of the nasal mucosa. The turbinates play a major role in the humidification and warming of inspired air (see Figure 1–1).

Beneath the superior and middle turbinates are the openings of the **paranasal sinuses**. The paranasal sinuses are air-filled cavities in the bones of the skull that communicate with the nasal cavity. The paranasal sinuses include the **maxillary, frontal, ethmoid**, and **sphenoid sinuses** (Figure 1–5, page 12). The paranasal sinuses provide mucus for the nasal cavity and act as resonating chambers for the production of sound. The receptors for the sense of smell are located in the **olfactory region**, which is near the superior and middle turbinates (see Figure 1–1). The two nasal passageways between the nares and the nasopharynx are also called the **choanae**.

Oral Cavity

The oral cavity is considered an accessory respiratory passage. It consists of the **vestibule**, which is the small outer portion between the teeth (and gums) and lips, and a larger section behind the teeth and gums that extends back to the oral pharynx (Figure 1–6, page 13). The oral cavity houses the anterior two-thirds of

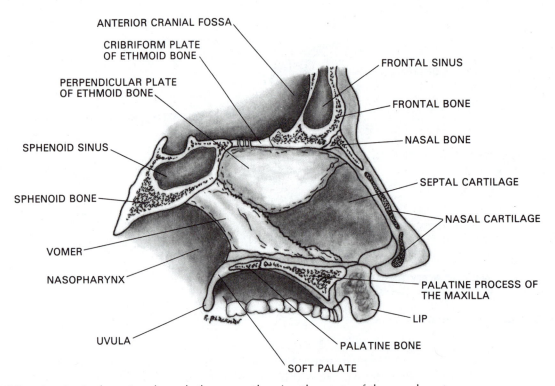

ANTERIOR CRANIAL FOSSA

CRIBRIFORM PLATE
OF ETHMOID BONE

PERPENDICULAR PLATE
OF ETHMOID BONE

SPHENOID SINUS

SPHENOID BONE

VOMER

NASOPHARYNX

UVULA

FRONTAL SINUS

FRONTAL BONE

NASAL BONE

SEPTAL CARTILAGE

NASAL CARTILAGE

PALATINE PROCESS OF
THE MAXILLA

LIP

PALATINE BONE

SOFT PALATE

FIGURE 1–3. Sagittal section through the nose, showing the parts of the nasal septum.

the tongue. The posterior one-third of the tongue is attached to the hyoid bone and
the mandible in the pharynx.

The roof the mouth is formed by the **hard** and **soft palate**. The hard palate is
composed of the **palatine process of the maxilla** and the **palatine bones** (see
Figure 1–3). The **soft palate** consists of a flexible mass of densely packed collagen
fiber that projects backward and downward, ending in the soft, fleshy structure
called the **uvula** (see Figure 1–6). The soft palate closes off the opening between
the nasal and oral pharynx by moving upward and backward during swallowing,
sucking, and blowing and during the production of certain speech sounds. The
levator veli palatinum muscle elevates the soft palate, and the **palatopharyngeal muscles** draw the soft palate forward and downward. The oral cavity is lined
with **stratified squamous epithelium** (nonciliated) (see Figure 1–4A).

Two folds of mucous membrane pass along the lateral borders of the
posterior portion of the oral cavity. These folds form the **palatoglossal arch** and
the **palatopharyngeal arch**, named after the muscles that they cover. Collectively, these arches are called the **palatine arches**. The **palatine tonsils** (faucial)
are located between the palatine arches on each side of the oral cavity. The palatine

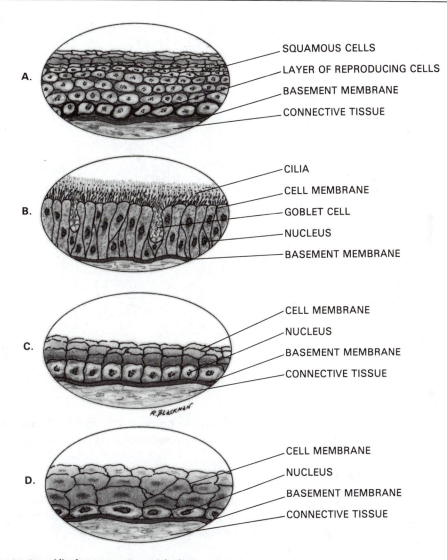

FIGURE 1–4. **A)** **Stratified squamous epithelium** consists of several layers of cells. This tissue is found in the anterior portion of the nasal cavity, oral cavity, oropharynx, and laryngopharynx. **B)** **Pseudostratified columnar epithelium** with cilia appears stratified, because the nuclei of the cells are located at different levels. These cells have microscopic hairlike projections called cilia that extend from the outer surface. Mucus-producing goblet cells are also found throughout this tissue. Pseudostratified columnar ciliated epithelium lines the posterior two-thirds of the nasal cavity and the tracheobronchial tree. **C)** **Simple cuboidal epithelium** consists of a single layer of cube-shaped cells. These cells are found in the bronchioles. **D)** **Simple squamous epithelium** consists of a single layer of thin, flattened cells with broad and thin nuclei. Substances such as oxygen and carbon dioxide readily pass through this type of tissue. These cells form the walls of the alveoli and the pulmonary capillaries that surround the alveoli.

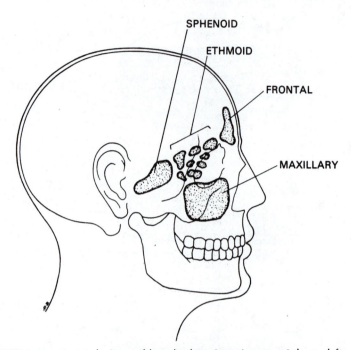

FIGURE 1–5. Lateral view of head, showing sinuses. Adapted from Short, *Essential Anatomies: Oral and Head/Neck,* © 1987 by Delmar Publishers Inc.

tonsils, like the pharyngeal tonsils or nasopharynx adenoids, are **lymphoid tissues** and are believed to serve certain protective functions (see Figure 1–6).

The Pharynx

After the inspired air passes through the nasal cavity, it enters the **pharynx**. The pharynx is divided into three parts: the **nasopharynx**, the **oropharynx**, and the **laryngopharynx** (see Figure 1–1).

Nasopharynx. The nasopharynx is located posterior to the nasal cavity and superior to the soft palate at the back of the oral cavity. The nasopharynx is lined with **pseudostratified ciliated columnar epithelium** (see Figure 1–4*B*). Lymphoid tissues called **pharyngeal tonsils**, or **adenoids**, are located in the posterior nasopharynx (see Figure 1–1). An opening for the **eustachian tube** (auditory tube) is located on the two lateral surfaces of the nasopharynx. The eustachian tube connects the nasopharynx to the middle ear and serves to equalize the pressure in the middle ear.

Oropharynx. The oropharynx lies between the soft palate superiorly and the base of the tongue inferiorly (see Figure 1–1). There is also a mass of lymphoid

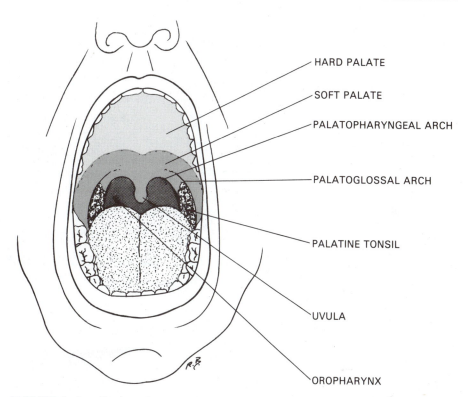

HARD PALATE

SOFT PALATE

PALATOPHARYNGEAL ARCH

PALATOGLOSSAL ARCH

PALATINE TONSIL

UVULA

OROPHARYNX

FIGURE 1–6. Oral cavity.

tissue located at the root of the tongue called the **lingual tonsil**. The mucosa of the oropharynx is composed of **stratified squamous epithelium** (nonciliated) (see Figure 1–4A).

Laryngopharynx. The laryngopharynx lies between the base of the tongue and the entrance to the **esophagus** (see Figure 1–1). The **epiglottis** is directly anterior to the laryngopharynx. The **aryepiglottic folds** form the lateral borders of the laryngopharynx. The laryngopharynx is lined with **stratified squamous epithelium** (nonciliated) (see Figure 1–4A).

THE LOWER AIRWAYS

The Larynx

The **larynx**, or voice box, is located between the base of the tongue and the upper end of the trachea (Figure 1–7). The larynx is commonly described as a

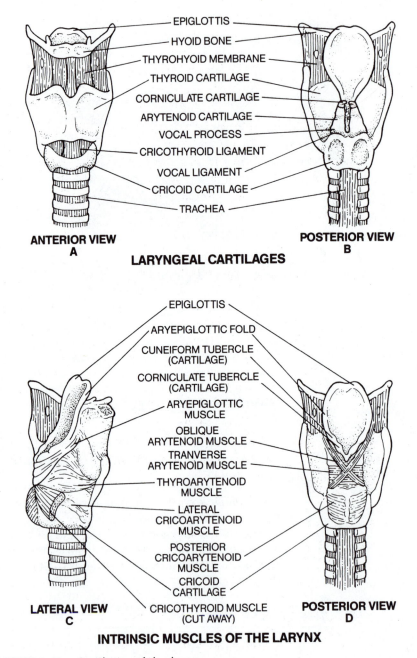

EPIGLOTTIS
HYOID BONE
THYROHYOID MEMBRANE
THYROID CARTILAGE
CORNICULATE CARTILAGE
ARYTENOID CARTILAGE
VOCAL PROCESS
CRICOTHYROID LIGAMENT
VOCAL LIGAMENT
CRICOID CARTILAGE
TRACHEA

ANTERIOR VIEW
A

POSTERIOR VIEW
B

LARYNGEAL CARTILAGES

EPIGLOTTIS
ARYEPIGLOTTIC FOLD
CUNEIFORM TUBERCLE
(CARTILAGE)
CORNICULATE TUBERCLE
(CARTILAGE)
ARYEPIGLOTTIC
MUSCLE
OBLIQUE
ARYTENOID MUSCLE
TRANVERSE
ARYTENOID MUSCLE
THYROARYTENOID
MUSCLE
LATERAL
CRICOARYTENOID
MUSCLE
POSTERIOR
CRICOARYTENOID
MUSCLE
CRICOID
CARTILAGE

LATERAL VIEW
C

CRICOTHYROID MUSCLE
(CUT AWAY)

POSTERIOR VIEW
D

INTRINSIC MUSCLES OF THE LARYNX

FIGURE 1–7. Cartilages of the larynx.

vestibule opening into the trachea from the pharynx. The larynx serves three functions: (1) it acts as a passageway of air between the pharynx and the trachea, (2) it works as a protective mechanism against the aspiration of solids and liquids, and (3) it generates sounds for speech.

Cartilages of the Larynx. The larynx consists of a framework of nine cartilages. Three are single cartilages: the **thyroid, cricoid cartilages**, and the **epiglottis**. Three are paired cartilages: the **arytenoid, corniculate**, and **cuneiform cartilages** (see Figure 1–7*A, B*). The cartilages of the larynx are held in position by ligaments, membranes, and **intrinsic** and **extrinsic muscles**. The interior of the larynx is lined with mucous membrane.

The **thyroid cartilage** (commonly called the Adam's apple) is the largest cartilage of the larynx. It is a double-winged structure that spreads over the anterior portion of the larynx. Along its superior border is a V-shaped notch, the **thyroid notch**. The upper portion of the thyroid cartilage is suspended from the horseshoe-shaped **hyoid bone** by the **thyrohyoid membrane**. Technically, the hyoid bone is not a part of the larynx.

The **epiglottis** is a broad, spoon-shaped fibrocartilaginous structure. Its base is attached to the medial surface of the thyroid cartilage, and it is free on its other borders. The epiglottis and the base of the tongue are connected by mucous membrane. The epiglottis prevents the aspiration of foods and liquids by covering the opening of the larynx during swallowing.

The **cricoid cartilage** is shaped like a signet ring. It is located inferior to the thyroid cartilage and forms a large portion of the posterior wall of the larynx. The inferior border of the cricoid cartilage is attached to the first C-shaped cartilage of the trachea.

The paired **arytenoid cartilages** are shaped like a three-sided pyramid. The base of each arytenoid cartilage rests on the superior surface of the posterior portion of the cricoid cartilage. The apex of each arytenoid cartilage curves posteriorly and medially and flattens for articulation with the corniculate cartilages. At the base of each arytenoid cartilage is a projection called the **vocal process**. The **vocal ligaments**, which form the medial portion of the vocal folds, attach to the vocal process.

The paired **cuneiform cartilages** and **corniculate cartilages** are small accessory cartilages that are closely associated with the arytenoid cartilages. The cuneiform cartilages are embedded within the aryepiglottic folds that extend from the apices of the arytenoid cartilages to the epiglottis. They probably act to stiffen the folds. The two corniculate cartilages lie on top of the arytenoid cartilages.

Interior of the Larynx. The interior portion of the larynx is lined by a mucous membrane that forms two pairs of folds that protrude inward. The upper pair are called the **false vocal folds**, since they play no role in vocalization. The lower pair functions as the **true vocal folds** (vocal cords). The medial border of each vocal fold is composed of a strong band of elastic tissue called the **vocal ligament**. Anteriorly, the vocal cords attach to the posterior surface of the thyroid cartilage. Posteriorly, the vocal folds attach to the vocal process of the arytenoid cartilage. The arytenoid cartilages can rotate about a vertical axis through the cricoarytenoid joint, allowing the medial border to move anteriorly or posteriorly. This action, in turn, loosens or tightens the true vocal cords.

The space between the true vocal cords is termed the **rima glottidis** or, for ease of reference, the **glottis** (Figure 1–8). In the adult the glottis is the narrowest point in the larynx. In the infant the cricoid cartilage is the narrowest point.

Above the vocal cords, the laryngeal mucosa is composed of **stratified squamous epithelium** (nonciliated) (see Figure 1–4A). Below the vocal cords, the laryngeal mucosa is covered by **pseudostratified columnar epithelium** (see Figure 1–4B).

Laryngeal Musculature.   The muscles of the larynx consist of the **extrinsic** and **intrinsic** muscle groups. The extrinsic muscles are subdivided into an **infrahyoid** and a **suprahyoid** group. The infrahyoid group consists of the **sternohyoid, sternothyroid, thyrohyoid**, and **omohyoid muscles**. These muscles pull the larynx and hyoid bone down to a lower position in the neck. The suprahyoid group consists of the **stylohyoid, mylohyoid, digastric, geniohyoid**, and **stylopharyngeus muscles**. These muscles pull the hyoid bone forward, upward, and

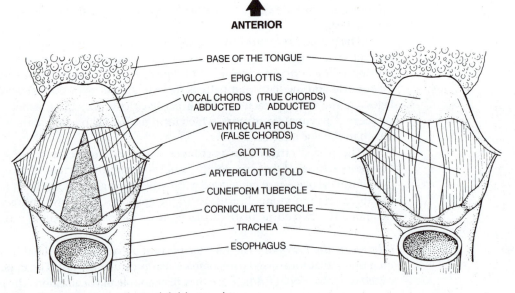

FIGURE 1–8.   Superior view of vocal folds (cords).

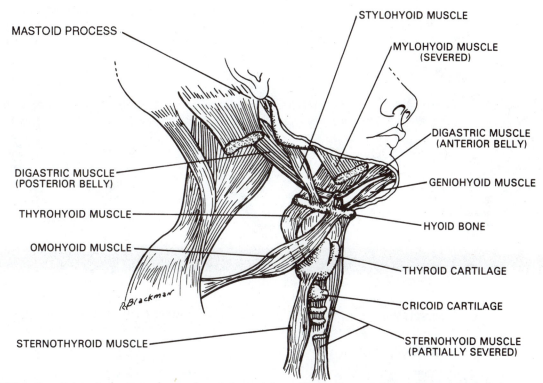

FIGURE 1–9. Extrinsic laryngeal muscles. Adapted from Short, *Essential Anatomies: Oral and Head/Neck*, © 1987 by Delmar Publishers Inc.

backward (Figure 1–9). The major **intrinsic muscles** that control the movement of the vocal folds are illustrated in Figure 1–7*C, D*. The action(s) of these muscles are described below.

Posterior Cricoarytenoid Muscles. These muscles pull inferiorly on the lateral angles of the arytenoids. This causes the vocal folds to move apart (abduct) and, thus, allows air to pass through (Figure 1–10*A*).

Lateral Cricoarytenoid Muscles. The action of these muscles is the opposite of the posterior cricoarytenoid muscles. These muscles pull laterally on the lateral angles of the arytenoids, causing the vocal folds to move together (adduct) (Figure 1–10*B*).

Transverse Arytenoid Muscles. These muscles pull the arytenoid cartilages together and, thereby, position the two vocal folds so that they vibrate as air passes between them during exhalation. Thus, the sounds for speech or singing are generated (Figure 1–10*C*).

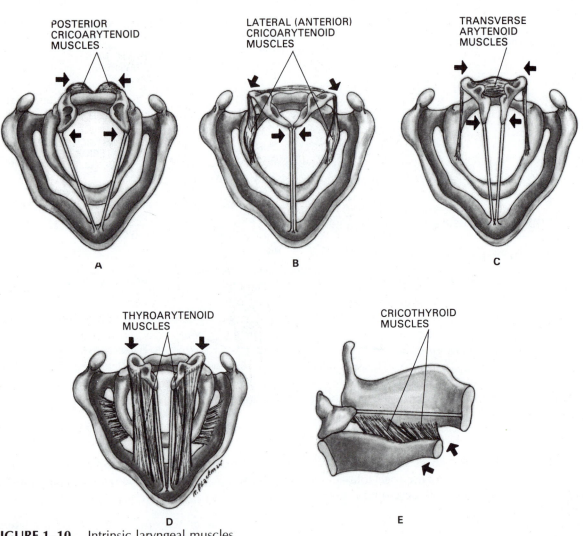

FIGURE 1–10. Intrinsic laryngeal muscles.

Thyroarytenoid Muscles. These muscles lie in the vocal folds lateral to the vocal ligaments. Contraction of the thyroarytenoid muscles pulls the arytenoid cartilages forward. This action loosens the vocal ligaments and allows a lower frequency of phonation (Figure 1–10D).

Cricothyroid Muscles. These muscles, which are located on the anterior surface of the larynx, can swing the entire thyroid cartilage anteriorly. This action provides an additional way to tense the vocal folds and, thereby, change the frequency of phonation (Figure 1–10E).

Ventilatory Function of the Larynx.   A primary function of the larynx is to ensure a free flow of air to and from the lungs. During a quiet inspiration, the vocal folds move apart *(abduct)* and widen the glottis. During exhalation, the vocal folds move toward the midline slightly *(adduct)*, but always maintain an open glottal airway.

A second vital function of the larynx is effort closure during exhalation, also known as **Valsalva's maneuver**. During this maneuver, there is a massive undifferentiated adduction of the laryngeal walls, including both the true and false vocal folds. As a result, the lumen of the larynx is tightly sealed, preventing air from escaping during physical work such as lifting, pushing, coughing, throat-clearing, vomiting, urination, defecation, and parturition.

The Tracheobronchial Tree

After passing through the larynx, inspired air enters the tracheobronchial tree, which is a series of branching airways commonly referred to as *generations*, or *orders*. These airways become progressively narrower, shorter, and more numerous as they branch throughout the lungs (Figure 1–11). Table 1–1 (page 21) lists the major subdivisions of the tracheobronchial tree.

In general, the airways exist in two major forms: (1) **cartilaginous airways** and (2) **noncartilaginous airways**. (The main structures of these airways are discussed in detail on pp. 26–31). The cartilaginous airways serve only to conduct air between the external environment and the sites of gas exchange. The noncartilaginous airways serve both as conductors of air and as sites of gas exchange. These will be discussed in detail below.

Histology of the Tracheobronchial Tree.   The tracheobronchial tree is composed of three major layers: an epithelial lining, the lamina propria, and a cartilaginous layer (Figure 1–12, page 22).

The Epithelial Lining.   The **epithelial lining** is predominantly composed of **pseudostratified ciliated columnar epithelium** interspersed with numerous mucous glands and separated from the lamina propria by a **basement membrane** (see Figure 1–12). Along the basement membrane of the epithelial lining are oval-shaped **basal cells**. These cells serve as a reserve supply of cells and replenish the superficial ciliated cells and mucous cells as needed.

The pseudostratified ciliated columnar epithelium extends from the trachea to the respiratory bronchioles. There are about 200 cilia per ciliated cell. The length of each cilium is about 5–7 μ (microns). As the bronchioles progressively become smaller, the columnar structure of the epithelium decreases in height and appears more cuboidal than columnar (see Figure 1–4C). The cilia progressively disappear in the terminal bronchioles and are completely absent in the respiratory bronchioles.

A mucus layer, commonly referred to as the **mucous blanket**, covers the epithelial lining of the tracheobronchial tree (Figure 1–13, page 23). In general,

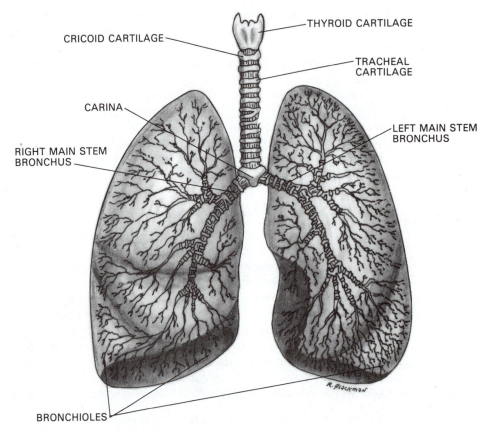

CRICOID CARTILAGE

THYROID CARTILAGE

TRACHEAL CARTILAGE

CARINA

LEFT MAIN STEM BRONCHUS

RIGHT MAIN STEM BRONCHUS

R. Blackman

BRONCHIOLES

FIGURE 1–11. Tracheobronchial tree.

the mucous blanket is composed of 95 percent water, with the remaining 5 percent consisting of glycoproteins, carbohydrates, lipids, DNA, some cellular debris, and foreign particles. The mucus is produced by (1) the **goblet cells**, and (2) the **submucosal**, or **bronchial, glands**. The goblet cells are located intermittently between the pseudostratified ciliated columnar cells and have been identified down to, and including, the terminal bronchioles. The submucosal glands, which produce most of the mucous blanket, extend deep into the lamina propria. These glands are innervated by the vagal parasympathetic nerve fibers (the tenth cranial nerve) and produce about 100 ml of bronchial secretions per day. Increased sympathetic activity decreases glandular secretions. The submucosal glands are particularly numerous in the medium-sized bronchi and disappear in the distal terminal bronchioles (see Figure 1–13).

The viscosity of the mucous blanket progressively increases from the epithelial lining to the inner luminal surface. The blanket has two distinct layers: (1) the **sol layer**, which is adjacent to the epithelial lining, and (2) the **gel layer**,

TABLE 1–1. Major Structures and Corresponding Generations of the Tracheobronchial Tree

	STRUCTURES OF THE LUNGS	GENERATIONS		
Conducting Zone	Trachea	0		Cartilaginous airways
	Main stem bronchi	1		
	Lobar bronchi	2		
	Segmental bronchi	3		
	Subsegmental bronchi	4–9		
	Bronchioles	10–15		Noncartilaginous airways
	Terminal bronchioles	16–19		
Respiratory Zone	Respiratory bronchioles	20–23		Sites of gas exchange
	Alveolar ducts	24–27		
	Alveolar sacs	28		

(Also called terminal respiratory units, primary lobule, lung parenchyma, acinus, and functional units)

NOTE: The precise number of generations between the subsegmental bronchi and the alveolar sacs is not known.

which is the more viscous layer adjacent to the inner luminal surface. Under normal circumstances, the cilia move in a wavelike fashion through the less viscous sol layer and continually strike the innermost portion of the gel layer (approximately 1500 times per minute). This action propels the mucus layer, along with any foreign particles stuck to the gel layer, toward the larynx at an estimated average rate of 2 cm per minute. Precisely what causes the cilia to move is unknown. At the larynx, the cough mechanism moves secretions beyond the larynx and into the oropharynx. This process is commonly referred to as the **mucociliary transport mechanism** or the **mucociliary escalator**, and is an important part of the cleansing mechanism of the tracheobronchial tree. Clinically, there are a number of factors that are now known to slow the rate of the mucociliary transport. Some common factors are:

- Cigarette smoke
- Dehydration
- Positive pressure ventilation

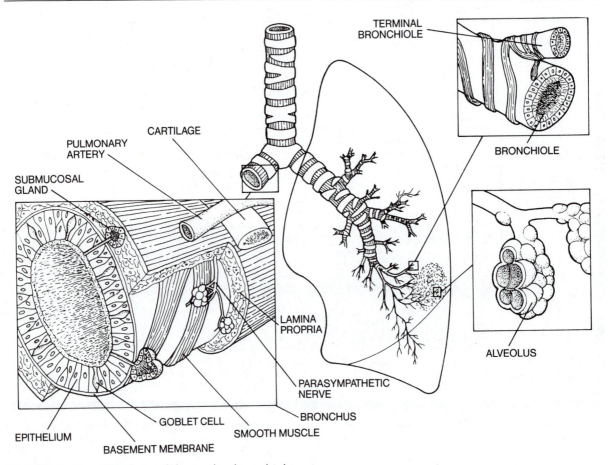
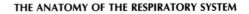

FIGURE 1–12.   Histology of the tracheobronchial tree.

- Endotracheal suctioning
- High inspired oxygen concentrations
- Hypoxia
- Atmospheric pollutants (e.g., sulfur dioxide, nitrogen dioxide, ozone)
- General anesthetics
- Parasympatholytics (e.g., atropine)

The Lamina Propria.   The **lamina propria** is the submucosal layer of the tracheobronchial tree. Within the lamina propria there is a loose, fibrous tissue that contains tiny blood vessels, lymphatic vessels, and branches of the vagus nerve. Also found within the lamina propria are two sets of smooth muscle fibers. These sets of muscles wrap around the tracheobronchial tree in fairly close spirals, one clockwise and the other counterclockwise. The smooth muscle fibers extend

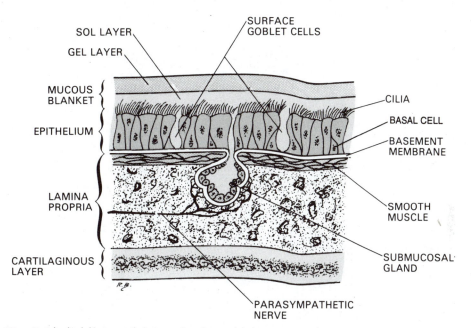

FIGURE 1–13. Epithelial lining of the tracheobronchial tree.

down to, and including, the alveolar ducts (see the section on sites of gas exchange in this chapter). The outer portion of the lamina propria is surrounded by a thin connective tissue called the **peribronchial sheath** (see Figure 1–16).

Mast Cells.   **Mast cells** play an important role in the immunologic mechanism. They are also found in the lamina propria—near the branches of the vagus nerve and blood vessels and scattered throughout the smooth muscle bundles, in the intra-alveolar septa, and as one of the cell constituents of the submucosal glands (Figure 1–14). Outside of the lungs, mast cells are found in loose connective tissue of skin and intestinal submucosa.

When they are activated, numerous substances are released from the mast cells which can significantly alter the diameter of the bronchial airways. Because of this fact, a basic understanding of how the mast cells function in the immunologic system is essential to the respiratory care practitioner.

There are two major immune responses: **cellular immunity** and **humoral immunity**. The *cellular immune response* involves the sensitized lymphocytes that are responsible for tissue rejection in transplants. This immune response is also termed a type IV, or delayed, type of hypersensitivity.

The *humoral immune response* involves the circulating antibodies that are involved in allergic responses such as allergic asthma. Antibodies (also called immunoglobulins) are serum globulins, or proteins, that defend against invading

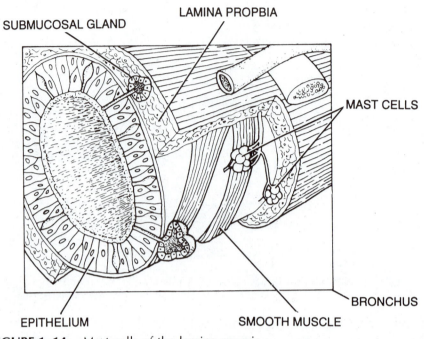

FIGURE 1–14. Mast cells of the lamina propria.

environmental antigens such as pollen, ragweed, animal dander, and feathers. Although five different immunoglobulins (IgG, IgA, IgM, IgD, and IgE) have been identified, the IgE (reaginic) antibody is basic to the allergic response. The mechanism of the IgE antibody-antigen reaction is as follows:

1. When a susceptible individual is exposed to a certain antigen, the lymphoid tissues release specific IgE antibodies. The newly formed IgE antibodies travel through the blood stream and attach to surface receptors on the mast cells. It is estimated that there are between 100,000 and 500,000 IgE receptor sites on the surface of each mast cell. Once the IgE antibodies attach to the mast cell, the individual (or more specifically, the mast cell) is said to be sensitive to the specific antigen (Figure 1–15A).
2. Each mast cell also has about 1000 secretory granules that contain several chemical mediators of inflammation (see below). Continued exposure, or reexposure, to the same antigen creates an IgE antibody-antigen reaction on the surface of the mast cell, which works to destroy or inactivate the antigen. This response, however, causes the mast cell to degranulate (break down) and to release the following chemical mediators (Figure 1–15B):
   a. Histamine
   b. Heparin

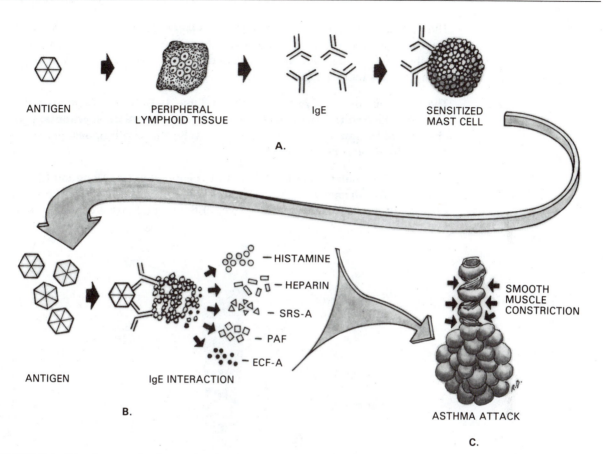

FIGURE 1–15. Immunologic mechanisms.

    c. Slow-reacting substance of anaphylaxis (SRS-A)
    d. Platelet-activating factor (PAF)
    e. Eosinophilic chemotactic factor of anaphylaxis (ECF-A)
3. The release of these chemical mediators causes increased vascular permeability, smooth muscle contraction, increased mucus secretion, and vasodilation with edema.

    Such a reaction in the lungs can be extremely dangerous and is seen in individuals during an allergic asthmatic episode. The production of IgE antibodies may be 20 times greater than normal in some asthmatic patients (the normal IgE antibody level in the serum is about 200 ng/ml). During an asthmatic attack, the patient demonstrates bronchial edema, bronchospasms and wheezing, increased mucus production, mucus plugging, air trapping, and lung hyperinflation (Figure 1–15C).

The Cartilaginous Layer.   The **cartilaginous layer**, which is the outermost layer of the tracheobronchial tree, progressively diminishes in size as the airways extend into the lungs. Cartilage is completely absent in bronchioles less than 1 millimeter (mm) in diameter (see Figure 1–12).

The Cartilaginous Airways.   As shown in Table 1–1, the cartilaginous airways consist of the **trachea, main stem bronchi, lobar bronchi, segmental bronchi**, and **subsegmental bronchi**. Collectively, the cartilaginous airways are referred to as the conducting zone.

Trachea.   The adult trachea is about 11 to 13 centimeters (cm) long and 1.5 to 2.5 centimeters in diameter (Figure 1–16). It extends vertically from the cricoid cartilage of the larynx to about the level of the second costal cartilage, or fifth

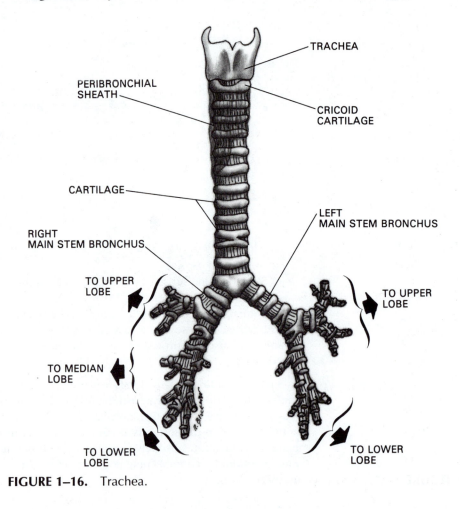

FIGURE 1–16.   Trachea.

thoracic vertebra. At this point, the trachea divides into the right and left main stem bronchi. The bifurcation of the trachea is known as the **carina**. Approximately 15 to 20 C-shaped cartilages support the trachea. These cartilages are incomplete posteriorly where the trachea and the esophagus share a fibroelastic membrane (Figure 1–17).

Main Stem Bronchi.   The right main stem bronchus branches off the trachea at about a 25-degree angle; the left main stem bronchus forms an angle of 40 to 60 degrees with the trachea. The right main stem bronchus is wider, more vertical, and about 5 centimeters shorter than the left main stem bronchus. Similar to the trachea, the main stem bronchi are supported by C-shaped cartilages. In the newborn, both the right and left main stem bronchi form about a 55-degree angle with the trachea. The main stem bronchi are the tracheobronchial tree's first generation.

Lobar Bronchi.   The right main stem bronchus divides into the upper, middle, and lower lobar bronchi. The left main stem bronchus branches into the upper and lower lobar bronchi. The lobar bronchi are the tracheobronchial tree's second generation. The C-shaped cartilages that support the trachea and the main stem bronchi progressively form cartilaginous plates around the lobar bronchi.

Segmental Bronchi.   A third generation of bronchi branch off the lobar bronchi to form the segmental bronchi. There are ten segmental bronchi in the right lung and

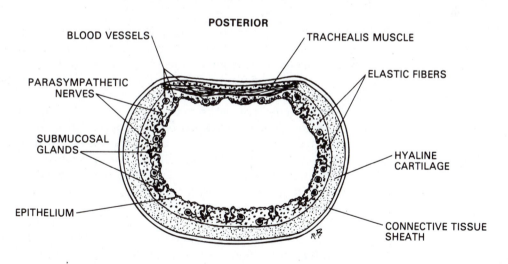

FIGURE 1–17.   Cross-section of trachea.

eight in the left lung. Each segmental bronchus is named according to its location within a particular lung lobe.

Subsegmental Bronchi.   The tracheobronchial tree continues to subdivide between the fourth and approximately the ninth generation into progressively smaller airways called subsegmental bronchi. These bronchi range in diameter from 1 to 4 mm. Peribronchial connective tissue containing nerves, lymphatics, and bronchial arteries surrounds the subsegmental bronchi to about the 1-mm diameter level. After this point, the connective tissue sheaths disappear.

The Noncartilaginous Airways.   The noncartilaginous airways are composed of the **bronchioles** and the **terminal bronchioles**.

Bronchioles.   When the bronchi decrease to less than 1 mm in diameter and are no longer surrounded by connective tissue sheaths, they are called bronchioles. The bronchioles are found between the tenth and fifteenth generations. At this level, cartilage is absent and the lamina propria is directly connected with the lung parenchyma (see lung parenchyma in the section on sites of gas exchange in this chapter). The bronchioles are surrounded by spiral muscle fibers and the epithelial cells are more cuboidal in shape (see Figure 1–12). The rigidity of the bronchioles is very low when compared with the cartilaginous airways. Because of this, the airway patency at this level may be substantially altered by intra-alveolar and intrapleural pressures and by alterations in the size of the lungs. This lack of airway support often plays a major role in respiratory disease.

Terminal Bronchioles.   The conducting tubes of the tracheobronchial tree end with the terminal bronchioles between the sixteenth and nineteenth generations. The average diameter of the terminal bronchioles is about 0.5 mm. At this point, the cilia and the mucous glands progressively disappear, the epithelium flattens and becomes cuboidal in shape (see Figures 1–4C and 1–12).

As the walls of the terminal bronchioles progressively become thinner, small channels, called the **canals of Lambert**, begin to appear between the inner luminal surface of the terminal bronchioles and the adjacent alveoli that surround them (Figure 1–18). Although specific information as to their function is lacking, it is believed that these tiny pathways may be important secondary avenues for collateral ventilation in patients with certain respiratory disorders (e.g., chronic obstructive pulmonary disease).

Also unique to the terminal bronchioles is the presence of **Clara cells**. These cells have thick protoplasmic extensions that bulge into the lumen of the terminal bronchioles. The precise function of the Clara cells is not known. They may have secretory functions that contribute to the extracellular liquid lining the bronchioles and alveoli. They may also contain enzymes that work to detoxify inhaled toxic substances.

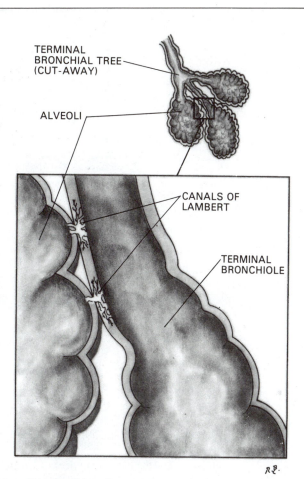

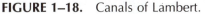

FIGURE 1–18. Canals of Lambert.

The anatomic structures beyond the terminal bronchioles are the normal sites of gas exchange and, although directly connected, are not considered part of the tracheobronchial tree.

Bronchial Cross-Sectional Area. The total cross-sectional area of the tracheobronchial tree steadily increases from the trachea to the terminal bronchioles. The total cross-sectional area increases significantly beyond the terminal bronchioles because of the many branches that occur at this level. The anatomic structures distal to the terminal bronchioles are, collectively, referred to as the **respiratory zone** (Figure 1–19).

Air flows down the tracheobronchial tree as a mass to about the level of the terminal bronchioles, similar to water flowing through a tube. Because the

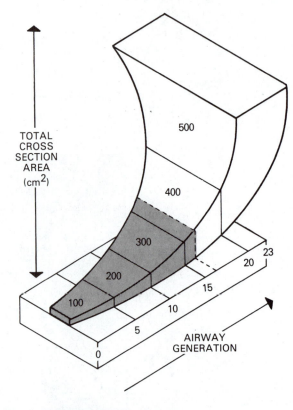

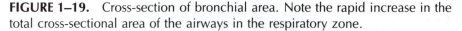
☒ CONDUCTING ZONE
☐ RESPIRATORY ZONE

FIGURE 1–19. Cross-section of bronchial area. Note the rapid increase in the total cross-sectional area of the airways in the respiratory zone.

cross-sectional area becomes so great beyond this point, however, the forward motion essentially stops and the natural molecular movement of gas becomes the dominant mechanism of ventilation.

Bronchial Blood Supply

The **bronchial arteries** nourish the tracheobronchial tree. The arteries arise from the aorta and follow the tracheobronchial tree as far as the terminal bronchioles. Beyond the terminal bronchioles, the bronchial arteries lose their identity and merge with the pulmonary arteries and capillaries, which are part of the pulmonary vascular system. The normal bronchial arterial blood flow is about 1 percent of the cardiac output. In addition to the tracheobronchial tree, the bronchial arteries nourish the mediastinal lymph nodes, the pulmonary nerves, some muscular pulmonary arteries and veins, a portion of the esophagus, and of the visceral pleura.

About one-third of the bronchial venous blood returns to the right atrium by way of the **azygos, hemiazygos**, and **intercostal veins**. Most of this blood comes from the first two or three generations of the tracheobronchial tree. The remaining two-thirds of the bronchial venous blood drains into the pulmonary circulation, via **bronchopulmonary anastomoses**, and then flows to the left atrium by way of the pulmonary veins. In effect, the bronchial venous blood, which is low in oxygen and high in carbon dioxide, mixes with blood that has just passed through the alveolar-capillary system, which is high in oxygen and low in carbon dioxide. The mixing of venous blood and freshly oxygenated blood is known as **venous admixture**. (The effects of venous admixture are discussed in greater detail in Chapter Seven.)

THE SITES OF GAS EXCHANGE

The anatomic structures distal to the terminal bronchioles are the functional units of gas exchange. They are composed of about three generations of **respiratory bronchioles**, followed by about three generations of **alveolar ducts**, and finally, ending in 15 to 20 grapelike clusters, the **alveolar sacs** (Figure 1–20). The respiratory bronchioles are characterized by alveoli budding from their walls. The walls of the alveolar ducts that arise from the respiratory bronchioles are completely composed of alveoli separated by septal walls that contain smooth muscle fibers. Most gas exchange takes place at the alveolar-capillary membrane (Figure 1–21, page 33). In the lungs of the adult male, there are approximately 300 million alveoli between 75 μ and 300 μ in diameter, and small pulmonary capillaries cover about 85 to 95 percent of the alveoli. This anatomic arrangement provides an average surface area of 70 square meters (about the size of a tennis court) available for gas exchange.

Collectively, the respiratory bronchioles, alveolar ducts, and alveolar clusters that originate from a single terminal bronchiole are referred to as a **primary lobule**. Each primary lobule is about 3.5 mm in diameter and contains about 2000 alveoli. It is estimated that there are approximately 130,000 primary lobules in the lung. Synonyms for primary lobule include **acinus, terminal respiratory unit, lung parenchyma**, and **functional units** (see Table 1–1).

Alveolar Epithelium

The alveolar epithelium is composed of two principal cell types: the **type I cell**, or **squamous pneumocyte**, and the **type II cell**, or **granular pneumocyte**.

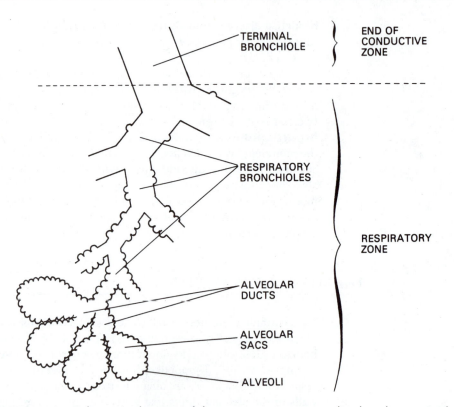

FIGURE 1–20. Schematic drawing of the anatomic structures distal to the terminal bronchioles; collectively, these are referred to as the primary lobule.

Type I cells are primarily composed of a cytoplasmic ground substance. They are broad, thin cells that form about 95 percent of the alveolar surface. They are between 0.1 μ and 0.5 μ thick and are the major sites of alveolar gas exchange.

Type II cells form the remaining 5 percent of the total alveolar surface. They have microvilli and are cuboidal in shape. They are believed to be the primary source of **pulmonary surfactant**. Surfactant molecules are situated at the air–liquid interface of the alveoli and play a major role in decreasing the surface tension of the fluid that lines the alveoli (see Figure 1–21).

Pores of Kohn

The **pores of Kohn** are small holes in the walls of the interalveolar septa (see Figure 1–21). They are between 3 μ and 13 μ in diameter and permit gas to move between adjacent alveoli. The formation of the pores may include one or more of the following processes: (1) the desquamation (i.e., shedding or peeling) of

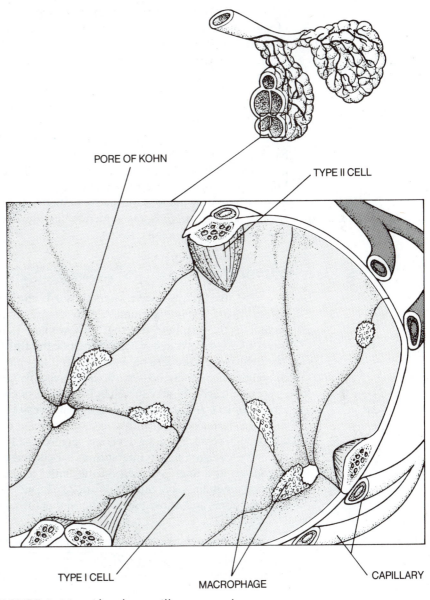

PORE OF KOHN

TYPE II CELL

TYPE I CELL

MACROPHAGE

CAPILLARY

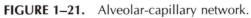

FIGURE 1–21.   Alveolar-capillary network.

epithelial cells due to disease, (2) the normal degeneration of tissue cells as a result of age, and (3) the movement of macrophages, which may leave holes in the alveolar walls. The formation of alveolar pores is accelerated by diseases involving the lung parenchyma, and the number and size of the pores increase progressively with age.

Alveolar Macrophages

Alveolar macrophages, or type III alveolar cells, play a major role in removing bacteria and other foreign particles that are deposited within the acini. Macrophages are believed to originate from stem cell precursors in the bone marrow. Then, as monocytes, they presumably migrate through the blood stream to the lungs, where they move about or are embedded in the extracellular lining of the alveolar surface. There is also evidence that the alveolar macrophages reproduce within the lung (see Figure 1–21).

Interstitium

The alveolar-capillary clusters are surrounded, supported, and shaped by the **interstitium**. The interstitium is a gellike substance composed of hyaluronic acid molecules that are held together by a weblike network of collagen fibers. The interstitium has two major compartments: the **tight space** and the **loose space**. The tight space is the area between the alveolar epithelium and the endothelium of the pulmonary capillaries—the area where most gas exchange occurs. The loose space is primarily the area that surrounds the bronchioles, respiratory bronchioles, alveolar ducts, and alveolar sacs. Lymphatic vessels and neural fibers are found in this area. Water content in this area can increase more than 30 percent before a significant pressure change develops (Figure 1–22).

The collagen in the interstitium is believed to limit alveolar distensibility. Expansion of a lung unit beyond the limits of the interstitial collagen can (1) occlude the pulmonary capillaries or (2) damage the structural framework of the collagen fibers and, subsequently, the wall of the alveoli.

PULMONARY VASCULAR SYSTEM

The pulmonary vascular system can be viewed as an independent vascular network with the sole purpose of delivering blood to and from the lungs for gas exchange. In addition to gas exchange, the pulmonary vascular system provides nutritional substances to the anatomic structures distal to the terminal bronchioles. Similar to the systemic vascular system, the pulmonary vascular system is composed of **arteries, arterioles, capillaries, venules**, and **veins**.

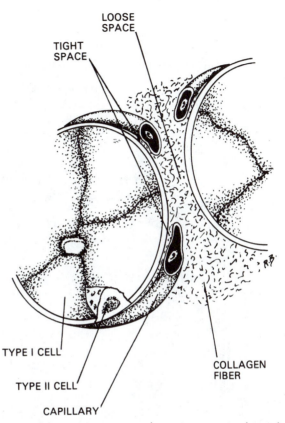

LOOSE
SPACE

TIGHT
SPACE

TYPE I CELL

TYPE II CELL

CAPILLARY

COLLAGEN
FIBER

FIGURE 1–22.   Interstitium. Most gas exchange occurs in the tight space area. The area around the bronchioles, respiratory bronchioles, alveolar ducts, and alveolar sacs is called the loose space.

Arteries

The right ventricle of the heart pumps deoxygenated blood into the **pulmonary artery**. Just beneath the aorta the pulmonary artery divides into the right and left branches (Figure 1–23). The branches then penetrate their respective lung through the hilum, which is that part of the lung where the main stem bronchi, vessels, and nerves enter. In general, the pulmonary artery follows the tracheobronchial tree in a posterolateral relation, branching or dividing as the tracheobronchial tree does.

The arteries have three layers of tissue in their walls (Figure 1–24, page 37). The inner layer is called the **tunica intima** and is composed of endothelium and a thin layer of connective and elastic tissue. The middle layer is called the **tunica media** and consists primarily of elastic connective tissue in large arteries and

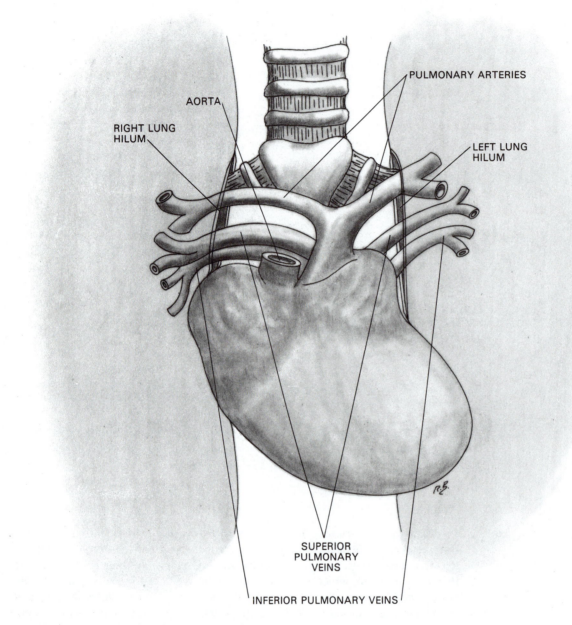

FIGURE 1–23. Major pulmonary vessels.

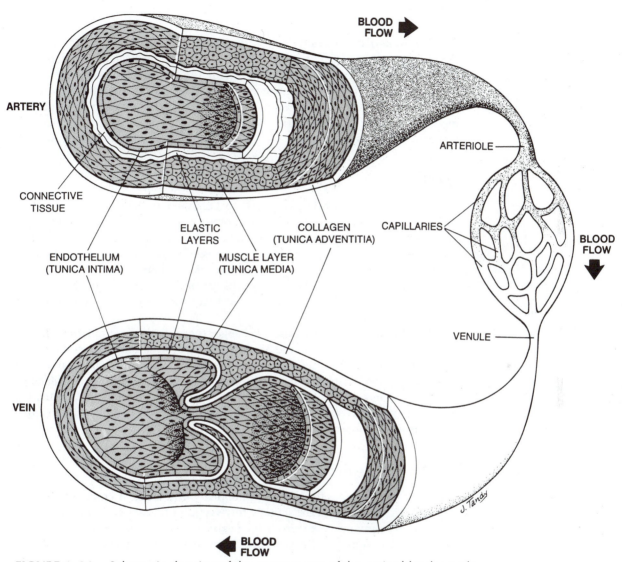

FIGURE 1–24.   Schematic drawing of the components of the major blood vessels.

smooth muscle in medium-sized to small arteries. The tunica media is the thickest layer in the arteries. The outermost layer is called the **tunica adventitia** and is composed of connective tissue. This layer also contains small vessels that nourish all three tissue layers. Because of the different layers, the arteries are relatively stiff vessels that are well suited for carrying blood under high pressures in the systemic system.

Arterioles

The walls of the arterioles consist of an endothelial layer, an elastic layer, and a layer of smooth muscle fibers (see Figure 1–24). The elastic and smooth muscle fibers gradually disappear just before entering the alveolar-capillary system. The pulmonary arterioles supply nutrients to the respiratory bronchioles, alveolar ducts, and alveoli. By virtue of their smooth muscle fibers, the arterioles play an important role in the distribution and regulation of blood and are called the **resistance vessels.**

Capillaries

The pulmonary arterioles give rise to a complex network of capillaries that surround the alveoli. The capillaries are composed of an endothelial layer (a single layer of squamous epithelial cells) (see Figure 1–24). The capillaries are essentially an extension of the inner lining of the larger vessels. The walls of the pulmonary capillaries are less than 0.1 μ thick and the external diameter of each vessel is about 10 μ. The capillaries are where gas exchange occurs. The pulmonary capillary endothelium also has a selective permeability to substances such as water, electrolytes, and sugars.

In addition to gas and fluid exchange, the pulmonary capillaries play an important biochemical role in the production and destruction of a broad range of biologically active substances. For example, serotonin, norepinephrine, and some prostaglandins are destroyed by the pulmonary capillaries. Some prostaglandins are produced and synthesized by the pulmonary capillaries, and some circulating inactive peptides are converted to their active form; for example, the inactive angiotensin I is converted to the active angiotensin II.

Venules and Veins

After blood moves through the pulmonary capillaries, it enters the pulmonary venules. The venules are actually tiny veins continuous with the capillaries. The venules empty into the veins, which carry blood back to the heart. Similar to the arteries, the veins usually have three layers of tissue in their walls (see Figure 1–24).

The veins differ from the arteries, however, in that the middle layer is poorly developed. As a result, the veins have thinner walls and contain less smooth muscle and less elastic tissue than the arteries. There are only two layers in the smaller veins, lacking a layer comparable to the tunica adventitia. In the systemic circulation, many medium- and large-sized veins (particularly those in the legs) contain one-way, flaplike valves that aid blood flow back to the heart. The valves open as long as the flow is toward the heart, but close if flow moves away from the heart.

The veins also differ from the arteries in that they are capable of collecting a large amount of blood with very little pressure change. Because of this unique feature, the veins are called **capacitance vessels**. Unlike the pulmonary arteries, which generally parallel the airways, the veins move away from the bronchi and take a more direct route out of the lungs. Ultimately, the veins in each lung merge into two large veins and exit through the lung hilum. The four pulmonary veins then empty into the left atrium of the heart (see Figure 1–23).

THE LYMPHATIC SYSTEM

Lymphatic vessels are found superficially around the lungs just beneath the visceral pleura and in the dense connective tissue wrapping of the bronchioles, bronchi, pulmonary arteries, and pulmonary veins. The primary function of the lymphatic vessels is to remove excess fluid and protein molecules that leak out of the pulmonary capillaries.

Deep within the lungs, the lymphatic vessels arise from the loose space of the interstitium. The vessels follow the bronchial airways, pulmonary arteries, and veins to the hilum of the lung (Figure 1–25). Single leaf, funnel-shaped valves are found in the lymphatic channels. These valves direct fluid toward the hilum. The larger lymphatic channels are surrounded by smooth muscle bands that actively produce peristaltic movements regulated by the autonomic nervous system. Both the smooth muscle activity and the normal, cyclic pressure changes generated in the thoracic cavity move lymphatic fluid toward the hilum. The vessels end in the pulmonary and bronchopulmonary **lymph nodes** located just inside and outside the lung parenchyma (Figure 1–26, page 41).

The lymph nodes are organized collections of lymphatic tissue interspersed along the course of the lymphatic stream. Lymph nodes produce lymphocytes and monocytes. The nodes act as filters, keeping particulate matter and bacteria from gaining entrance to the blood stream.

There are no lymphatic vessels in the walls of the alveoli. Some alveoli, however, are strategically located immediately adjacent to peribronchovascular lymphatic vessels. These vessels are called **juxta-alveolar lymphatics** and are thought to play an active role in the removal of excess fluid and other foreign material that gain entrance into the interstitial space of the lung parenchyma.

Superficially, there are more lymphatic vessels on the surface of the lower lung lobes than on that of the upper or middle lobes. The lymphatic channels on the left lower lung lobe are more numerous and larger in diameter than the lymphatic vessels on the surface of the right lower lung lobe (Figure 1–27, page 42). This anatomic difference provides a possible explanation why patients with **bilateral effusion** (i.e., the escape of fluid from the blood vessels from both lungs) commonly have more fluid in the lower right lung than in the lower left.

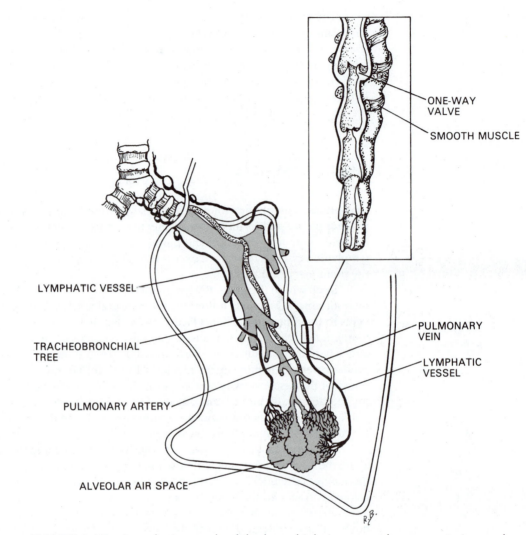

FIGURE 1–25. Lymphatic vessels of the bronchial airways, pulmonary arteries, and veins.

NEURAL CONTROL OF THE LUNGS

The balance, or tone, of the bronchial and arteriolar smooth muscle of the lungs is controlled by the **autonomic nervous system**. The autonomic nervous system is the part of the nervous system that regulates involuntary vital functions, including the activity of the cardiac muscle, the smooth muscle, and glands. It has two

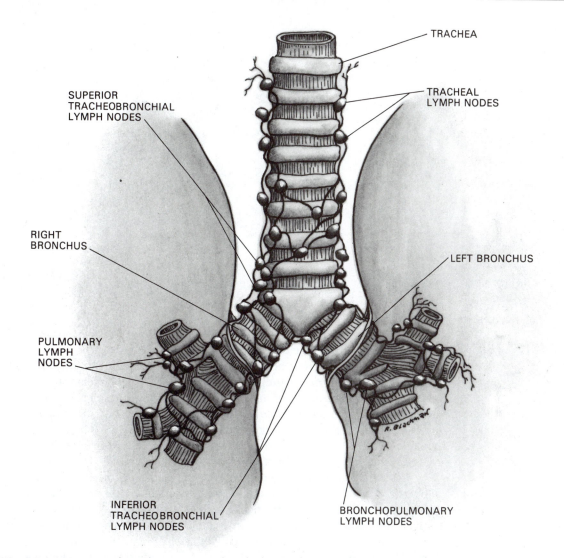

TRACHEA

TRACHEAL
LYMPH NODES

SUPERIOR
TRACHEOBRONCHIAL
LYMPH NODES

RIGHT
BRONCHUS

LEFT BRONCHUS

PULMONARY
LYMPH
NODES

INFERIOR
TRACHEOBRONCHIAL
LYMPH NODES

BRONCHOPULMONARY
LYMPH NODES

FIGURE 1–26.   Lymph nodes associated with the trachea and the right and left main stem bronchi.

divisions: (1) the **sympathetic nervous system**, which accelerates the heart rate, constricts blood vessels, relaxes bronchial smooth muscles, and raises blood pressure; and (2) the **parasympathetic nervous system**, which slows the heart rate, constricts bronchial smooth muscles, and increases intestinal peristalsis and gland activity. Table 1–2 (page 43) lists some effects of the two divisions of the autonomic nervous system.

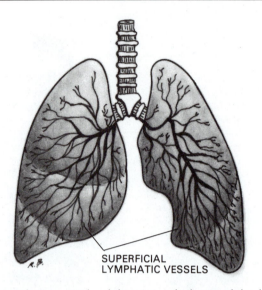

SUPERFICIAL
LYMPHATIC VESSELS

FIGURE 1–27. Lymphatic vessels of the visceral pleura of the lungs.

The neural fibers of the sympathetic and parasympathetic nervous systems control the smooth muscle tone in the following way.

When the sympathetic nervous system is activated, neural transmitters, such as **epinephrine** and **norepinephrine**, are released. These agents stimulate (1) the **beta$_2$ receptors** in the bronchial smooth muscles, causing relaxation of the airway musculature, and (2) the **alpha receptors** of the smooth muscles of the arterioles, causing the pulmonary vascular system to constrict. When the parasympathetic nervous system is activated, the neutral transmitter **acetylcholine** is released, causing constriction of the bronchial smooth muscle.

Inactivity of either the sympathetic or the parasympathetic nervous system allows the action of the other to dominate the bronchial smooth muscle response. For example, if a beta$_2$ blocking agent such as **propranolol** is administered to a patient, the parasympathetic nervous system becomes dominant and bronchial constriction ensues. In contrast, if a patient receives a parasympathetic blocking agent such as **atropine**, the sympathetic nervous system becomes dominant and bronchial relaxation occurs.

THE LUNGS

The apex of each lung is somewhat pointed and the base is broad and concave to accommodate the convex diaphragm (Figures 1–28 and 1–29, page 44). As shown in Figure 1–30 (page 45), the apices of the lungs rise to about the level of the first rib. The base extends anteriorly to about the level of the sixth rib (xiphoid process

TABLE 1–2. Some Effects of Autonomic Nervous System Activity

EFFECTOR SITE	SYMPATHETIC NERVOUS SYSTEM	PARASYMPATHETIC NERVOUS SYSTEM
Heart	Increases rate Increases strength of contraction	Decreases rate Decreases strength of contraction
Bronchial smooth muscle	Relaxation	Constriction
Bronchial glands	Decreases secretions	Increases secretions
Salivary glands	Decreases secretions	Increases secretions
Stomach	Decreases motility	Increases motility
Intestines	Decreases motility	Increases motility
Eye	Widens pupils	Constricts pupils

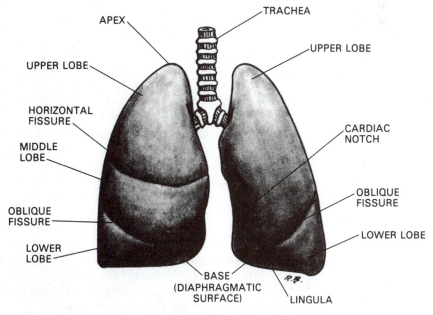

FIGURE 1–28. Anterior view of the lungs.

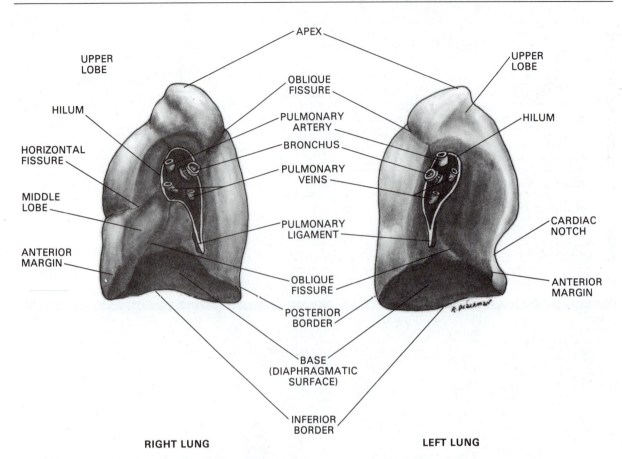

FIGURE 1–29.   Medial view of the lungs.

level), and posteriorly to about the level of the eleventh rib (four ribs below the inferior angle of the scapula). The **mediastinal border** of each lung is concave to fit the heart and other mediastinal structures. At the center of the mediastinal border is the **hilum**, where the right and left main stem bronchi, blood vessels, lymph vessels, and various nerves enter and exit the lungs.

The **right lung** is larger and heavier than the left. It is divided into the **upper, middle**, and **lower lobes** by the **oblique** and the **horizontal fissures**. The oblique fissure extends from the costal to the mediastinal borders of the lung and separates the upper and middle lobes from the lower lobe. The horizontal fissure extends horizontally from the oblique fissure to about the level of the fourth costal cartilage and separates the middle from the upper lobe.

The **left lung** is divided into only two lobes—the **upper** and the **lower**. These two lobes are separated by the **oblique fissure**, which extends from the costal to the mediastinal borders of the lung.

ANTERIOR VIEW   POSTERIOR VIEW

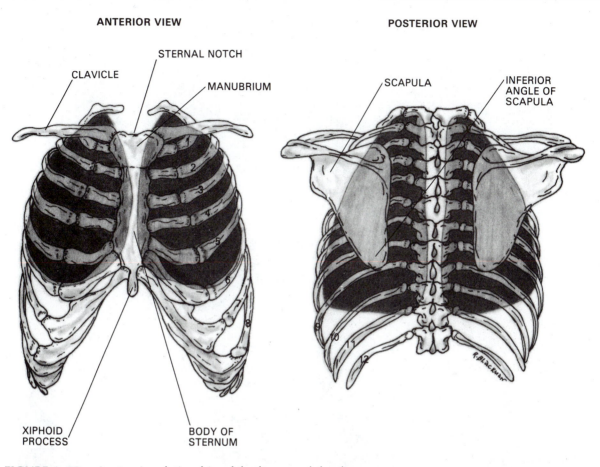

FIGURE 1–30. Anatomic relationship of the lungs and the thorax.

All lobes are further subdivided into **bronchopulmonary segments**. In Figure 1–31, the segments are numbered to demonstrate their relationship.

THE MEDIASTINUM

The **mediastinum** is a cavity that contains organs and tissues in the center of the thoracic cage between the right and left lungs (Figure 1–32, page 47). It is bordered anteriorly by the sternum and posteriorly by the thoracic vertebrae. The mediastinum contains the trachea, the heart, the major blood vessels (commonly known as the great vessels) that enter and exit from the heart, various nerves, portions

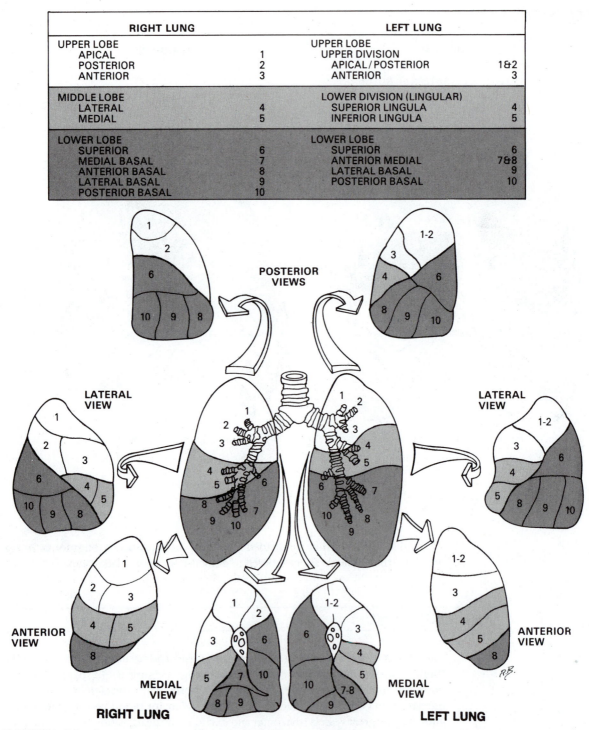

RIGHT LUNG		LEFT LUNG	
UPPER LOBE		**UPPER LOBE**	
APICAL	1	UPPER DIVISION	
POSTERIOR	2	APICAL/POSTERIOR	1&2
ANTERIOR	3	ANTERIOR	3
MIDDLE LOBE		**LOWER DIVISION (LINGULAR)**	
LATERAL	4	SUPERIOR LINGULA	4
MEDIAL	5	INFERIOR LINGULA	5
LOWER LOBE		**LOWER LOBE**	
SUPERIOR	6	SUPERIOR	6
MEDIAL BASAL	7	ANTERIOR MEDIAL	7&8
ANTERIOR BASAL	8	LATERAL BASAL	9
LATERAL BASAL	9	POSTERIOR BASAL	10
POSTERIOR BASAL	10		

POSTERIOR VIEWS

LATERAL VIEW

LATERAL VIEW

ANTERIOR VIEW

ANTERIOR VIEW

MEDIAL VIEW

MEDIAL VIEW

RIGHT LUNG

LEFT LUNG

FIGURE 1–31. Lung segments. Although the segment subdivisions of the right and left lungs are similar, there are some slight anatomic differences, which are noted by combined names and numbers. Because of these slight variations, some workers consider that, technically, there are only eight segments in the left lung and that the apical-posterior segment is number 1 and the anteromedial is number 6.

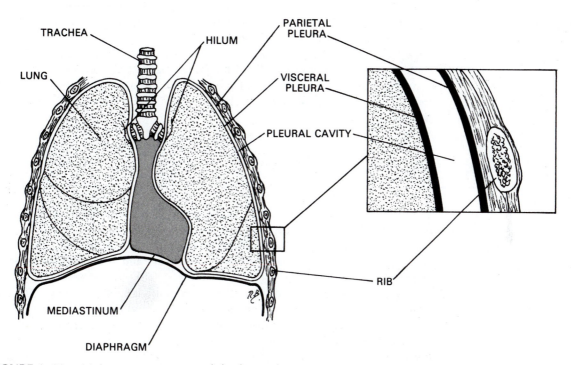

FIGURE 1–32. Major structures around the lungs.

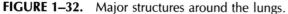

of the esophagus, the thymus gland, and lymph nodes. If the mediastinum is compressed or distorted, it can severely compromise the cardiopulmonary system.

THE PLEURAL MEMBRANES

Two moist, slick-surfaced membranes, called the **visceral** and **parietal pleurae**, are closely associated with the lungs. The visceral pleura is firmly attached to the outer surface of each lung and extends into each of the interlobar fissures. The parietal pleura lines the inside of the thoracic walls, the thoracic surface of the diaphragm, and the lateral portion of the mediastinum. The potential space between the visceral and parietal pleurae is called the **pleural cavity**.

The visceral and parietal pleurae are held together by a thin film of serous fluid—somewhat like two flat, moistened pieces of glass. This fluid layer allows the two pleural membranes to glide over each other during inspiration and expiration. Thus, during inspiration the pleural membranes hold the lung tissue to the inner surface of the thorax and diaphragm, causing the lungs to expand (see Figure 1–32).

Because the lungs have a natural tendency to collapse and the chest wall has a natural tendency to expand, a negative or subatmospheric pressure (negative intrapleural pressure) normally exists between the parietal and visceral pleurae. Should air or gas be introduced into the pleural cavity (e.g., as a result of a chest puncture wound), the intrapleural pressure rises to atmospheric pressure and causes the pleural membranes to separate. This condition is called a **pneumothorax**.

THE THORAX

The **thorax** houses and protects the organs of the cardiopulmonary system. Twelve **thoracic vertebrae** form the posterior midline border of the thoracic cage. The **sternum** forms the anterior border of the chest. The sternum is composed of the **manubrium sterni**, the **body**, and the **xyphoid process** (Figure 1–33).

The twelve pairs of ribs form the lateral boundary of the thorax. The ribs attach directly to the vertebral column posteriorly and indirectly by way of the costal cartilage anteriorly to the sternum. The first seven ribs are referred to as **true ribs**, since they are attached directly to the sternum by way of their costal cartilage. Because the cartilage of the eighth, ninth, and tenth ribs attaches to the cartilage of the ribs above, they are referred to as **false ribs**. Ribs eleven and twelve float freely anteriorly and are called **floating ribs**. There are eleven intercostal spaces between the ribs; these spaces contain blood vessels, intercostal nerves, and the external and internal intercostal muscles (Figure 1–34, page 50).

THE DIAPHRAGM

The **diaphragm** is the major muscle of ventilation (Figure 1–35, page 51). It is a domeshaped musculofibrous partition located between the thoracic cavity and the abdominal cavity. Although the diaphragm is generally referred to as one muscle, it is actually composed of two separate muscles known as the **right** and **left hemidiaphragms**. Each hemidiaphragm arises from the lumbar vertebrae, the costal margin, and the xyphoid process. The two muscles then merge together at the midline into a broad connective sheet called the **central tendon**. The diaphragm is pierced by the esophagus, the aorta, several nerves, and the inferior vena cava. Terminal branches of the **phrenic nerves**, which leave the spinal cord between the third and fifth cervical segments, supply the primary motor innervation to each hemidiaphragm. The **lower thoracic nerves** also contribute to the motor innervation of each hemidiaphragm.

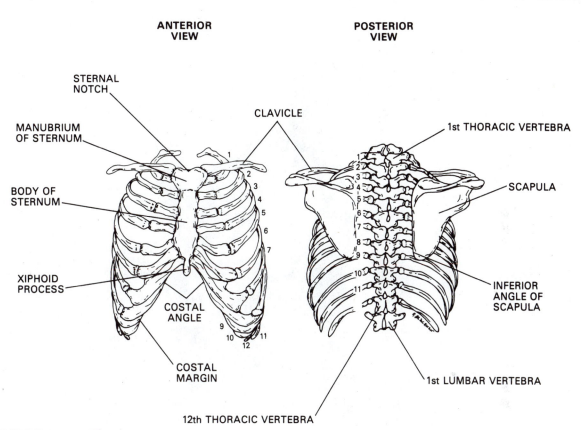

FIGURE 1–33. The thorax.

When stimulated to contract, the diaphragm moves downward and the lower ribs move upward and outward. This action increases the volume of the thoracic cavity, which, in turn, lowers the intrapleural and intra-alveolar pressures in the thoracic cavity. As a result, gas from the atmosphere flows into the lungs. During expiration, the diaphragm relaxes and domes upward into the thoracic cavity. This action increases the intra-alveolar and intrapleural pressures, causing gas to flow out of the lungs.

The Accessory Muscles of Ventilation

During normal ventilation by a healthy person, the diaphragm alone can manage the task of moving gas in and out of the lungs. During vigorous exercise, however, and during the advanced stages of chronic obstructive pulmonary disease, the accessory muscles of inspiration and expiration are activated to assist the diaphragm.

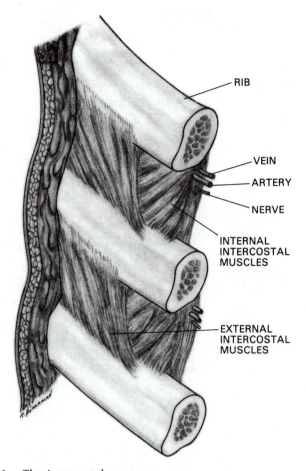

RIB

VEIN

ARTERY

NERVE

INTERNAL
INTERCOSTAL
MUSCLES

EXTERNAL
INTERCOSTAL
MUSCLES

FIGURE 1–34.   The intercostal space.

The Accessory Muscles of Inspiration

The accessory muscles of inspiration are those muscles that are recruited to assist the diaphragm in creating a subatmospheric pressure in the lungs to enable adequate inspiration. Following are the major accessory muscles of inspiration:

- Scalene muscles
- Sternocleidomastoid muscles
- Pectoralis major muscles
- Trapezius muscles
- External intercostal muscles

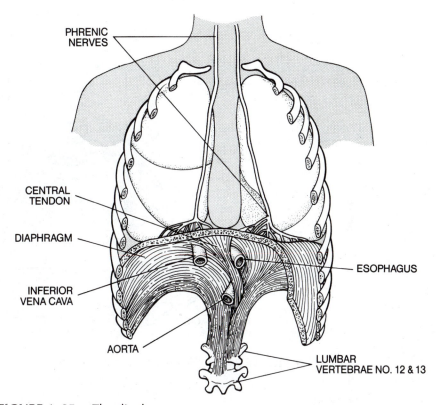

PHRENIC
NERVES

CENTRAL
TENDON

DIAPHRAGM

INFERIOR
VENA CAVA

AORTA

ESOPHAGUS

LUMBAR
VERTEBRAE NO. 12 & 13

FIGURE 1–35.   The diaphragm.

Scalene Muscles.   The **scalene muscles** are three separate muscles that function as a unit. They are known as the **anterior**, the **medial**, and the **posterior** scalene muscles. They originate on the transverse processes of the second to the sixth cervical vertebrae and insert into the first and second ribs (Figure 1–36). The primary function of these muscles is to flex the neck. When used as accessory muscles for inspiration, they elevate the first and second ribs. This action works to decrease the intrapleural pressure.

Sternocleidomastoid Muscles.   The **sternocleidomastoid muscles** are located on each side of the neck (Figure 1–37, page 53). They originate from the sternum and the clavicle and insert into the mastoid process and occipital bone of the skull. Normally the sternocleidomastoid muscle pulls from its sternoclavicular origin and rotates the head to the opposite side and turns it upward. When the sternocleidomastoid muscle functions as an accessory muscle of inspiration, the head and neck are fixed by other muscles and the sternocleidomastoid pulls from

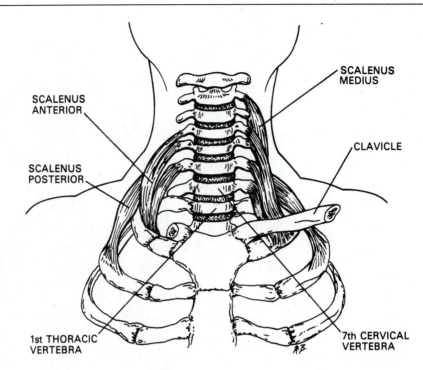

FIGURE 1–36.   Scalenus muscles.

its insertion on the skull and elevates the sternum. This action increases the anteroposterior diameter of the chest.

Pectoralis Major Muscles.   The **pectoralis major muscles** are powerful, fan-shaped muscles located on each side of the upper chest. They originate from the clavicle and the sternum and insert into the upper part of the humerus.

   Normally, the pectoralis majors pull from their sternoclavicular origin and bring the upper arm to the body in a hugging motion (Figure 1–38). When functioning as accessory muscles of inspiration, they pull from the humeral insertion and elevate the chest, resulting in an increased anteroposterior diameter. It is common to observe patients with chronic obstructive pulmonary disease bracing their arms against something stationary and using their pectoralis majors to increase the diameter of their chests (Figure 1–39, page 54).

Trapezius Muscles.   The **trapezius muscles** are large, flat, triangular muscles that are situated superficially in the upper back and the back of the neck. They originate from the occipital bone, the ligamentum nuchae, and the spinous processes of the seventh cervical vertebra and all the thoracic vertebrae. They

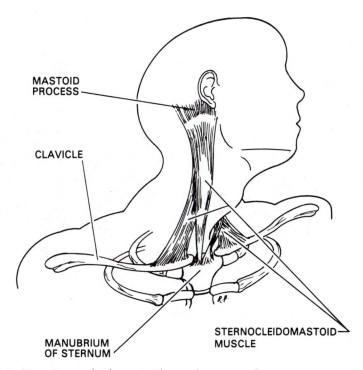

MASTOID
PROCESS

CLAVICLE

MANUBRIUM
OF STERNUM

STERNOCLEIDOMASTOID
MUSCLE

FIGURE 1–37. Sternocleidomastoid muscle.

insert into the spine of the scapula, the acromion process, and the lateral third of the clavicle (Figure 1–40, page 55).

Normally, the trapezius muscles rotate the scapula, raise the shoulders, and abduct and flex the arms. Their action is typified in shrugging of the shoulders (Figure 1–41, page 56). When used as accessory muscles of inspiration, the trapezius muscles help to elevate the thoracic cage.

External Intercostal Muscles. The **external intercostal muscles** arise from the lower border of each rib (the upper limit of an intercostal space), and insert into the upper border of the rib below. Anteriorly, the fibers run downward and medially. Posteriorly, the fibers run downward and laterally (Figure 1–42, page 57). The external intercostal muscles contract during inspiration and pull the ribs upward and outward, increasing both the lateral and anteroposterior diameters of the thorax (an antagonist action to the internal intercostal muscles). This action increases lung volume and prevents intercostal space retractions during an excessively forceful inspiration.

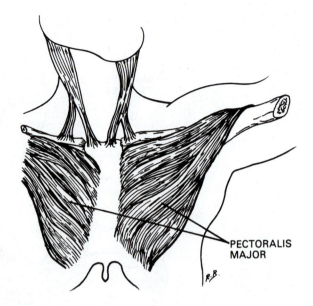
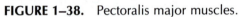

PECTORALIS
MAJOR

FIGURE 1–38.   Pectoralis major muscles.

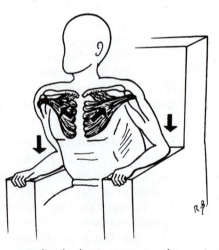

FIGURE 1–39.   How an individual may appear when using the pectoralis major muscles for inspiration.

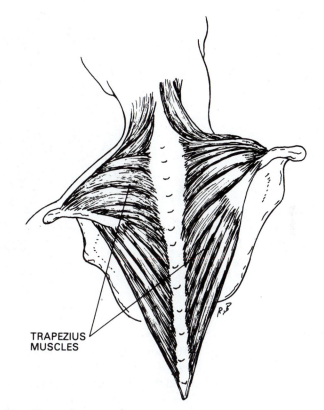

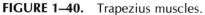

FIGURE 1–40. Trapezius muscles.

The Accessory Muscles of Expiration

The accessory muscles of expiration are those muscles that are recruited to assist in exhalation when airway resistance becomes significantly elevated. When these muscles contract, they increase the intrapleural pressure and offset the increased airway resistance. Following are the major accessory muscles of exhalation:

- Rectus abdominis muscles
- External abdominis obliquus muscles
- Internal abdominis obliquus muscles
- Transversus abdominis muscles
- Internal intercostal muscles

Rectus Abdominis Muscles.   The **rectus abdominis muscles** are a pair of muscles that extend the entire length of the abdomen. Each muscle forms a vertical

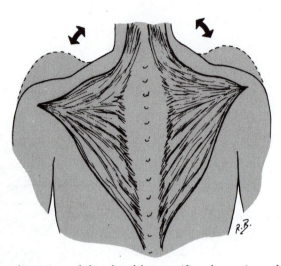

FIGURE 1–41. Shrugging of the shoulders typifies the action of the trapezius muscles.

mass about four inches wide and is separated from the other by the *linea alba*. The muscles arise from the iliac crest and pubic symphysis and insert into the xyphoid process and the fifth, sixth, and seventh ribs.

When contracted, the rectus abdominis muscles assist in compressing the abdominal contents. This compression, in turn, pushes the diaphragm into the thoracic cage (Figure 1–43*A*, page 58), thereby assisting in exhalation.

External Abdominis Oblique Muscles. The **external abdominis obliquus muscles** are broad, thin, muscles positioned on the anterolateral sides of the abdomen. They are the longest and the most superficial of all the anterolateral abdominal muscles. They arise by eight digitations from the lower eight ribs and the abdominal aponeurosis and insert into the iliac crest and the linea alba.

When contracted, the external abdominis obliquus muscles assist in compressing the abdominal contents, which, in turn, push the diaphragm into the thoracic cage (Figure 1–43*B*), thereby assisting in exhalation.

Internal Abdominis Oblique Muscles. Smaller and thinner than the external abdominis obliques, the **internal abdominis obliquus muscles** are located in the lateral and ventral parts of the abdominal wall directly under the external abdominis obliquus muscles. They arise from the inguinal ligament, the iliac crest, and the lower portion of the lumbar aponeurosis. They insert into the last four ribs and into the linea alba.

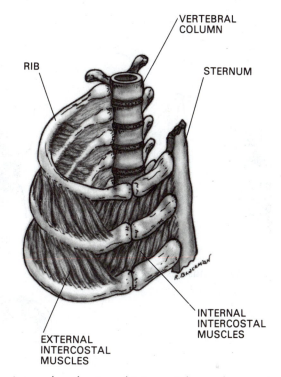

FIGURE 1–42.   Internal and external intercostal muscles.

The internal abdominis obliquus muscles also assist in exhalation by compressing the abdominal contents and in pushing the diaphragm into the thoracic cage (Figure 1–43C).

Transversus Abdominis Muscles.   The **transversus abdominis muscles** are found immediately under the internal abdominis obliquus muscles. These muscles arise from the inguinal ligament, the iliac crest, the thoracolumbar fascia, and the lower six ribs, and insert into the linea alba. When activated, they also help to constrict the abdominal contents (Figure 1–43D).

When all four pairs of accessory muscles of exhalation contract, the abdominal pressure increases and drives the diaphragm into the thoracic cage. As the diaphragm moves into the thoracic cage during exhalation, the intrapleural pressure increases, enhancing the amount of gas flow (Figure 1–44).

Internal Intercostal Muscles.   The **internal intercostal muscles** run between the ribs immediately beneath the external intercostal muscles. The muscles arise from the inferior border of each rib and insert into the superior border of the rib below. Anteriorly, the fibers run in a downward and lateral direction. Posteriorly,

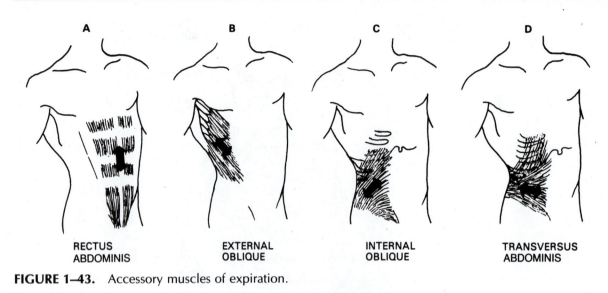

FIGURE 1–43.   Accessory muscles of expiration.

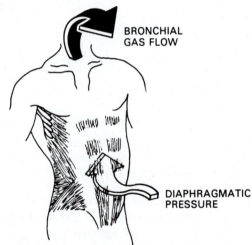

FIGURE 1–44.   The collective action of the accessory muscles of expiration causes the intrapleural pressure to increase, the chest to move outward, and bronchial gas flow to increase.

the fibers run downward and in a medial direction (see Figure 1–42). The internal intercostal muscles contract during expiration and pull the ribs downward and inward, decreasing both the lateral and anteroposterior diameters of the thorax (an antagonist action to the external intercostal muscles). This action decreases lung volume and offsets intercostal bulging during excessive expiration.

SELF-ASSESSMENT QUESTIONS

1. Which of the following line the anterior one third of the nasal cavity?
     a. Stratified squamous epithelium
     b. Simple cuboidal epithelium
     c. Type I cells
     d. Pseudostratified ciliated columnar epithelium
     e. Simple squamous epithelium

2. Which of the following form(s) the nasal septum?
     I. Frontal process of the maxilla bone
     II. Ethmoid bone
     III. Nasal bones
     IV. Vomer
        a. I only
        b. III only
        c. IV only
        d. I and III only
        e. II and IV only

3. Which of the following prevents the aspiration of foods and liquids?
     a. Epiglottis
     b. Cricoid cartilage
     c. Arytenoid cartilages
     d. Thyroid cartilages
     e. Corniculate cartilages

4. The canals of Lambert are found in the
     a. trachea
     b. terminal bronchioles
     c. alveoli
     d. main stem bronchi
     e. alveolar ducts

5. The eustachian tubes are found in the
     a. nasopharynx
     b. oropharynx
     c. laryngopharynx
     d. oral cavity
     e. tracheobronchial tree

6. The inferior portion of the larynx is composed of the
     a. arytenoid cartilage
     b. thyroid cartilage
     c. hyoid bone
     d. glottis
     e. cricoid cartilage

7. Which of the following has the greatest cross-sectional area?
    a. Terminal bronchioles
    b. Main stem bronchi
    c. Lobar bronchi
    d. Trachea
    e. Segmental bronchi

8. The left main stem bronchus angles off from the carina at about
    a. 5 to 10 degrees from the carina
    b. 10 to 20 degrees from the carina
    c. 20 to 30 degrees from the carina
    d. 30 to 40 degrees from the carina
    e. 40 to 60 degrees from the carina

9. Ninety-five percent of the alveolar surface is composed of which of the following?
    I. Type I cells
    II. Granular pneumocytes
    III. Type II cells
    IV. Squamous pneumocytes
        a. I only
        b. II only
        c. III only
        d. I and IV only
        e. II and IV only

10. Which of the following is/are released when the parasympathetic nerve fibers are stimulated?
    I. Norepinephrine
    II. Atropine
    III. Epinephrine
    IV. Acetylcholine
        a. II only
        b. IV only
        c. I and III only
        d. I, II, and III only
        e. I, II, III and IV

11. Which of the following is/are released when the sympathetic nerve fibers are stimulated?
    I. Norepinephrine
    II. Propranolol
    III. Acetylcholine
    IV. Epinephrine
        a. I only
        b. II only

    c. I and IV only

    d. II, III, and IV only

    e. I, II, III and IV

12. Pseudostratified ciliated columnar epithelium lines which of the following?

    I. Oropharynx

    II. Trachea

    III. Nasopharynx

    IV. Oral cavity

    V. Laryngopharynx

      I only

      II only

      IV only

      II and III only

      I, II, III, and V only

13. Which of the following is/are accessory muscles of inspiration?

    I. Trapezius muscles

    II. Internal abdominis obliquus muscles

    III. Scalene muscles

    IV. Transversus abdominis muscles

      a. I only

      b. II only

      c. I and III only

      d. II and IV only

      e. II, III, and IV only

14. The horizontal fissure separates the

      a. middle and upper lobes of the right lung

      b. upper and lower lobes of the left lung

      c. middle and lower lobes of the right lung

      d. oblique fissure of the left lung

      e. oblique fissure of the right lung

15. Which of the following supply the motor innervation of each hemidiaphragm?

    I. Vagus nerve (tenth cranial nerve)

    II. Phrenic nerve

    III. Lower thoracic nerves

    IV. Glossopharyngeal nerve (ninth cranial nerve)

      a. I only

      b. II only

      c. IV only

      d. I and IV only

      e. II and III only

16. The lung segment called the superior lingula is found in the

      a. left lung, lower division of the upper lobe

      b. right lung, lower lobe

      c. left lung, upper division of the upper lobe

      d. right lung, upper lobe

      e. left lung, lower lobe

17. Cartilage is found in which of the following structures of the tracheobronchial tree?

      I. Bronchioles

      II. Respiratory bronchioles

      III. Segmental bronchi

      IV. Terminal bronchioles

        a. I only

        b. III only

        c. IV only

        d. I and IV only

        e. I, II, and IV only

18. The bronchial arteries nourish the tracheobronchial tree down to, and including, which of the following?

      a. Respiratory bronchioles

      b. Subsegmental bronchi

      c. Alveolar ducts

      d. Terminal bronchioles

      e. Segmental bronchi

19. Which of the following elevates the soft palate?

      a. Palatoglossal muscle

      b. Levator veli palatine muscle

      c. Transverse arytenoid muscle

      d. Stylopharyngeus muscles

      e. Palatopharyngeal muscle

20. Which of the following are called the resistance vessels?

      a. Arterioles

      b. Veins

      c. Capillaries

      d. Venules

      e. Arteries

Answers appear in Appendix VII.

CHAPTER 2

VENTILATION

OBJECTIVES

By the end of this chapter, the student should be able to:

1. Define ventilation.
2. Differentiate between the following pressure differences across the lungs:
   —Driving pressure
   —Transairway pressure
   —Transpulmonary pressure
   —Transthoracic pressure
3. Describe the role of the diaphragm in ventilation.
4. Explain how the excursion of the diaphragm affects the intrapleural pressure, intra-alveolar pressure, and bronchial gas flow during
   —inspiration
   —end-inspiration
   —expiration
   —end-expiration
5. Define the term static.
6. Define lung compliance.
7. Calculate lung compliance.
8. Explain how Hooke's law can be applied to the elastic properties of the lungs.
9. Define surface tension.
10. Describe the physical principles of Laplace's law.
11. Describe how Laplace's law can be applied to the alveolar fluid lining.
12. Explain how pulmonary surfactant offsets alveolar surface tension.
13. List respiratory disorders that cause a deficiency of pulmonary surfactant.
14. Define the term dynamic.
15. Describe how Poiseuille's law arranged for flow relates to the radius of the bronchial airways.
16. Describe how Poiseuille's law arranged for pressure relates to the radius of the bronchial airways.
17. Describe how Poiseuille's law can be rearranged to simple proportionalities.
18. Define airway resistance and explain how it relates to
    —laminar flow
    —turbulent flow

19. Calculate airway resistance.
20. Define time constants and explain how they relate to alveolar units with
    —increased airway resistance
    —decreased compliance
21. Define dynamic compliance and explain how it relates to
    —increased airway resistance
    —frequency dependence
22. Describe how the following relates to the normal ventilatory pattern:
    —Tidal volume (V_T)
    —Ventilatory rate
    —I : E ratio
23. Differentiate between alveolar ventilation and deadspace ventilation, and include an explanation of the following:
    —Anatomic deadspace
    —Alveolar deadspace
    —Physiologic deadspace
24. Describe how the following affect the total alveolar ventilation:
    —Depth of breathing
    —Rate of breathing
25. Calculate an individual's total alveolar ventilation in one minute (minute ventilation) when given the following information:
    —Alveolar ventilation
    —Deadspace ventilation
    —Breaths per minute
26. Describe how the normal intrapleural pressure differences cause regional differences in normal lung ventilation.
27. Describe how the following alter the ventilatory pattern (i.e., the respiratory rate and tidal volume):
    —Decreased lung compliance
    —Increased airway resistance
28. Define the following specific ventilatory patterns:
    —Apnea
    —Eupnea
    —Biot's breathing
    —Hyperpnea
    —Hyperventilation
    —Hypoventilation
    —Tachypnea
    —Cheyne-Stokes breathing
    —Kussmaul breathing
    —Orthopnea
    —Dyspnea
29. Complete the self-assessment questions at the end of this chapter.

The term **ventilation** is defined as the process that exchanges gases between the external environment and the alveoli. It is the mechanism by which oxygen is carried from the atmosphere to the alveoli and by which carbon dioxide (delivered to the lungs in mixed venous blood) is carried from the alveoli to the atmosphere.

To understand the process of ventilation, the respiratory care practitioner must understand (1) how the excursion of the diaphragm changes the intra-alveolar and intrapleural pressures, (2) the static characteristics of the lungs, (3) the dynamic characteristics of the lungs, and (4) the characteristics of normal and abnormal ventilatory patterns.

PRESSURE DIFFERENCES ACROSS THE LUNGS

Understanding the following pressure differences across the lungs is an essential building block in the study of ventilation.

Driving Pressure is the pressure difference between two points in a tube or vessel; it is the force moving gas or fluid through the tube or vessel. For example, if the gas pressure at the beginning of a tube is 20 mm Hg, and the pressure at the end of the same tube is 5 mm Hg, the driving pressure is 15 mm Hg. In other words, the force required to move the gas through the tube is 15 mm Hg.

Transairway Pressure (P_{ta}) is the barometric pressure difference between the mouth pressure (P_m) and the alveolar pressure (P_{alv}).

$$P_{ta} = P_m - P_{alv}$$

For example, if the P_{alv} is 757 mm Hg and the P_m is 760 mm Hg during inspiration, the P_{ta} is 3 mm Hg (Figure 2–1A).

$$P_{ta} = P_m - P_{alv}$$
$$= 760 \text{ mm Hg} - 757 \text{ mm Hg}$$
$$= 3 \text{ mm Hg}$$

Or, if the P_{alv} is 763 mm Hg and the P_m is 760 mm Hg during expiration, the P_{ta} is −3 mm Hg. Gas in this example, however, is moving in the opposite direction (Figure 2–1B). In essence, the P_{ta} represents the driving pressure (the pressure difference between the mouth and the alveolus) that forces gas in or out of the lungs.

Transpulmonary Pressure (P_{tp}) is the difference between the alveolar pressure (P_{alv}) and the pleural pressure (P_{pl}).

$$P_{tp} = P_{alv} - P_{pl}$$

For example, if the P_{pl} is 755 mm Hg and the P_{alv} is 760 mm Hg (e.g., inspiration), the P_{tp} is 5 mm Hg (Figure 2–2A).

$$P_{tp} = P_{alv} - P_{pl}$$
$$= 760 \text{ mm Hg} - 755 \text{ mm Hg}$$
$$= 5 \text{ mm Hg}$$

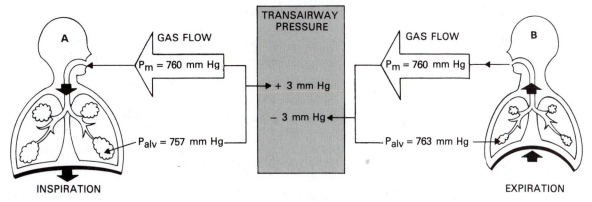

FIGURE 2–1. Transairway pressure: The difference between the pressure at the mouth (P_m) and the alveolar pressure (P_{alv}). Even though gas is moving in opposite directions in *A* and *B*, the transairway pressure is 3 mm Hg in both examples. Note: In this illustration, the pressure of the mouth (P_m) is equal to the barometric pressure (BP).

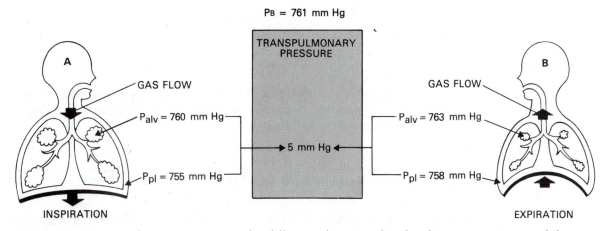

FIGURE 2–2. Transpulmonary pressure: The difference between the alveolar pressure (P_{alv}) and the pleural pressure (P_{pl}). This illustration assumes a barometric pressure (BP) of 761 mm Hg.

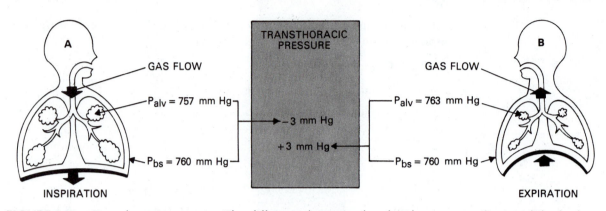

FIGURE 2–3. Transthoracic pressure: The difference between the alveolar pressure (P_{alv}) and the body surface pressure (P_{bs}). Note: In this illustration, the body surface pressure (P_{bs}) is equal to the barometric pressure (BP).

Or, if the P_{alv} is 763 mm Hg and the P_{pl} is 758 mm Hg (e.g., expiration), the P_{tp} is 5 mm Hg (Figure 2–2*B*).

Transthoracic Pressure (P_{tt}) is the difference between the alveolar pressure (P_{alv}) and the body surface pressure (P_{bs}).

$$P_{tt} = P_{alv} - P_{bs}$$

For example, if the P_{alv} is 757 mm Hg and the P_{bs} is 760 mm Hg (e.g., inspiration), the P_{tt} is −3 mm Hg (Figure 2–3*A*).

$$P_{tt} = P_{alv} - P_{bs}$$

$$= 757 \text{ mm Hg} - 760 \text{ mm Hg}$$

$$= -3 \text{ mm Hg}$$

Or, if the P_{alv} is 763 mm Hg and the P_{bs} is 760 mm Hg (e.g., expiration), the P_{tt} is 3 mm Hg (Figure 2–3*B*).

Technically, there is no real difference between the transairway pressure (P_{ta}) and the transthoracic pressure (P_{tt}). The P_{tt} is merely another way to view the pressure differences across the lungs.

ROLE OF THE DIAPHRAGM IN VENTILATION

The flow of gas in and out of the lungs is caused by the transpulmonary and transairway pressure changes that occur in response to the action of the diaphragm (Figure 2–4). When stimulated to contract during inspiration, diaphragmatic

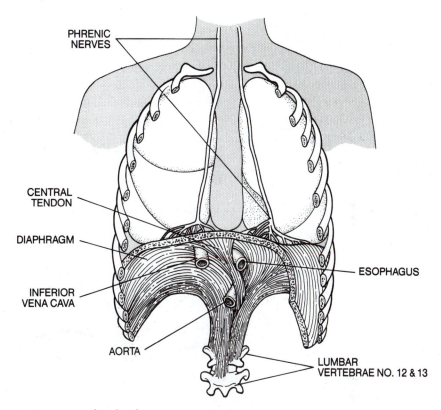

PHRENIC
NERVES

CENTRAL
TENDON

DIAPHRAGM

INFERIOR
VENA CAVA

AORTA

ESOPHAGUS

LUMBAR
VERTEBRAE NO. 12 & 13

FIGURE 2–4. The diaphragm.

leaves move downward, causing the thoracic volume to increase and the intrapleural and intra-alveolar pressures to decrease (see Boyle's law, Chapter Three). Because the intra-alveolar pressure is less than the barometric pressure during this period, gas from the atmosphere moves down the tracheobronchial tree until the intra-alveolar pressure and the barometric pressure are in equilibrium. This equilibrium point is known as **end-inspiration** (pre-expiration).

During expiration, each diaphragmatic leaf relaxes and moves upward, causing the thoracic volume to decrease and the intrapleural and intra-alveolar pressures to increase. During this period, the intra-alveolar pressure is greater than the barometric pressure and gas flows out of the lungs until the intra-alveolar pressure and the barometric pressure are once again in equilibrium. This equilibrium point is known as **end-expiration** (pre-inspiration). The intrapleural pressure during normal inspiration and expiration is always less than the barometric pressure (Figure 2–5).

At rest, the normal excursion (movement) of the diaphragm is about 1.5 cm, and the normal intrapleural pressure change is about 3 to 6 cm H_2O pressure (2 to

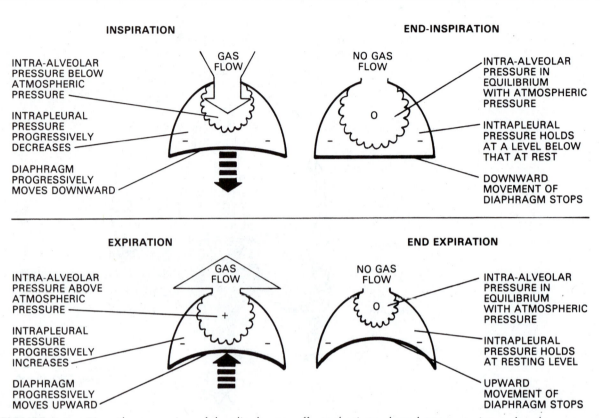

FIGURE 2–5. How the excursion of the diaphragm affects the intrapleural pressure, intra-alveolar pressure, and bronchial gas flow during inspiration and expiration.

4 mm Hg). During a deep inspiration, however, the diaphragm may move as much as 6 to 10 cm, a fact which can cause the average intrapleural pressure to drop as low as 50 cm H_2O subatmospheric. During a forced expiration, the intrapleural pressure may climb between 70 and 100 cm H_2O above atmospheric.

STATIC CHARACTERISTICS OF THE LUNGS

The term **static** refers to the study of matter at rest and the forces bringing about or maintaining equilibrium. Normally, the lungs have a natural tendency to recoil inward, or to collapse. In contrast, the chest wall has a natural tendency to move outward, or to expand. Because of these two opposing forces, the lungs are at their resting volume (**functional residual capacity**) when the inward recoil force of the lungs is equal to the outward, or expanding, force of the chest wall. In other words, the functional residual capacity is the volume remaining in the lungs when the recoil pressure of the lungs and the outward pressure generated by the chest wall cancel each other out.

There are two major static forces in the lungs that cause an inflated lung to recoil inward: (1) the elastic properties of the lung tissue itself and (2) the surface tension produced by the layer of fluid that lines the inside of the alveoli.

Elastic Properties of the Lung

How readily the elastic force of the lungs accepts a volume of inspired air is known as **lung compliance** (C_L). C_L is defined as the change in lung volume (ΔV) per unit pressure change (ΔP). Mathematically, C_L is expressed in liters per centimeters of water pressure (L/cm H_2O). In other words, compliance determines how much air, in liters (L), the lungs will accommodate for each centimeter of water pressure change (cm H_2O) (e.g., each transpulmonary pressure change).

For example, if an individual generates a negative intrapleural pressure change of 5 cm H_2O during inspiration, and the lungs accept a new volume of .75 L of gas, the C_L of the lungs would be expressed as .15 L/cm H_2O:

$$C_L = \frac{\Delta V \, (L)}{\Delta P \, (cm \, H_2O)}$$

$$= \frac{.75 \, L \, of \, gas}{5 \, cm \, H_2O}$$

$$= .15 \, L/cm \, H_2O \, (or, \, 150 \, ml/cm \, H_2O)$$

It is irrelevant whether the change in driving pressure is in the form of a positive or negative pressure. In other words, a negative 5 cm H_2O pressure generated in the intrapleural space around the lungs will produce the same volume change as a positive 5 cm H_2O pressure generated at the airway (e.g., by means of a mechanical ventilator) (Figure 2–6).

At rest, the average C_L for each breath is about 0.1 L/cm H_2O. In other words, approximately 100 ml of air is delivered into the lungs per 1 cm H_2O pressure change (see Figure 2–6). When lung compliance is increased, the lungs accept a greater volume of gas per unit of pressure change. When C_L is decreased, the lungs accept a smaller volume of gas per unit of pressure change. This relationship is also illustrated by the volume-pressure curve in Figure 2–7 (page 73).

Finally, it should be noted that C_L—both in the normal and abnormal lung—progressively decreases as the alveoli approach their total filling capacity. This occurs because the elastic force of the alveoli steadily increases as the lungs expand, which, in turn, reduces the ability of the lungs to accept an additional volume of gas (see Figure 2–7).

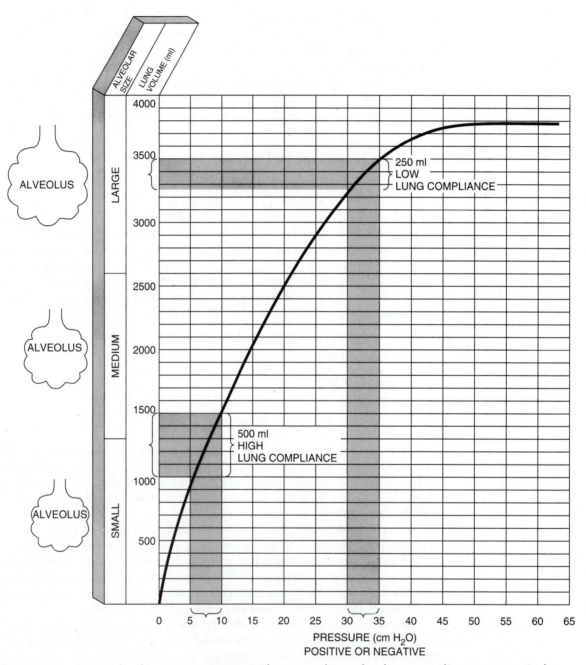

FIGURE 2–6. Normal volume-pressure curve. The curve shows that lung compliance progressively decreases as the lungs expand in response to more volume. For example, note the greater volume change between 5 and 10 cm H$_2$O (small/medium alveoli) than between 30 and 35 cm H$_2$O (large alveoli).

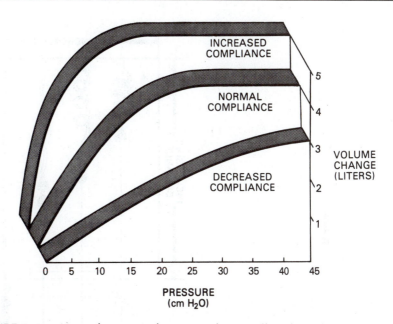

FIGURE 2–7. How changes in lung compliance affect the volume-pressure curve. When lung compliance decreases, the volume-pressure curve shifts to the right. When lung compliance increases, the volume-pressure curve shifts to the left.

Hooke's Law. Hooke's law provides another way to conceptualize the meaning of compliance by describing the physical properties of an elastic substance. **Elastance** is the natural ability of matter to respond directly to force and to return to its original resting position or shape after the external force no longer exists. In pulmonary physiology, elastance is defined as the change in pressure per change in volume:

$$\text{Elastance} = \frac{\Delta P}{\Delta V}$$

Elastance is the reciprocal (opposite) of compliance. Thus, lungs with high compliance (greater ease of filling) have low elastance; lungs with low compliance (lower ease of filling) have high elastance.

Hooke's law states that when a truly elastic body, like a spring, is acted on by 1 unit of force, the elastic body will stretch 1 unit of length, and when acted on by 2 units of force it will stretch 2 units of length, and so forth. This phenomenon is only true, however, within the elastic body's normal functional range. That is, when the force goes beyond the elastic limit of the substance, the ability of length to directly increase in response to force ceases. Should the force continue to rise, the elastic substance will ultimately break (Figure 2–8).

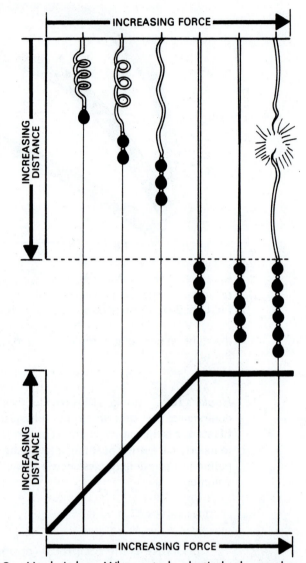

FIGURE 2–8. Hooke's law. When a truly elastic body—such as the spring in this illustration—is acted on by 1 unit of force, the elastic body will stretch 1 unit of length; when acted on by 2 units of force, it will stretch 2 units of length; and so forth. When the force goes beyond the elastic limit of the substance, however, the ability of length to increase in response to force quickly ceases.

When Hooke's law is applied to the elastic properties of the lungs, *volume* is substituted for *length*, and *pressure* is substituted for *force*. Thus, over the normal physiologic range of the lungs, volume varies directly with pressure. The lungs behave in a manner similar to the spring, and once the elastic limit of the lung unit is reached, little or no volume change occurs in response to pressure changes. Should the change in pressure continue to rise, the lung unit will rupture (Figure 2–9).

Clinically, this phenomenon explains a hazard associated with mechanical ventilation. That is, if the pressure during mechanical ventilation (positive pressure breath) causes the lung unit to expand beyond its elastic capability, the lung unit could rupture—allowing alveolar gas to move into the intrapleural space causing the lungs to collapse. This condition is called a **pneumothorax**.

Surface Tension and Its Effect on Lung Expansion

In addition to the elastic properties of the lungs, the normal fluid (primarily H_2O) that lines the inner surface of the alveoli can profoundly resist lung expansion. To understand how the liquid coating the intra-alveolar surface can hinder lung expansion, an understanding of the following is essential: (1) the meaning of surface tension, (2) the physical principles of Laplace's law, and (3) how the substance called pulmonary surfactant offsets alveolar surface tension.

Surface Tension. When liquid molecules are completely surrounded by identical molecules, the molecules are mutually attracted toward one another and, therefore, move freely in all directions (Figure 2–10A, page 77). When a liquid–gas interface exists, however, the liquid molecules at the liquid–gas interface are strongly attracted to the liquid molecules within the liquid mass (Figure 2–10B). This molecular, cohesive force at the liquid–gas interface is called *surface tension*. It is the surface tension, for example, that maintains the shape of a water droplet, or makes it possible for an insect to move or stay afloat on the surface of a pond.

The quantitative measurement of surface tension is expressed in dynes per centimeter. One dyne/cm is the force necessary to cause a tear 1 centimeter long in the surface layer of a liquid, similar to using two hands to pull a thin piece of cloth apart until a split 1 centimeter in length is formed (1 cm H_2O pressure equals 980 dynes/cm). The liquid film that lines the interior surface of the alveoli has the potential to exert a force in excess of 70 dynes/cm, a force that can easily cause complete alveolar collapse.

Laplace's Law. Laplace's law describes how the *distending pressure* of a liquid bubble (not an alveolus) is influenced by (1) the surface tension of the bubble and (2) the size of the bubble itself. When Laplace's law is applied to a sphere with one liquid–gas interface (e.g., a bubble completely submerged in a liquid), the equation is written as follows:

$$P = \frac{2\,ST}{r}$$

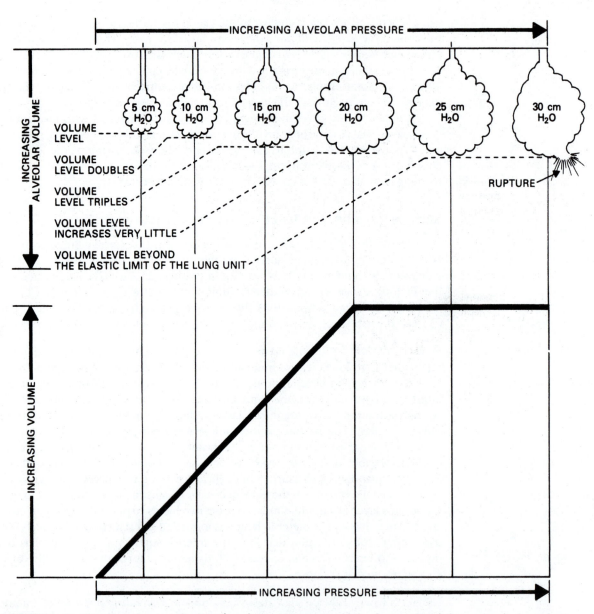

FIGURE 2–9. Hooke's law applied to the elastic properties of the lungs. Over the normal physiologic range of the lungs, volume changes vary directly with pressure changes. Once the elastic limit is reached, however, little or no volume change occurs in response to pressure changes.

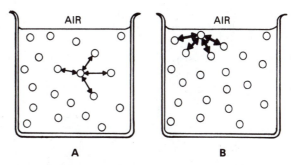

FIGURE 2–10. In model *A*, the liquid molecules in the middle of the container are mutually attracted toward each other and, therefore, move freely in all directions. In model *B*, the liquid molecules near the surface (liquid–gas interface) are strongly attracted to the liquid molecules within the liquid mass. This molecular force at the liquid–gas interface is called surface tension.

where P is the pressure difference (dynes/cm^2), ST is surface tension (dynes/cm), and r is the radius of the liquid sphere (cm); the factor 2 is required when the law is applied to a liquid sphere with one liquid–gas interface.

When the law is applied to a bubble with two liquid–gas interfaces (e.g., a soap bubble blown on the end of a tube has a liquid–gas interface both on the inside and on the outside of the bubble), the numerator contains the factor 4 rather than 2:

$$P = \frac{4\,ST}{r}$$

The mathematical arrangement of Laplace's law shows that the *distending pressure* of a liquid sphere is (1) directly proportional to the surface tension of the liquid and (2) inversely proportional to the radius (size) of the sphere.

In other words, the numerator of Laplace's law shows that (a) as the surface tension of a liquid bubble increases, the distending pressure necessary to hold the bubble open increases, or (b) the opposite—when the surface tension of a liquid bubble decreases, the distending pressure of the bubble decreases (Figure 2–11). The denominator of Laplace's law shows that (a) when the size (radius) of a liquid bubble increases, the distending pressure necessary to hold the bubble open decreases, or (b) the opposite—when the size of the bubble decreases, the distending pressure of the bubble increases (Figure 2–12, page 79). Because of this interesting physical phenomenon, when two different size bubbles—having the same surface tension—are in direct communication, the greater pressure in the smaller bubble will cause the smaller bubble to empty into the larger bubble (Figure 2–13, page 80).

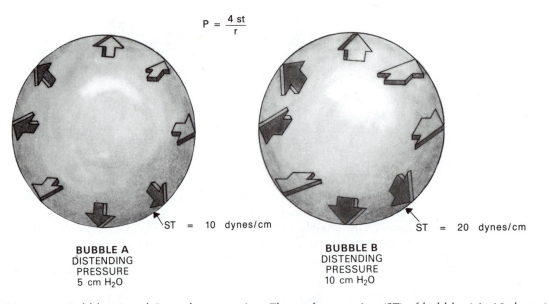

$$P = \frac{4\ st}{r}$$

ST = 10 dynes/cm

ST = 20 dynes/cm

BUBBLE A
DISTENDING
PRESSURE
5 cm H_2O

BUBBLE B
DISTENDING
PRESSURE
10 cm H_2O

FIGURE 2–11.   Bubbles *A* and *B* are the same size. The surface tension (ST) of bubble *A* is 10 dynes/cm and requires a distending pressure (P) of 5 cm H_2O to maintain its size. The surface tension of bubble *B* is 20 dynes/cm H_2O (twice the surface tension of bubble *A*) and requires a distending pressure of 10 cm H_2O (twice that of bubble *A*) to maintain its size (r = radius).

During the formation of a new bubble (e.g., a soap bubble blown on the end of a tube), the principles of Laplace's law do not come into effect until the distending pressure of the liquid sphere goes beyond what is called the *critical opening pressure*. As shown in Figure 2–14 (page 81), the critical opening pressure is the high pressure (with little volume change) that is initially required to overcome the liquid molecular force during the formation of a new bubble— similar to the high pressure first required to blow up a new balloon. Figure 2–14 also shows that, prior to the critical opening pressure, the distending pressure must progressively increase to enlarge the size of the bubble. In other words, the distending pressure is *directly proportional* to the radius of the bubble (the opposite of what Laplace's law states).

Once the critical opening pressure is reached, however, the distending pressure progressively decreases as the bubble increases in size—the distending pressure, as described by Laplace's law, is *inversely proportional* to the radius of the bubble. The distending pressure will continue to decrease until the bubble enlarges to its breaking point and ruptures. It is interesting to note that just before the bubble breaks, the distending pressure is at its lowest level (see Figure 2–14).

Conversely: Laplace's law shows that as an inflated bubble decreases in size, the distending pressure proportionally increases until the pressure reaches what is called the *critical closing pressure* (actually the same pressure as the critical

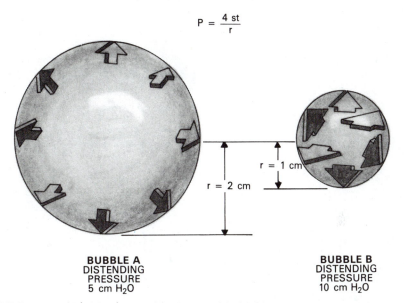

$$P = \frac{4 \text{ st}}{r}$$

r = 1 cm

r = 2 cm

BUBBLE A
DISTENDING
PRESSURE
5 cm H$_2$O

BUBBLE B
DISTENDING
PRESSURE
10 cm H$_2$O

FIGURE 2–12.   The surface tension (ST) of bubbles *A* and *B* is identical. The radius (r) of bubble *A* is 2 cm, and it requires a distending pressure (P) of 5 cm H$_2$O to maintain its size. The radius of bubble *B* is 1 cm (one-half that of bubble *A*), and it requires a distending pressure of 10 cm H$_2$O (twice that of bubble *A*) to maintain its size.

opening pressure). When the size of the bubble decreases beyond this point, the liquid molecular force of the bubble becomes greater than the distending pressure and the bubble collapses (see Figure 2–14).

It should be emphasized that Laplace's law does not state that the surface tension varies with the size of the bubble. To the contrary, the law shows that as a liquid bubble changes in size, it is the *distending pressure*, not the *surface tension*, that varies inversely with the radius. In fact, as the radius of the sphere increases, the surface tension remains the same until the size of the bubble goes beyond its natural elastic limit and ruptures.

The fact that the surface tension remains the same while the radius of a liquid sphere changes can be illustrated mathematically by rearranging Laplace's law as follows:

a. Since surface tension is a property of the fluid and is constant for any specific fluid, Laplace's law can be restated as:

$$P = \frac{k}{r}$$

where k is a constant (in this case, the constant k equals surface tension) and P (pressure) is inversely proportional to r (radius).

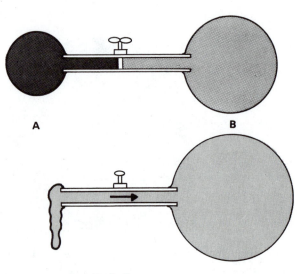

$P_A > P_B$

FIGURE 2–13. Bubbles *A* and *B* have the same surface tension. When the two bubbles are in direct communication, the higher pressure in the smaller bubble (*A*) causes it to empty into the large bubble (*B*).

b. The equation $P = k/r$ can be rearranged as follows:

$$Pr = k$$

The formula now shows that the variable quantities (Pr) are inversely proportional and that their product is a constant (k). Thus, as one variable increases, the other must decrease to maintain a constant product (k).

To demonstrate this concept, consider taking a 400-mile automobile trip. With the formula distance = rate × time ($d = rt$), which represent product (d) and variable quantities (rt), we have:

$$400 = rt \ (d = 400 \text{ miles})$$

or

$$\frac{400}{r} = t$$

On such a trip, assume that we travel at 50 miles per hour (mi/h) and that the trip takes 8 hours (400/50 = 8). If we travel by train and increase the speed to 100 mi/h, the time of the trip decreases to 4 hours. If, however, we decrease

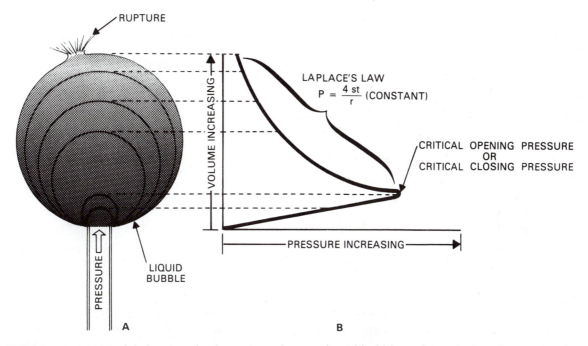

FIGURE 2–14. *A*) Model showing the formation of a new liquid bubble at the end of a tube. *B*) Graph showing the distending pressure required to maintain the bubble's size (volume) at various stages. Initially, a very high pressure, with little volume change, is required to inflate the bubble. Once the critical opening pressure (same as critical closing pressure) is reached, however, the distending pressure progressively decreases as the size of the bubble increases. Thus, between the critical opening pressure and the point at which the bubble ruptures, the bubble behaves according to Laplace's law. In essence, Laplace's law applies to the normal functional size range of the bubble.

the speed to 25 mi/h, the time increases to 16 hours (400/25 = 16). In other words, as the speed increases the time decreases and vice versa, but the product (d) remains a constant 400 miles, which is determined by the length of the trip.

c. Thus, when two variables are inversely proportional, such as rt = 400 or t = 400/r, the time increases as the rate decreases, and time decreases as the rate increases (Figure 2–15). Note the similarity of the graph in Figure 2–15 to the portion of the graph that represents Laplace's law in Figure 2–14*B*.

Laplace's Law Applied to the Alveolar Fluid Lining. Since the liquid film that lines the alveolus resembles a bubble or sphere, according to Laplace's law, when the alveolar fluid is permitted to behave according to its natural tendency, a high transpulmonary pressure must be generated to keep the small alveoli open (see

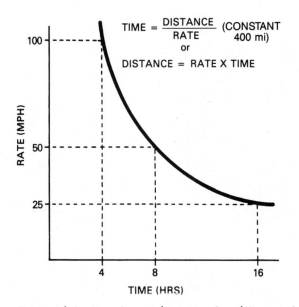

FIGURE 2–15. Rate and time are inversely proportional (as rate increases, time decreases; and as rate decreases, time increases).

Figure 2–14). Fortunately, in the healthy lung the natural tendency for the smaller alveoli to collapse is offset by a fascinating substance called **pulmonary surfactant**.

How Pulmonary Surfactant Offsets Alveolar Surface Tension. Pulmonary surfactant is a phospholipid (dipalmitoyl phosphatidyl choline) produced by the alveolar Type II cells (see Figure 1–21). The surfactant molecule has both a hydrophobic end (water insoluble) and a hydrophilic end (water soluble). This unique hydrophobic/hydrophilic characteristic causes the surfactant molecule to position itself at the alveolar gas–liquid interface so that the hydrophilic end is in the liquid phase and the hydrophobic end is in the gas phase. The interruption of the alveolar fluid caused by the surfactant hydrophilic/hydrophobic ends has the ability to profoundly lower the alveolar surface tension as described below.

The presence of pulmonary surfactant at the alveolar gas–liquid interface causes surface tension to decrease in proportion to the ratio of surfactant to alveolar surface area. That is, when the alveolus decreases in size (decreased volume), the proportion of surfactant to alveolar surface area increases. This mechanism, in turn, increases the physiologic effect of the pulmonary surfactant and causes the alveolar surface tension to decrease (Figure 2–16A).

On the other hand, as the alveolus increases in size (increased volume), the relative amount of surfactant to alveolar surface area decreases (since the number

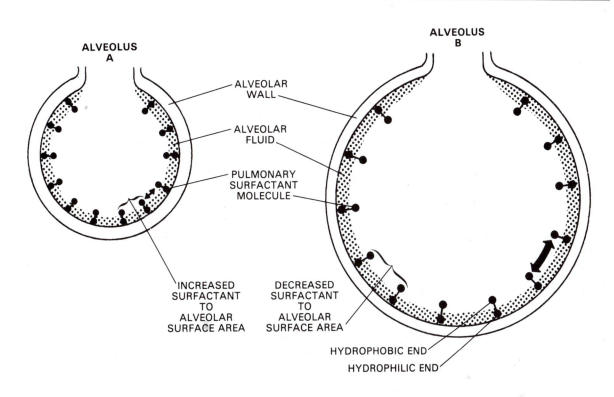

FIGURE 2–16.   In the normal lung, the surface tension is low in the small alveolus (*A*) because the ratio of surfactant to alveolar surface is high. As the alveolus enlarges (*B*), the surface tension steadily increases because the ratio of surfactant to alveolar surface decreases.

of surfactant molecules does not change when the size of the alveolus changes). This mechanism, in turn, decreases the physiologic effect of pulmonary surfactant and causes the alveolar surface tension to increase (Figure 2–16*B*). In fact, as the alveolus enlarges, the surface tension will progressively increase to the value it would naturally have in the absence of pulmonary surfactant. Clinically, however, the fact that surface tension increases as the alveolus enlarges is non-significant— since, as Laplace's law demonstrates, the distending pressure required to maintain a bubble size progressively decreases as the size of the bubble increases (see Figure 2–14).

It is estimated that the surface tension of the average alveolus varies from 1 to 5 dynes/cm (when the alveolus is very small) to about 50 dynes/cm (when the alveolus is fully distended) (Figure 2–17). Because pulmonary surfactant has the

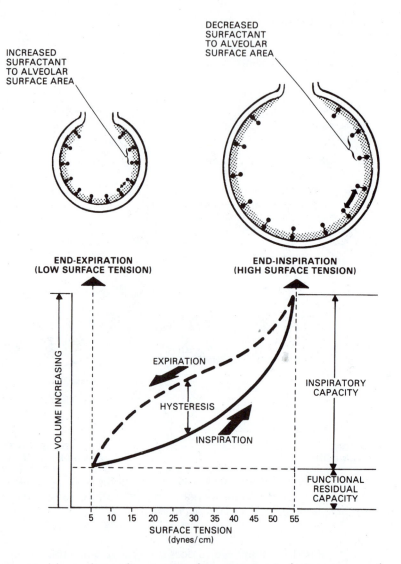

FIGURE 2–17. In the normal lung, the surface tension force progressively increases as the alveolar size increases. Similarly, as the alveolar size decreases, the surface tension force progressively decreases. Note that, because of the alveolar surface tension, the actual physical change of the alveolus lags behind the pressure applied to it. When such a phenomenon occurs in the field of physics (i.e., a physical manifestation lagging behind a force), a *hysteresis* is said to exist. When this lung characteristic is plotted on a volume-pressure curve, the alveolus is shown to deflate along a different curve than that inscribed during inspiration and the curve has a looplike appearance. The hysteresis loop shows graphically that at any given pressure the alveolar volume is less during inspiration than it is during expiration. This alveolar hysteresis is virtually eliminated when the lungs are inflated experimentally with saline; such an experimental procedure removes the alveolar liquid–gas interface and, therefore, the alveolar surface tension. *Inspiratory capacity* is the volume of air that can be inhaled after a normal exhalation. *Functional residual capacity* is the volume of air remaining in the lungs after a normal exhalation.

ability to reduce the surface tension of the small alveoli (the numerator in Laplace's law), the high distending pressure that would otherwise be required to offset the critical closing pressure of the small alveoli is virtually eliminated.

In the absence of pulmonary surfactant, however, the alveolar surface tension increases to the force it would naturally have (50 dynes/cm), and the distending pressure necessary to overcome the recoil forces of the liquid film that coats the small alveoli is very high. In short, the distending pressure required to offset the recoil force of the alveolar fluid behaves according to the principles of Laplace's law. As a result, when the distending pressure of the small alveoli falls below the critical closing pressure, the liquid molecular force snaps the alveolar walls together (see Figure 2–14). Once the liquid walls of the alveolus come in contact with one another, a mutual liquid bond develops that strongly resists the re-expansion of the alveolus. Complete alveolar collapse is called **atelectasis**.

Table 2–1 lists some respiratory disorders that cause pulmonary surfactant deficiency.

Summary of the Static Characteristics of the Lungs. There are two major static forces in the lungs that cause an inflated lung to recoil inward: (1) the elastic properties of the lungs and (2) the surface tension of the liquid film that lines the alveolus.

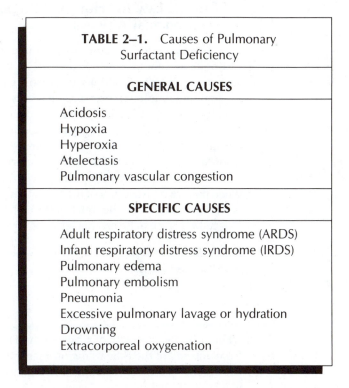

TABLE 2–1. Causes of Pulmonary Surfactant Deficiency
GENERAL CAUSES
Acidosis Hypoxia Hyperoxia Atelectasis Pulmonary vascular congestion
SPECIFIC CAUSES
Adult respiratory distress syndrome (ARDS) Infant respiratory distress syndrome (IRDS) Pulmonary edema Pulmonary embolism Pneumonia Excessive pulmonary lavage or hydration Drowning Extracorporeal oxygenation

In the healthy lung, both the elastic tension and the degree of surface tension are low in the small alveoli. As the alveoli increase in size, both the elastic tension and the degree of surface tension progressively increase. The elastic tension, however, is the predominant force, particularly in the large alveoli (Figure 2–18, page 87).

In the absence of pulmonary surfactant, the alveolar fluid lining behaves according to Laplace's law—that is, a high intrapleural pressure must be generated to keep the small alveoli open. When such a condition exists, the surface tension force predominates in the small alveoli (see Figure 2–18).

DYNAMIC CHARACTERISTICS OF THE LUNGS

The term **dynamic** refers to the study of forces in action. In the lungs, dynamic refers to the movement of gas in and out of the lungs and the pressure changes required to move the gas. The dynamic features of the lung are best explained by (1) Poiseuille's law for flow and pressure and (2) the airway resistance equation.

Poiseuille's Law for Flow and Pressure Applied to the Bronchial Airways

During a normal inspiration, intrapleural pressure decreases from its normal resting level (about −3 to −6 cm H_2O pressure), which causes the bronchial airways to lengthen and to increase in diameter (*passive dilation*). During expiration, intrapleural pressure increases (or returns to its normal resting state), which causes the bronchial airways to decrease in length and in diameter (*passive constriction*) (Figure 2–19, page 88). Under normal circumstances, such anatomic changes of the bronchial airways are not remarkable. In certain respiratory disorders (e.g., emphysema or chronic bronchitis), however, bronchial gas flow and intrapleuralpressure may change significantly, particularly during expiration, when passive constriction of the tracheobronchial tree occurs. The reason for this is best explained in the relationship of factors described in Poiseuille's law. Poiseuille's law can be arranged for either flow or pressure.

Poiseuille's Law Arranged for Flow. When Poiseuille's law is arranged for flow, it is written as follows:

$$\dot{V} = \frac{\Delta P r^4 \pi}{8 l \eta}$$

where η = the viscosity of a gas (or fluid), Δ (Delta) P = the change of pressure from one end of the tube to the other, r = the radius of the tube, l = the length of the tube, $\dot{V}$ = the gas (or fluid) flowing through the tube; $\pi/8$ = constants, which will be excluded from the discussion.

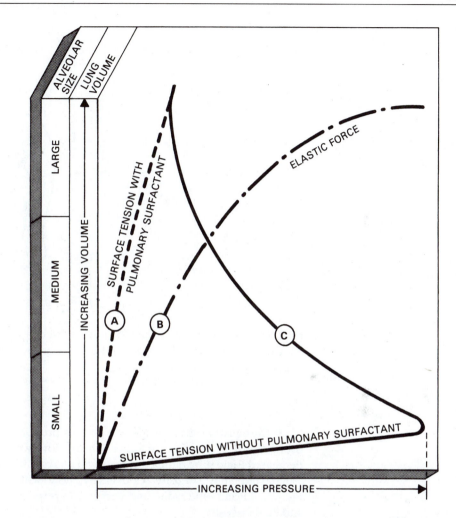

FIGURE 2–18. In the normal lung, both the surface tension force (*A*) and the elastic force (*B*) progressively increase as the alveolus enlarges. The elastic force is the predominant force in both the small and the large alveoli. In the absence of pulmonary surfactant, the surface tension force (*C*) predominates in the small alveoli. The elastic force (*B*) still predominates in the large alveoli. Note that, as the alveolus enlarges, the pressure required to offset the "abnormal" surface tension force (*C*) ultimately decreases to the same pressure required to offset the "normal" surface tension force (*B*). Thus, it can be seen that when there is a deficiency of pulmonary surfactant, the surface tension of the small alveoli creates a high recoil force. If a high pressure is not generated to offset this surface tension force, the alveoli will collapse.

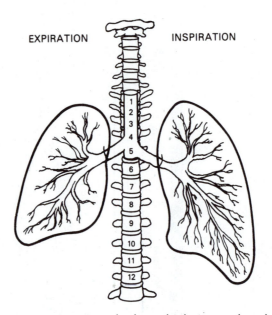

EXPIRATION   INSPIRATION

FIGURE 2–19.   During inspiration, the bronchial airways lengthen and increase in diameter. During expiration, the bronchial airways decrease in length and diameter.

The equation states that flow is directly proportional to P and r^4 and inversely proportional to l and η. In other words, flow will decrease in response to a decreased P and tube radius, and flow will increase in response to a decreased tube length and fluid viscosity. Conversely, flow will increase in response to an increased P and tube radius and decrease in response to an increased tube length and fluid viscosity.

It should be emphasized that flow is profoundly affected by the radius of the tube. As Poiseuille's law illustrates, $\dot{V}$ is a function of the fourth power of the radius (r^4). In other words, assuming that pressure (P) remains constant, decreasing the radius of a tube by one-half reduces the gas flow to 1/16 of its original flow.

For example, if the radius of a bronchial tube through which gas flows at a rate of 16 ml per second is reduced to one-half its original size because of mucosal swelling, the flow rate through the bronchial tube would decrease to 1 ml/sec (1/16 the original flow rate) (Figure 2–20).

Similarly, decreasing a tube radius by 16 percent decreases gas flow to one-half its original rate. For instance, if the radius of a bronchial tube through which gas flows at a rate of 16 ml/second is decreased by 16 percent (because of mucosal swelling, for example), the flow rate through the bronchial tube would decrease to 8 ml/second (one-half the original flow rate) (Figure 2–21, page 90).

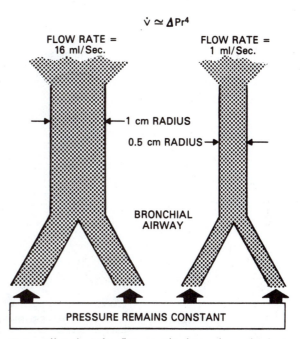

$$\dot{V} \simeq \Delta Pr^4$$

FLOW RATE = 16 ml/Sec.

FLOW RATE = 1 ml/Sec.

← 1 cm RADIUS

0.5 cm RADIUS →

BRONCHIAL AIRWAY

PRESSURE REMAINS CONSTANT

FIGURE 2–20. Poiseuille's law for flow applied to a bronchial airway with its radius reduced 50 percent.

Poiseuille's Law Arranged for Pressure. When Poiseuille's law is arranged for pressure, it is written as follows:

$$P = \frac{\dot{V}8l\eta}{r^4\pi}$$

The equation now states that pressure is directly proportional to $\dot{V}$, l, and η and inversely proportional to r^4. In other words, pressure will increase in response to a decreased tube radius and decrease in response to a decreased flow rate, tube length, or viscosity. The opposite is also true: pressure will decrease in response to an increased tube radius, and increase in response to an increased flow rate, tube length, or viscosity.

Pressure is a function of the radius to the fourth power and therefore is profoundly affected by the radius of a tube. In other words, if flow ($\dot{V}$) remains constant, decreasing a tube radius to one-half of its previous size requires an increase in pressure to 16 times its original level.

For example, if the radius of a bronchial tube with a driving pressure of 1 cm H_2O is reduced to one-half its original size because of mucosal swelling, the driving pressure through the bronchial tube would have to increase to 16 cm H_2O ($16 \times 1 = 16$) to maintain the same flow rate (Figure 2–22, page 91).

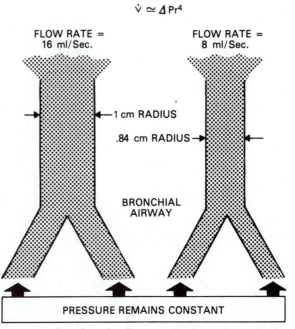

FIGURE 2–21. Poiseuille's law for flow applied to a bronchial airway with its radius reduced 16 percent.

Similarly, decreasing the bronchial tube radius by 16 percent increases the pressure to twice its original level. For instance, if the radius of a bronchial tube with a driving pressure of 10 cm H_2O is decreased by 16 percent because of mucosal swelling, the driving pressure through the bronchial tube would have to increase to 20 cm H_2O (twice its original pressure) to maintain the same flow (Figure 2–23, page 92).

Poiseuille's Law Rearranged to Simple Proportionalities. When Poiseuille's law is applied to the tracheobronchial tree during spontaneous breathing, the two equations can be rewritten as simple proportionalities:

$$\dot{V} \approx Pr^4$$

$$P \approx \frac{\dot{V}}{r^4}$$

Based on the proportionality for flow, it can be stated that since gas flow varies directly with r^4 of the bronchial airway, flow must diminish during exhalation because the radius of the bronchial airways decreases. Stated differently, assuming that the pressure remains constant as the radius (r) of the bronchial airways decreases, gas flow ($\dot{V}$) also decreases. During normal spontaneous breathing, however, the gas flow reduction during exhalation is negligible.

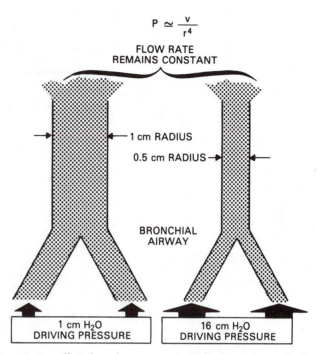

FIGURE 2–22. Poiseuille's law for pressure applied to a bronchial airway with its radius reduced 50 percent.

In terms of the proportionality for pressure ($P \approx \dot{V}/r^4$), if gas flow is to remain constant during exhalation, the transthoracic pressure must vary inversely with the fourth power of the radius of the airway. In other words, as the radius of the bronchial airways decreases during exhalation, the driving pressure must increase to maintain a constant gas flow.*

During normal spontaneous breathing, the need to increase the transairway pressure during exhalation in order to maintain a certain gas flow is not significant. However, in certain respiratory disorders (e.g., emphysema and bronchitis), gas flow reductions and transthoracic pressure increases may be substantial as a result of the bronchial narrowing that develops in such disorders.

Airway Resistance

Airway resistance (R_{aw}) is defined as the pressure difference between the mouth and the alveoli (*transairway pressure*) divided by flow rate. In other words, the rate at which a certain volume of gas flows through the bronchial airways is a

---

*See Mathematical Discussion of Poiseuille's Law in Appendix III.

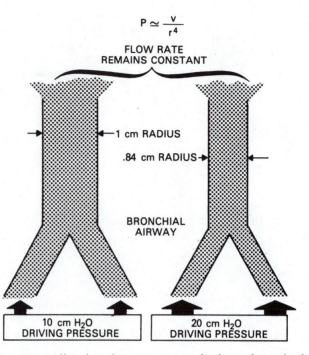

FIGURE 2–23.   Poiseuille's law for pressure applied to a bronchial airway with its radius reduced 16 percent.

function of the pressure gradient and the resistance created by the airways to the flow of gas. Mathematically, R_{aw} is measured in centimeters of water per liter per second (L/sec), according to the following equation:

$$R_{aw} = \frac{\Delta P \, (cm \, H_2O)}{\dot{V}(L/sec)}$$

For example, if an individual produces a flow rate of 4 L/sec during inspiration by generating a transairway pressure of 4 cm H_2O, R_{aw} would equal 1 cm H_2O/L/sec:

$$R_{aw} = \frac{\Delta P}{\dot{V}}$$

$$= \frac{4 \, cm \, H_2O}{4 \, L/sec}$$

$$= 1 \, cm \, H_2O/L/sec$$

Normally, the R_{aw} in the tracheobronchial tree is about 1.0 to 2.0 cm H_2O/L/sec. However, in chronic obstructive pulmonary diseases (e.g., emphysema or asthma), R_{aw} may be very high.

The movement of gas through a tube (or bronchial airway) can be classified as (1) laminar flow, or (2) turbulent flow (Figure 2–24).

Laminar Flow. Laminar gas flow refers to a gas flow that is streamlined. The gas molecules move through the tube in a pattern parallel to the sides of the tube. This flow pattern occurs at low flow rates and at low pressure gradients.

Turbulent Flow. Turbulent gas flow refers to gas molecules that move through a tube in a random manner. Gas flow encounters resistance from both the sides of the tube and from the collision with other gas molecules. This flow pattern occurs at high flow rates and at high pressure gradients.

Time Constants

A product of airway resistance (R_{aw}) and lung compliance (C_L) is a phenomenon called **time constant**. Time constant is defined as the time (in seconds) necessary to inflate a particular lung region to 60 percent of its potential filling capacity. For example, lung regions that have either an increased R_{aw} or an increased C_L require more time to inflate. These alveoli are said to have a *long time constant*. In contrast, lung regions that have either a decreased R_{aw} or a decreased C_L require less time to inflate. These alveoli are said to have a *short time constant*.

Mathematically, the time constant (T_C) is arranged as follows:

$$T_C\,(\text{sec}) = \underbrace{\frac{\Delta P\,(\text{cm H}_2\text{O})}{\dot{V}\,(\text{L/sec})}}_{(R_{aw})} \times \underbrace{\frac{\Delta V\,(\text{L})}{\Delta P\,(\text{cm H}_2\text{O})}}_{(C_L)}$$

$$= \frac{\text{cm H}_2\text{O} \times \text{L}}{\text{L/sec} \times \text{cm H}_2\text{O}}$$

LAMINAR

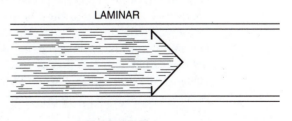

TURBULENT

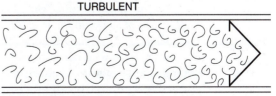

FIGURE 2–24. Types of gas flow.

This equation shows that as R_{aw} increases, the value for pressure (P) (in cm H_2O) in the numerator increases. Or, when C_L decreases, the value for volume (V) in liters (L) in the numerator decreases.

Thus, assuming that all other variables remain constant, if the R_{aw} of a specific lung region doubles, the time constant will also double (i.e., the lung unit will take twice as long to inflate). In contrast, if the C_L is reduced by half, the time constant will also be reduced by half—and, it is important to note, the potential filling capacity of the lung region is also reduced by half. To help illustrate this concept, consider the time constants illustrated in Figure 2–25.

In Figure 2–25A, two alveolar units have identical R_{aw} and C_L. Thus, the two alveoli require the same amount of time to inflate—they have the same time constants. Figure 2–25B shows two alveolar units with the same R_{aw} but with two different C_L. Because the C_L in Unit B is one-half the C_L of Unit A, Unit B (low compliance) receives one-half the volume of Unit A (high compliance). It is important to realize that (1) Unit B has a shorter time constant than Unit A, and (2) Unit B receives only one-half the volume received by Unit A.

In Figure 2–25C, the two alveolar units have the same compliance, but two different R_{aw}. Because the R_{aw} leading to Unit B is two times greater than the R_{aw} leading to Unit A, Unit B (high R_{aw}) requires twice the time to fill to the same volume as Unit A (low R_{aw}). It is important to note that the two alveolar units do not have the same time constant—the time constant for Unit B is two times longer than that of Unit A. Thus, it is also important to note that as the breathing frequency increases, the time necessary to fill Unit B may not be adequate. Clinically, how readily a lung region fills during a period of gas flow is called **dynamic compliance**.

Dynamic Compliance

The measurement called dynamic compliance is a product of the time constants. Dynamic compliance is defined as the change in the volume of the lungs divided by the change in the transpulmonary pressure (obtained via a partially swallowed esophageal pressure balloon) during the time required for one breath. Dynamic compliance is distinctively different from the static lung compliance (C_L) defined earlier in this chapter as the change in lung volume (ΔV) per unit pressure change (ΔP) (see Figure 2–6). In short, static compliance is determined during a period of no gas flow; whereas dynamic compliance is measured during a period of gas flow.

In the healthy lung, the dynamic compliance is about equal to static compliance at all breathing frequencies (the ratio of dynamic compliance to static compliance is 1) (Figure 2–26, page 96).

In patients with partially obstructed airways, however, the ratio of dynamic compliance to static compliance falls significantly as the breathing frequency rises (see Figure 2–26). In other words, the alveoli distal to the obstruction do

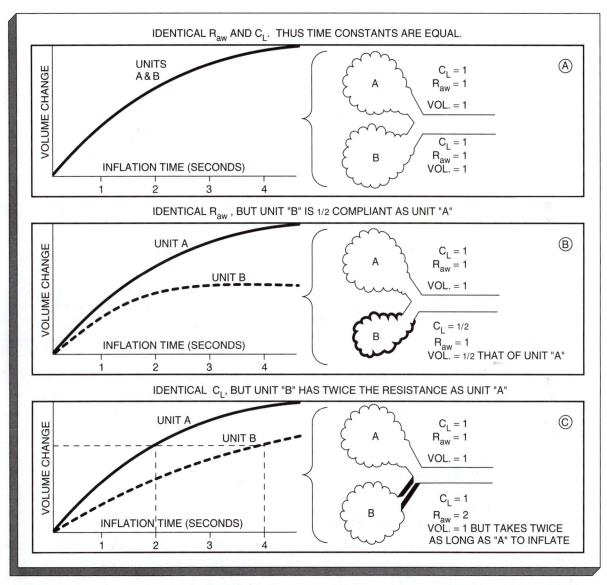

FIGURE 2–25. Time constants for hypothetical alveoli with differing lung compliances (C_L), supplied by airways with differencing resistances (R_{aw}).

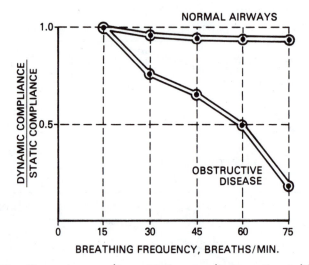

FIGURE 2–26. Dynamic compliance/static compliance ratio at different breathing frequencies. In normal subjects there is essentially no ratio change. In individuals with obstructive disorders, however, the ratio decreases dramatically as the respiratory rate increases.

not have enough time to fill to their potential filling capacity as the breathing frequency increases. The compliance of such alveoli is said to be **frequency dependent.**

VENTILATORY PATTERNS

The Normal Ventilatory Pattern

The ventilatory pattern consists of (1) the tidal volume (V_T), (2) the ventilatory rate, and (3) the time relationship between inhalation and exhalation (I : E ratio).

Tidal volume is defined as the volume of air that normally moves into and out of the lungs in one quiet breath. Normally, V_T is about 7 to 9 ml/kg (3 to 4 ml/lb) of ideal body weight. The normal adult ventilatory rate is about 15 breaths per minute. The I : E ratio is usually about 1 : 2. That is, the time required to inhale a normal breath is about one-half the time required to exhale the same breath.

Technically, though, the time required to inhale and exhale while at rest is about equal (a 1 : 1 ratio) in terms of "true" gas flow. The reason exhalation is considered twice as long as inhalation in the I : E ratio is that the ratio includes the

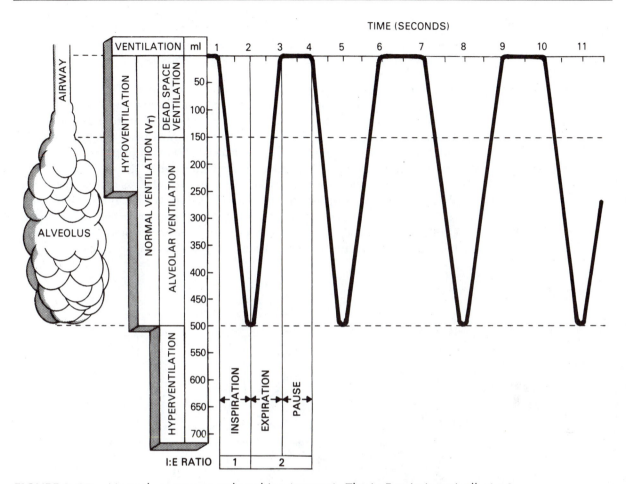

FIGURE 2–27. Normal, spontaneous breathing (eupnea). The I : E ratio is typically 1 : 2.

normal pause, during which there is no gas flow, that typically occurs at end-expiration as part of the exhalation phase (Figure 2–27).

This normal pause that occurs at end-exhalation is usually about equal, in terms of time, to either the inspiratory or expiratory phase. Thus, when an individual is at rest, the time required for a normal ventilatory cycle consists of approximately three equal phases: (1) the inspiratory phase, (2) the expiratory phase, and (3) the pause phase at end-expiration (see Figure 2–27).

Alveolar Ventilation Versus Deadspace Ventilation

Only the inspired air that reaches the alveoli is physiologically effective in terms of gas exchange. This portion of the inspired gas is referred to as **alveolar ventilation**. The volume of inspired air that does not reach the alveoli is not physiologically effective. This portion of gas is referred to as **deadspace ventilation** (Figure 2–28). There are three types of deadspace: (1) **anatomic deadspace**, (2) **alveolar deadspace**, and (3) **physiologic deadspace**.

Anatomic Deadspace.   Anatomic deadspace is the volume of gas in the conducting airways: the nose, mouth, pharynx, larynx, and lower airways down to, but not including, the respiratory bronchioles. The volume of anatomic deadspace is approximately equal to 1 ml/lb (2.2 ml/kg) of normal body weight. Thus, if an individual weighs 150 pounds, approximately 150 ml of inspired gas would be anatomic deadspace gas (or physiologically ineffective).

Because of the anatomic deadspace, moreover, the gas that does enter the alveoli during each inspiration (alveolar ventilation) is actually a combination of (1) anatomic deadspace gas (non-fresh gas) and (2) gas from the atmosphere (fresh gas). To visualize this, consider the inspiration and expiration of 450 ml (V_T) in an individual with an anatomic deadspace of 150 ml (Figure 2–29).

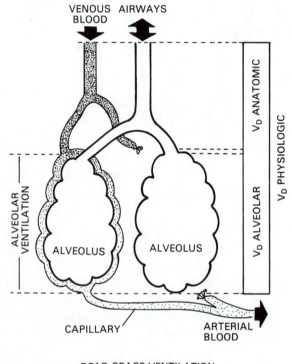

DEAD SPACE VENTILATION
(V_D)

FIGURE 2–28.   Deadspace ventilation (V_D).

Inspiration. As shown in Figure 2–29A, 150 ml of gas fill the anatomic deadspace at pre-inspiration. This gas was the last 150 ml of gas to leave the alveoli during the previous exhalation. Thus, as shown in Figure 2–29B, the first 150 ml of gas to enter the alveoli during inspiration are from the anatomic deadspace (non-fresh gas). The next 300 ml of gas to enter the alveoli are from the atmosphere (fresh gas). The last 150 ml of fresh gas inhaled fill the anatomic deadspace (see Figure 2–29B). Thus, of the 450 ml of gas that enter the alveoli, 150 ml come from the conducting airways (non-fresh gas) and 300 ml come from the atmosphere (fresh gas).

Expiration. As shown in Figure 2–29C, 450 ml of gas are forced out of the alveoli during expiration. The first 150 ml of gas exhaled are from the anatomic dead-space. This gas was the last 150 ml that entered the conducting airways during the previous inspiration (see Figure 2–29B). The next 300 ml of gas exhaled come from the alveoli. The last 150 ml of gas to leave the alveoli fill the anatomic deadspace. During the next inspiration, the last 150 ml of gas exhaled from the alveoli will, again, reenter the alveoli, thus diluting the oxygen concentration of any atmospheric gas that enters the alveoli (see Figure 2–29A).

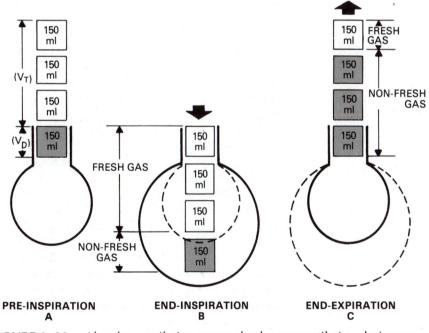

FIGURE 2–29. Alveolar ventilation versus deadspace ventilation during one ventilatory cycle. (See text for explanation.)

Therefore minute alveolar ventilation ($\dot{V}_A$) is equal to the tidal volume (V_T) minus the deadspace ventilation (V_D) multiplied by the breaths per minute (frequency):

$$\dot{V}_A = (V_T - V_D) \times \text{breaths/min}$$

For example, if:

$$V_T = 450 \text{ ml}$$

$$V_D = 150 \text{ ml}$$

Breaths/min = 12

then minute alveolar ventilation would be computed as follows:

$$\dot{V}_A = V_T - V_D \times \text{breaths/min}$$

$$= 450 \text{ ml} - 150 \text{ ml} \times 12$$

$$= 300 \times 12$$

$$= 3600 \text{ ml}$$

Finally, an individual's breathing pattern (depth and rate of breathing) can profoundly alter the total alveolar ventilation. For example, Table 2–2 shows three different subjects, each having a total minute ventilation (MV) of 6000 ml and each having an anatomic deadspace volume of 150 ml. Each subject, however, has a different tidal volume and breathing frequency. Subject A has a tidal volume of 150 ml and a breathing frequency of 40 breaths/min. Even though gas rapidly moves in and out of the lungs, the actual alveolar ventilation is zero. Subject A is merely moving 150 ml of gas in and out of the anatomic deadspace at a rate of 40 times per minute. Clinically, this subject would become unconscious in a few minutes.

Subject B has a tidal volume of 500 ml and a breathing frequency of 12 breaths/min. This subject has an alveolar ventilation of 4200 ml. Subject C has a tidal volume of 1000 ml and a frequency of 6 breaths/min. This subject has an alveolar ventilation of 5100 ml.

The important deduction to be drawn from Table 2–2 is that an **increased depth of breathing is far more effective than an equivalent increase in breathing rate in increasing an individual's total alveolar ventilation.** Or, conversely, a decreased depth of breathing can lead to a significant and, perhaps, a critical reduction of alveolar ventilation. This is because the anatomic deadspace volume represents a fixed volume (normally about one-third), and the fixed volume will make up a larger portion of a decreasing tidal volume. This fraction increases as the tidal volume decreases until, as demonstrated by subject A, it represents the entire tidal volume. On the other hand, any increase in the tidal volume beyond the anatomic deadspace goes entirely toward increasing alveolar ventilation.

TABLE 2–2. Effect of Breathing Depth and Frequency on Alveolar Ventilation

SUBJECT	BREATHING DEPTH (V_T) (ml)	BREATHING FREQUENCY (BREATHS/MIN)	TOTAL MV* (ml/MIN)	$V_D^\dagger$ (ml/MIN)	$V_A^\ddagger$ (ml/MIN)
A	150	40	6000	150 × 40 = 6000	0
B	500	12	6000	150 × 12 = 1800	4200
C	1000	6	6000	150 × 6 = 900	5100

*Total pulmonary ventilation, or minute ventilation (MV), is the product of breathing depth, or tidal volume (V_T), times breathing frequency, or breaths per minute.

†Total deadspace ventilation (V_D) is the product of anatomic deadspace volume (150 ml in each subject) times breathing frequency.

‡V_A = alveolar ventilation.

Alveolar Deadspace.   Alveolar deadspace occurs when an alveolus is ventilated but not perfused with pulmonary blood. Thus, the air that enters the alveolus is not physiologically effective in terms of gas exchange, since there is no pulmonary capillary blood flow. The amount of alveolar deadspace is unpredictable.

Physiologic Deadspace.   Physiologic deadspace is the sum of the anatomic deadspace and alveolar deadspace. Since neither of these two forms of deadspace is physiologically effective in terms of gas exchange, the two forms are combined and are referred to as physiologic deadspace.

HOW NORMAL INTRAPLEURAL PRESSURE DIFFERENCES CAUSE REGIONAL DIFFERENCES IN NORMAL LUNG VENTILATION

As discussed earlier, the diaphragm moves air in and out of the lungs by changing the intrapleural and intra-alveolar pressures. Ordinarily, the intrapleural pressure is always below atmospheric pressure during both inspiration and expiration (see Figure 2–5).

The intrapleural pressure, however, is not evenly distributed within the thorax. In the normal individual in the upright position, there is a natural intrapleural pressure gradient from the upper lung region to the lower. The negative intrapleural pressure at the apex of the lung is normally greater (from −7 to -10 cm H_2O pressure) than at the base (from -2 to -3 cm H_2O pressure). This gradient is gravity dependent and is thought to be due to the normal weight distribution of the lungs above and below the hilum. In other words, because the lung is suspended from the hilum, and because the lung base weighs more than the apex (primarily due to the increased blood flow in the lung base), the lung base requires more pressure for support than the lung apex. This causes the negative intrapleural pressure around the lung base to be less.

Because of the greater negative intrapleural pressure in the upper lung regions, the alveoli in those regions are expanded more than the alveoli in the lower regions. In fact, many of the alveoli in the upper lung regions may be close to, or at, their total filling capacity. This means, therefore, that the compliance of the alveoli in the upper lung regions is normally less than the compliance of the alveoli in the lower lung regions in the normal person in the upright position. As a result, during inspiration the alveoli in the upper lung regions are unable to accommodate as much gas as the alveoli in the lower lung regions. Thus, in the normal individual in the upright position, ventilation is usually much greater and more effective in the lower lung regions (Figure 2–30).

THE EFFECT OF AIRWAY RESISTANCE AND LUNG COMPLIANCE ON VENTILATORY PATTERNS

As already mentioned, the respiratory rate and tidal volume presented by an individual is known as the *ventilatory pattern*. The normal ventilatory pattern is a respiratory rate of about 15 breaths per minute and a tidal volume of about 500 ml. Although the precise mechanism is not clear, it is well documented that these ventilatory patterns frequently develop in response to changes in lung compliance and airway resistance.

When lung compliance decreases, the patient's ventilatory rate generally increases while, at the same time, the tidal volume decreases. When airway resistance increases, the patient's ventilatory frequency usually decreases while, at the same time, the tidal volume increases (Figure 2–31).

The ventilatory pattern adopted by the patient is thought to be based on minimum work requirements rather than ventilatory efficiency. In physics, work is defined as the force applied multiplied by the distance moved (work = force $\times$ distance). In respiratory physiology, the changes in transpulmonary pressure (force) multiplied by the change in lung volume (distance) may be used to quantitate the amount of work required to breathe (work = pressure $\times$ volume). Normally, about 5 percent of an individual's total energy output goes to the work of breathing.

Thus, because the patient may adopt a ventilatory pattern based on the **expenditure of energy** rather than the **efficiency of ventilation**, it cannot be

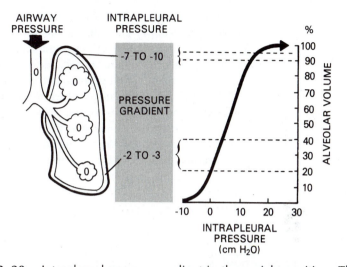

FIGURE 2–30. Intrapleural pressure gradient in the upright position. The negative intrapleural pressure is normally greater in the upper lung regions as compared to the lower lung regions. Because of this, the alveoli in the upper lung regions expand more than the alveoli in the lower lung regions. This condition causes alveolar compliance to be lower in the upper lung regions, and ventilation to be greater in the lower lung regions.

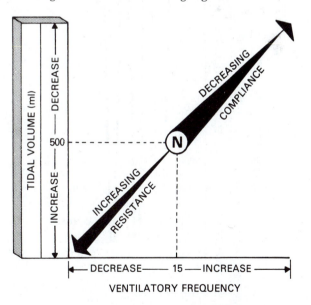

FIGURE 2–31. The effects of increased airway resistance and decreased lung compliance on ventilatory frequency and tidal volume.

assumed that the ventilatory pattern acquired by the patient in response to a certain respiratory disorder is the most efficient in terms of physiologic gas exchange. Such ventilatory patterns are usually seen in the more severe pulmonary disorders that cause lung compliance to decrease or airway resistance to increase.

The patient's adopted ventilatory pattern is frequently not seen in the clinical setting because of secondary heart or lung problems. For example, a patient with chronic emphysema, who has adopted a decreased ventilatory rate and an increased tidal volume because of increased R_{aw}, may demonstrate an increased ventilatory rate and a decreased tidal volume in response to a lung infection or pneumonia that causes lung compliance to decrease.

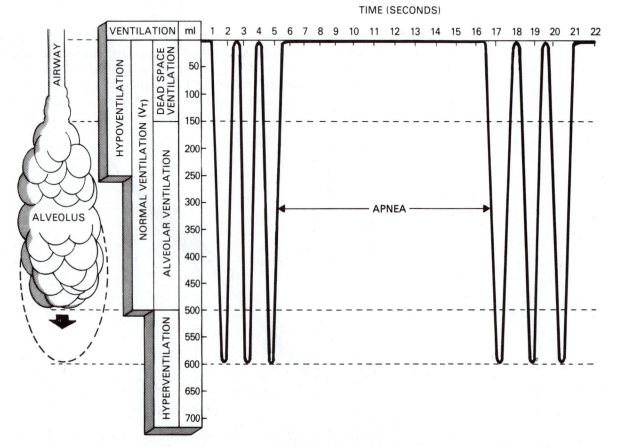

FIGURE 2–32. Biot's breathing: Short episodes of rapid, uniformly deep inspirations, followed by 10 to 30 seconds of apnea. (See Biot's breathing, page 106)

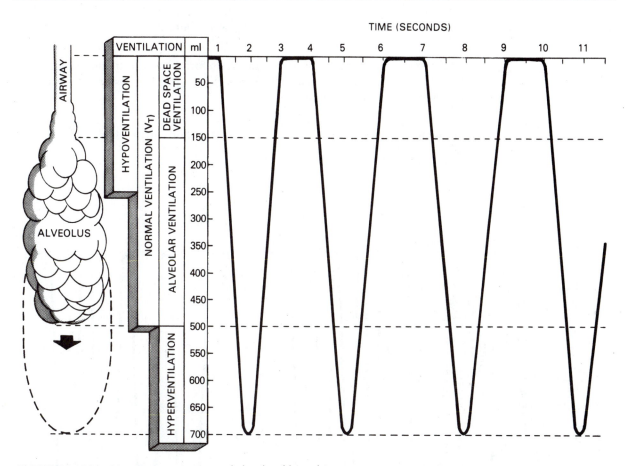

FIGURE 2–33. Hyperpnea: Increased depth of breathing.

OVERVIEW OF SPECIFIC VENTILATORY PATTERNS

The following are ventilatory patterns frequently seen by the respiratory care practitioner in the clinical setting.

Apnea. Complete absence of spontaneous ventilation. This causes the $P_{A_{O_2}}$* and Pa_{O_2}† to rapidly decrease and the $P_{A_{CO_2}}$‡ and Pa_{CO_2}§ to increase. Death will ensue in minutes.

---

*$P_{A_{O_2}}$ = alveolar oxygen tension
†Pa_{O_2} = arterial oxygen tension
‡$P_{A_{CO_2}}$ = alveolar carbon dioxide tension
§Pa_{CO_2} = arterial carbon dioxide tension

Eupnea. Normal, spontaneous breathing (see Figure 2–27).

Biot's Breathing. Short episodes of rapid, uniformly deep inspirations, followed by 10 to 30 seconds of apnea (Figure 2–32). This pattern was first described in patients suffering from meningitis.

Hyperpnea. Increased depth (volume) of breathing with or without an increased frequency (Figure 2–33).

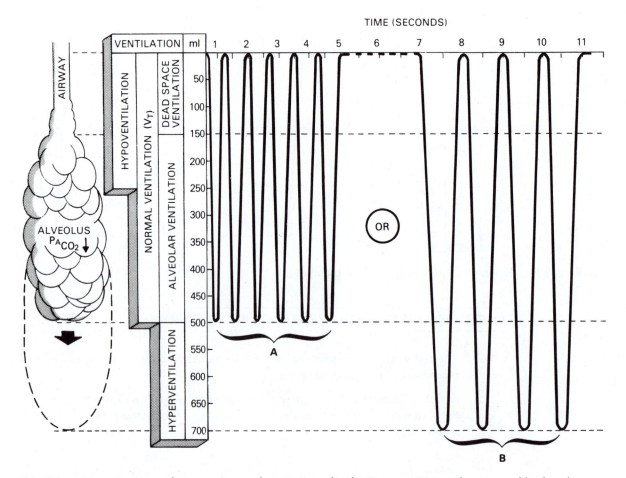

FIGURE 2–34. Hyperventilation: Increased rate (A) or depth (B), or some combination of both, of breathing that causes the $P_{A_{CO_2}}$ and, therefore, the Pa_{CO_2} to decrease.

Hyperventilation.   Increased alveolar ventilation (produced by any ventilatory pattern that causes an increase in either the ventilatory rate or the depth of breathing) that causes the $P_{A_{CO_2}}$ and, therefore, the Pa_{CO_2} to decrease (Figure 2–34).

Hypoventilation.   Decreased alveolar ventilation (produced by any ventilatory pattern that causes a decrease in either the ventilatory rate or the depth of breathing) that causes the $P_{A_{CO_2}}$ and, therefore, the Pa_{CO_2} to increase (Figure 2–35).

Tachypnea.   A rapid rate of breathing.

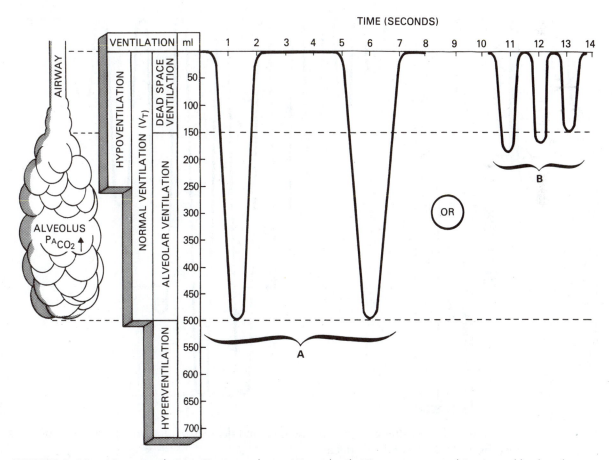

FIGURE 2–35.   Hypoventilation: Decreased rate (*A*) or depth (*B*), or some combination of both, of breathing that causes the $P_{A_{CO_2}}$, therefore, the Pa_{CO_2} to increase.

Cheyne-Stokes Breathing. 10 to 30 seconds of apnea, followed by a gradual increase in the volume and frequency of breathing, followed by a gradual decrease in the volume of breathing until another period of apnea occurs (Figure 2–36). As the depth of breathing increases, the $P_{A_{O_2}}$ and Pa_{O_2} rise and the $P_{A_{CO_2}}$ and Pa_{CO_2} fall. As the depth of breathing decreases, the $P_{A_{O_2}}$ and Pa_{O_2} fall and the $P_{A_{CO_2}}$ and Pa_{CO_2} rise. Cheyne-Stokes breathing is associated with cerebral disorders.

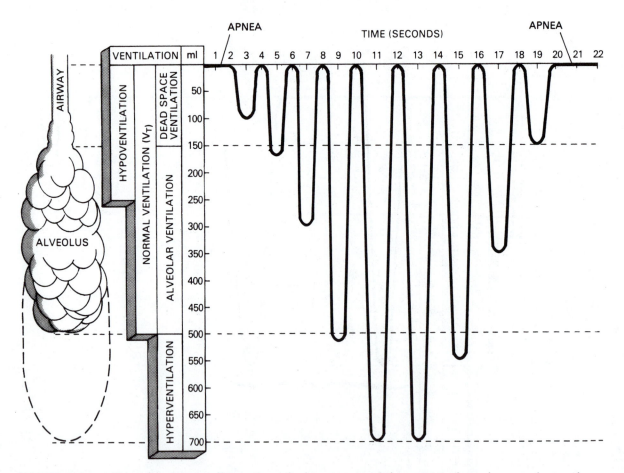

FIGURE 2–36. Cheyne-Stokes breathing: A gradual increase and decrease in the volume and rate of breathing, followed by 10 to 30 seconds of apnea.

Kussmaul Breathing. Both an increased depth (hyperpnea) and rate of breathing (Figure 2–37). This ventilatory pattern causes the $P_{A_{CO_2}}$ and Pa_{CO_2} to decline and the $P_{A_{O_2}}$ and Pa_{O_2} to increase. Kussmaul breathing is commonly associated with diabetic acidosis (ketoacidosis).

Orthopnea. A condition in which an individual is able to breathe most comfortably only in the upright position.

Dyspnea. Difficulty in breathing, of which the individual is aware.

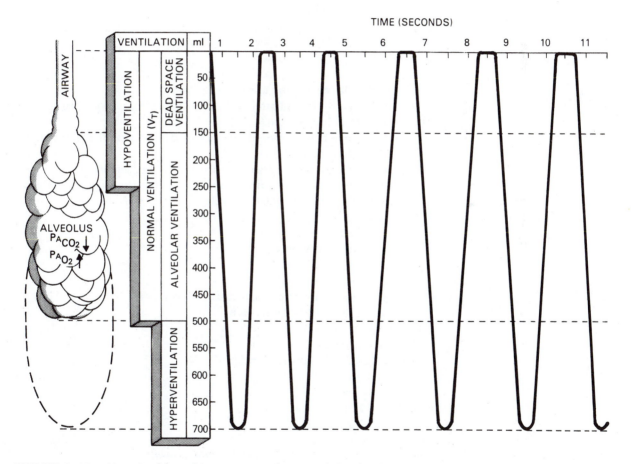

FIGURE 2–37. Kussmaul breathing: Increased rate and depth of breathing. This breathing pattern causes the $P_{A_{CO_2}}$ and Pa_{CO_2} to decrease and $P_{A_{O_2}}$ and Pa_{O_2} to increase.

SELF-ASSESSMENT QUESTIONS

1. The average compliance of the lungs and chest wall combined is
   a. 0.1 L/cm H_2O
   b. 0.2 L/cm H_2O
   c. 0.3 L/cm H_2O
   d. 0.4 L/cm H_2O
   e. 0.5 L/cm H_2O

2. Normally, the airway resistance in the tracheobronchial tree is about
   a. 0.5 to 1.0 cm H_2O/L/sec
   b. 1.0 to 2.0 cm H_2O/L/sec
   c. 2.0 to 3.0 cm H_2O/L/sec
   d. 3.0 to 4.0 cm H_2O/L/sec
   e. 4.0 to 5.0 cm H_2O/L/sec

3. In the normal individual in the upright position
   I. the negative intrapleural pressure is greater (i.e., more negative) in the upper lung regions
   II. the alveoli in the lower lung regions are larger than the alveoli in the upper lung regions
   III. ventilation is more effective in the lower lung regions
   IV. the intrapleural pressure is always below atmospheric pressure during a normal ventilatory cycle
   a. I and II only
   b. II and III only
   c. II, III, and IV only
   d. I, III, and IV only
   e. I, II, III and IV

4. When lung compliance decreases, the patient commonly has
   I. an increased ventilatory rate
   II. a decreased tidal volume
   III. an increased tidal volume
   IV. a decreased ventilatory rate
   a. I only
   b. II only
   c. III only
   d. I and II only
   e. II and IV only

5. When arranged for flow ($\dot{V}$), Poiseuille's law states that $\dot{V}$ is
   I. inversely proportional to r^4
   II. directly proportional to P
   III. inversely proportional to η

        IV. directly proportional to l
- a. I only
- b. II only
- c. II and III only
- d. III and IV only
- e. II, III, and IV only

6. During a normal exhalation, the
   - I. intra-alveolar pressure is greater than the atmospheric pressure
   - II. intrapleural pressure is less than the atmospheric pressure
   - III. intra-alveolar pressure is in equilibrium with the atmospheric pressure
   - IV. intrapleural pressure progressively decreases
     - a. I only
     - b. IV only
     - c. I and II only
     - d. II and IV only
     - e. II and III only

7. At rest, the normal intrapleural pressure change during quiet breathing is about
   - a. 0–2 mm Hg
   - b. 2–4 mm Hg
   - c. 4–6 mm Hg
   - d. 6–8 mm Hg
   - e. 8–10 mm Hg

8. Normally, an individual's tidal volume is about
   - a. 1–2 ml/lb
   - b. 3–4 ml/lb
   - c. 5–6 ml/lb
   - d. 7–8 ml/lb
   - e. 9–10 ml/lb

9. A rapid and shallow ventilatory pattern is called
   - a. Hyperpnea
   - b. Apnea
   - c. Alveolar hyperventilation
   - d. Tachypnea
   - e. Kussmaul breathing

10. Assuming that pressure remains constant, if the radius of a bronchial airway through which gas flows at a rate of 400 L/min is reduced to one-half of its original size, the flow through the bronchial airway would change to
    - a. 10 L/min
    - b. 25 L/min
    - c. 100 L/min

     d. 200 L/min

     e. 300 L/min

11. The difference between the alveolar pressure and the pleural pressure is called the

     a. transpulmonary pressure

     b. transthoracic pressure

     c. driving pressure

     d. transairway pressure

     e. transmural pressure

12. According to Laplace's law, if a bubble with a radius of 4 cm and a distending pressure of 10 cm H_2O is reduced to a radius of 2 cm, the new distending pressure of the bubble will be

     a. 5 cm H_2O

     b. 10 cm H_2O

     c. 15 cm H_2O

     d. 20 cm H_2O

     e. 25 cm H_2O

13. If alveolar Unit A has one-half the compliance of alveolar Unit B, the

     I. time constant of Unit A is essentially the same as Unit B

     II. volume in Unit B is two times greater than Unit A

     III. time constant of Unit B is twice as long as Unit A

     IV. volume in Unit B is essentially the same as the volume of Unit A

     a. I only

     b. III only

     c. IV only

     d. II and III only

     e. III and IV only

14. If a patient weighs 175 pounds and has a tidal volume of 550 ml and a respiratory rate of 17 breaths per minute, what is the patient's minute alveolar ventilation?

Answer: _____

15. Lung compliance study

Part I: If a patient generates a negative intrapleural pressure change of −8 cm H_2O during inspiration, and the lungs accept a new volume of 630 ml, what is the compliance of the lungs?

Answer: _____

Part II: If the same patient, 6 hours later, generates an intrapleural pressure of −12 cm H_2O during inspiration, and the lungs accept a new volume of 850 ml, what is the compliance of the lungs?

Answer: _____

Part III: In comparing Part II to Part I, the patient's lung compliance is
    a. increasing
    b. decreasing

16. If a patient produces a flow rate of 5 L/second during inspiration by generating a transairway pressure of 20 cm H_2O, what is the patient's R_{aw}?
    a. 1 cm H_2O/L/sec
    b. 2 cm H_2O/L/sec
    c. 3 cm H_2O/L/sec
    d. 4 cm H_2O/L/sec
    e. 5 cm H_2O/L/sec

17. As R_{aw} increases, the patient commonly manifests:
    I. a decreased ventilatory rate
    II. an increased tidal volume
    III. a decreased tidal volume
    IV. an increased ventilatory rate
    a. I only
    b. II only
    c. IV only
    d. III and IV only
    e. I and II only

18. If the radius of a bronchial airway, which has a driving pressure of 2 mm Hg, is reduced by 16% of its original size, what will be the new driving pressure required to maintain the same gas flow through the bronchial airway?
    a. 4 mm Hg
    b. 8 mm Hg
    c. 12 mm Hg
    d. 16 mm Hg
    e. 20 mm Hg

19. In the healthy lung, when the alveolus decreases in size during a normal exhalation, the:
    I. Surface tension decreases
    II. Surfactant to alveolar surface area increases
    III. Surface tension increases
    IV. Surfactant to alveolar surface area decreases
    a. I only
    b. III only
    c. IV only
    d. I and II only
    e. III and IV only

20. At end expiration, P_{ta} is:
    a. 0 mm Hg
    b. 2 mm Hg
    c. 4 mm Hg
    d. 6 mm Hg
    e. 8 mm Hg

Answers appears in Appendix VII.

CHAPTER 3

THE DIFFUSION OF PULMONARY GASES

OBJECTIVES

By the end of this chapter, the student should be able to:

1. Define *diffusion*.
2. State the following gas laws:
   —Boyle's law
   —Charles' law
   —Gay-Lussac's law
   —Dalton's law
3. Identify the percentage and partial pressure of the gases that compose the *barometric pressure:*
   —Nitrogen
   —Oxygen
   —Argon
   —Carbon dioxide
4. Identify the partial pressure of the gases in the *air*, *alveoli*, and *blood:*
   —Oxygen (P_{O_2})
   —Carbon dioxide (P_{CO_2})
   —Nitrogen (P_{N_2})
   —Water (P_{H_2O})
5. Calculate the *ideal alveolar gas equation*.
6. Name the nine major structures of the *alveolar-capillary membrane* that a gas molecule must diffuse through.
7. Describe how oxygen and carbon dioxide normally diffuse across the alveolar-capillary membrane.
8. Explain how *Fick's law* relates to gas diffusion.
9. Describe how the following relate to the *diffusion constants* in Fick's law:
   —Henry's law
   —Graham's law
10. Describe how Fick's law can be applied to certain clinical conditions.

11. Define the meaning of *perfusion limited*, and explain how it relates to a gas like nitrous oxide.
12. Define the meaning of *diffusion limited*, and explain how it relates to a gas like carbon monoxide.
13. Describe how oxygen can be classified as perfusion or diffusion limited.
14. Complete the self-assessment questions at the end of this chapter.

As discussed in Chapter Two, the mass movement of air in and out of the lungs occurs by virtue of transpulmonary and transairway pressure changes that are generated by the action of the diaphragm. This mechanism carries oxygen from the atmosphere to the alveoli and carbon dioxide from the alveoli to the external environment. The process of ventilation, however, merely moves gases from one point to another (e.g., from the atmosphere to the alveoli); it does not move gas molecules across the alveolar-capillary membrane. This process occurs by means of **passive diffusion**.

Diffusion is defined as the movement of gas molecules from an area of relatively high concentration of gas to one of low concentration. Different gases each move according to their own individual partial pressure gradients. Diffusion continues until all the gases in the two areas are in equilibrium.

To aid in the understanding of how gases transfer (diffuse) across the alveolar-capillary membrane, a brief review of the physical principles governing the behavior of gases (gas laws) and the partial pressures of the atmospheric gases is appropriate.

GAS LAWS

The behavior of gases surrounding the earth is described in a mathematical relationship known as the *ideal gas law:*

$$PV = nRT$$

where P is pressure, V is volume, T is temperature on the Kelvin (K) scale,* n is the number of moles of gas molecules present, and R is the gas constant, which has a fixed value of 0.0821.

Assuming that the amount of gas remains constant (i.e., n remains unchanged), the ideal gas law can be used to predict specific changes of temperature, pressure, and volume under different conditions. In other words, if nR remains constant, then:

$$\frac{P_1 \times V_1}{T_1} = \frac{P_2 \times V_2}{T_2}$$

Thus, when any one of the above variables (P, V, T) is held constant while one of the others changes in value, the new value of the third variable can be calculated. The following three laws illustrate the interrelationship of P, V, and T:

Boyle's Law $(P_1 \times V_1 = P_2 \times V_2)$.   Boyle's law states that if temperature remains constant, pressure will vary inversely to volume. For example, if an air-tight container, which has a volume of 200 ml and a pressure of 10 cm H_2O, has its volume reduced 50 percent (100 ml), the new pressure in the container can be computed as follows:

$$P_2 = \frac{P_1 \times V_1}{V_2}$$

$$= \frac{10 \text{ cm } H_2O \times 200 \text{ ml}}{100 \text{ ml}}$$

$$= 20 \text{ cm } H_2O$$

Charles' Law $(V_1/T_1 = V_2/T_2)$.   Charles' law states that if pressure remains constant, volume and temperature will vary directly. That is, if the temperature of the gas in a 3-liter balloon is increased from 250 K (Kelvin) to 300 K, the resulting volume of the balloon can be calculated as follows:

$$V_2 = \frac{V_1 \times T_2}{T_1}$$

$$= \frac{3 \text{ L} \times 300 \text{ K}}{250 \text{ K}}$$

$$= 3.6 \text{ L}$$

---

*Whenever the temperature of gases is involved in calculations, all temperatures must be converted to the Kelvin scale. Fahrenheit (°F) is converted first to Celsius (°C) as follows: 5/9 (F − 32). Celsius is converted to Kelvin (K) by adding 273 to the Celsius temperature (e.g., 37°C + 273 = 310 K).

Gay-Lussac's Law $(P_1/T_1 = P_2/T_2)$.   Gay-Lussac's law states that if the volume remains constant, pressure and temperature will vary directly. For instance, if the temperature of the gas in a closed container, having a pressure of 50 cm H_2O, is increased from 275 K to 375 K, the resulting pressure in the container can be calculated as follows:

$$P_2 = \frac{P_1 \times T_2}{T_1}$$

$$= \frac{50 \text{ cm } H_2O \times 375 \text{ K}}{275 \text{ K}}$$

$$= \frac{18750}{275}$$

$$= 68 \text{ cm } H_2O$$

Dalton's Law.   Since the earth's atmosphere consists of several kinds of gases, it is essential to understand how these gases behave when they are mixed together. This is described by Dalton's law, which states that in a mixture of gases, the total pressure is equal to the sum of the partial pressures of each separate gas. In other words, if 10 molecules of gas are enclosed in a container, the total pressure may be expressed as 10; if 5 molecules of a different gas are enclosed in another container of equal volume, the total pressure may be expressed as 5; if both these gases are enclosed in a container of equal volume, the total pressure may be expressed as 15 (Figure 3–1).

It should be stressed that the pressure produced by a particular gas is completely unaffected by the presence of another gas. In short, each gas in a mixture will individually contribute to the total pressure created by the mixture of gas.

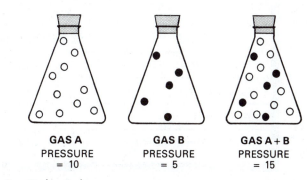

GAS A
PRESSURE
= 10

GAS B
PRESSURE
= 5

GAS A + B
PRESSURE
= 15

FIGURE 3–1. Dalton's law.

THE PARTIAL PRESSURES OF ATMOSPHERIC GASES

The atmospheric gases that surround the earth exert a force on the earth's surface called the *barometric pressure*. At sea level the barometric pressure is about 760 mm Hg and is a function of Dalton's law. The barometric pressure is primarily derived from the gases listed in Table 3–1.

The pressure between the external atmosphere and the alveoli is in equilibrium, except for slight changes (3–6 cm H_2O) that take place during inspiration or expiration. Within the circulatory system, however, the sum of the partial pressures is reduced, since the venous blood, which has a reduced P_{O_2} because of cellular metabolism, is not in equilibrium with the atmosphere.

It should also be noted that the barometric pressure decreases with an increase in altitude. For example, as one ascends a mountain, the barometric pressure steadily decreases. This is because the density of the different gas molecules surrounding the earth decreases with increased altitude. As the density of the various gases decreases, the partial pressure exerted by each gas also decreases. It should also be pointed out that, even though the barometric pressure varies with the altitude, the percent concentration of the atmospheric gases is the same at both high and low elevations (see Table 3–1). Table 3–2 shows the partial pressure of gases in dry air, alveolar air, arterial blood, and venous blood.

Note that even though the total barometric pressure is the same in the atmosphere and in the alveoli, the partial pressure of oxygen in the atmosphere (159 mm Hg) is significantly higher than the partial pressure of oxygen in the alveoli (100 mm Hg). This is because alveolar oxygen must mix—or compete in terms of partial pressures—with alveolar CO_2 pressure ($P_{A_{CO_2}} = 40$ mm Hg) and alveolar water vapor pressure ($P_{H_2O} = 47$ mm Hg), which are not nearly as high in the atmosphere. In short, by the time the oxygen molecules reach the alveoli, they

TABLE 3–1.   Gases that Compose the Barometric Pressure

GAS	% OF ATMOSPHERE	PARTIAL PRESSURE (mm Hg)
Nitrogen (N_2)	78.08	593
Oxygen (O_2)	20.95	159
Argon (Ar)	0.93	7
Carbon Dioxide (CO_2)	0.03	0.2

TABLE 3–2.   Partial Pressure (in mm Hg) of Gases in the Air, Alveoli, and Blood*

GASES	DRY AIR	ALVEOLAR GAS	ARTERIAL BLOOD	VENOUS BLOOD
P_{O_2}	159.0	100.0	95.0	40.0
P_{CO_2}	0.2	40.0	40.0	46.0
P_{H_2O} (water vapor)	0.0	47.0	47.0	47.0
P_{N_2} (and other gases in minute quantities)	600.8	573.0	573.0	573.0
Total	760.0	760.0	755.0	706.0

*The values shown are based upon standard pressure and temperature.

are diluted by the addition of CO_2 and H_2O molecules. This must lead to a decrease in the partial pressure of oxygen in the alveoli ($P_{A_{O_2}}$).

Water Vapor Pressure.   Depending on the surrounding temperature and pressure, water can exist as a liquid, gas, or solid. Water in the gaseous form is called *water vapor*, or *molecular water*. When water vapor is present in a volume of gas, it behaves according to the gas laws and exerts a partial pressure. Since alveolar gas is 100 percent humidified (saturated) at body temperature, the alveolar gas is assumed to have an *absolute humidity* of 44 mg/L, and a *water vapor pressure* (P_{H_2O}) of 47 mm Hg—regardless of the humidity of the inspired air (Table 3–3).

THE IDEAL ALVEOLAR GAS EQUATION

Clinically, the alveolar oxygen tension $P_{A_{O_2}}$ can be computed from the **ideal alveolar gas equation**. A useful clinical approximation of the ideal alveolar gas equation is as follows:

$$P_{A_{O_2}} = [P_B - P_{H_2O}]F_{I_{O_2}} - Pa_{CO_2}(1.25)$$

where $P_{A_{O_2}}$ is the partial pressure of oxygen in the alveoli, P_B is the barometric pressure, P_{H_2O} is the partial pressure of water vapor in the alveoli ($P_{H_2O} = 47$ mm Hg), $F_{I_{O_2}}$ is the fractional concentration of inspired oxygen, and Pa_{CO_2} is the partial pressure of arterial carbon dioxide. The number 1.25 is a factor that adjusts for

TABLE 3–3. Relationship Between Temperature, Absolute Humidity, and Water Vapor Pressure*

TEMPERATURE	ABSOLUTE (MAXIMUM) HUMIDITY	WATER VAPOR PRESSURE
37°C	44.0 mg/L	47.0 mm Hg
35°C	39.6 mg/L	42.2 mm Hg
30°C	30.4 mg/L	31.8 mm Hg
27°C	25.8 mg/L	26.7 mm Hg
25°C	23.0 mg/L	23.8 mm Hg
20°C	17.3 mg/L	17.5 mm Hg

*At sea level (760 mm Hg).

alterations in oxygen tension due to variations in the *respiratory exchange ratio* (RR), which is the ratio of the amount of oxygen that moves into the pulmonary capillary blood to the amount of carbon dioxide that moves out of the pulmonary blood and into the alveoli. Normally, about 200 ml/minute of carbon dioxide move into the alveoli while about 250 ml/minute of oxygen move into the pulmonary capillary blood, making the respiratory exchange ratio about 0.8.

Thus, if a patient is receiving an $F_{I_{O_2}}$ of .40 on a day when the barometric pressure is 755 mm Hg, and if the Pa_{CO_2} is 55 mm Hg, the patient's alveolar oxygen tension ($P_{A_{O_2}}$) can be calculated as follows:

$$P_{A_{O_2}} = [P_B - P_{H_2O}]F_{I_{O_2}} - Pa_{CO_2}(1.25)$$

$$= [755 - 47].40 - 55(1.25)$$

$$= [708].40 - 68.75$$

$$= [283.2] - 68.75$$

$$= 214.45$$

Clinically, when the Pa_{CO_2} is under 60 mm Hg, and when the patient is receiving oxygen therapy, the following simplified version of the alveolar gas equation may be used:

$$P_{A_{O_2}} = [P_B - P_{H_2O}]F_{I_{O_2}} - Pa_{CO_2}$$

THE DIFFUSION OF PULMONARY GASES

The process of diffusion is the passive movement of gas molecules from an area of high partial pressure to an area of low partial pressure until both areas are equal in pressure. Once gas equilibrium occurs, gas diffusion ceases.

In the lungs, a gas molecule must diffuse through the alveolar-capillary membrane, which is composed of (1) the liquid lining the intra-alveolar membrane, (2) the alveolar epithelial cell, (3) the basement membrane of the alveolar epithelial cell, (4) loose connective tissue (the interstitial space), (5) the basement membrane of the capillary endothelium, (6) the capillary endothelium, (7) the plasma in the capillary blood, (8) the erythrocyte membrane, and (9) the intracellular fluid in the erythrocyte until a hemoglobin molecule is encountered. Added together, the thickness of these physical barriers is between 0.36 and 2.5 μ. Under normal circumstances, this is a negligible barrier to the diffusion of oxygen and carbon dioxide (Figure 3–2).

OXYGEN AND CARBON DIOXIDE DIFFUSION ACROSS THE ALVEOLAR-CAPILLARY MEMBRANE

In the healthy resting individual, venous blood entering the alveolar-capillary system has an average oxygen tension (Pv_{O_2}) of 40 mm Hg, and an average carbon dioxide tension (Pv_{CO_2}) of 46 mm Hg. As blood passes through the capillary, the average alveolar oxygen tension (PA_{O_2}) is about 100 mm Hg, and the average alveolar carbon dioxide tension (PA_{CO_2}) is about 40 mm Hg (see Table 3–2).

Thus, when venous blood enters the alveolar-capillary system, there is an oxygen pressure gradient of about 60 mm Hg and a carbon dioxide pressure gradient of about 6 mm Hg. As a result, oxygen molecules diffuse across the alveolar-capillary membrane into the blood while, at the same time, carbon dioxide molecules diffuse out of the capillary blood and into the alveoli (Figure 3–3, page 125).

The diffusion of oxygen and carbon dioxide will continue until equilibrium is reached between the two gases; this is usually accomplished in about 0.25 second. Under normal resting conditions, the total transit time for blood to move through the alveolar-capillary system is about 0.75 second. Thus, the diffusion of oxygen and carbon dioxide is completed in about one-third of the time available (Figure 3–4, page 126).

In exercise, however, blood passes through the alveolar-capillary system at a much faster rate and, therefore, the time for gas diffusion decreases (i.e., the time available for gas diffusion is less than 0.75 second). In the healthy lung, oxygen equilibrium usually occurs in the alveolar-capillary system during exercise—in spite of the shortened transit time (Figure 3–5, page 127). In the presence of

ALVEOLAR—CAPILLARY MEMBRANE

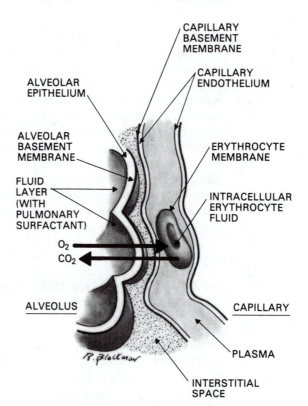

FIGURE 3–2. The major barriers of the alveolar-capillary membrane through which a gas molecule must diffuse.

certain pulmonary diseases, however, the time required to achieve oxygen equilibrium in the alveolar-capillary system may not be adequate. Such diseases include alveolar fibrosis, alveolar consolidation, and pulmonary edema (Figure 3–6, page 128).

FICK'S LAW AND GAS DIFFUSION

The diffusion of gas takes place according to Fick's law, which is written as follows:

$$\dot{V}\,gas \; \alpha \; \frac{A.D.\,(P_1 - P_2)}{T}$$

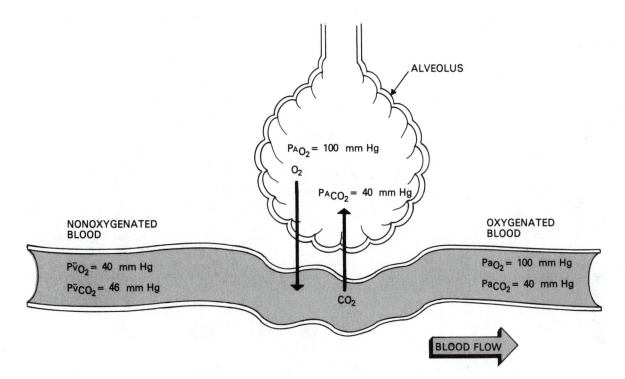

FIGURE 3–3. Normal gas pressures for oxygen and carbon dioxide as blood moves through the alveolar-capillary membrane. Pv_{O_2} = partial pressure of oxygen in mixed venous blood; $P\bar{v}_{CO_2}$ = partial pressure of carbon dioxide in mixed venous blood; PA_{O_2} = partial pressure of oxygen in alveolar gas; PA_{CO_2} = partial pressure of carbon dioxide in alveolar gas; Pa_{O_2} = partial pressure of oxygen in arterial blood; Pa_{CO_2} = partial pressure of carbon dioxide in arterial blood.

where $\dot{V}$ gas is the amount of gas that diffuses from one point to another, A is surface area, D is diffusion constants, $P_1 - P_2$ is the difference in partial pressure between two points, and T is thickness.

The law states that the rate of gas transfer across a sheet of tissue is directly proportional to the surface area of the tissue, to the diffusion constants, and to the difference in partial pressure of the gas between the two sides of the tissue and is inversely proportional to the thickness of the tissue (Figure 3–7, page 129).

The diffusion constants (D) noted in Fick's law are determined by Henry's law and Graham's law.

Henry's Law. Henry's law states that the amount of a gas that dissolves in a liquid at a given temperature is proportional to the partial pressure of the gas. The amount of gas that can be dissolved by 1 ml of a given liquid at standard pressure (760 mm Hg) and specified temperature is known as the *solubility coefficient*

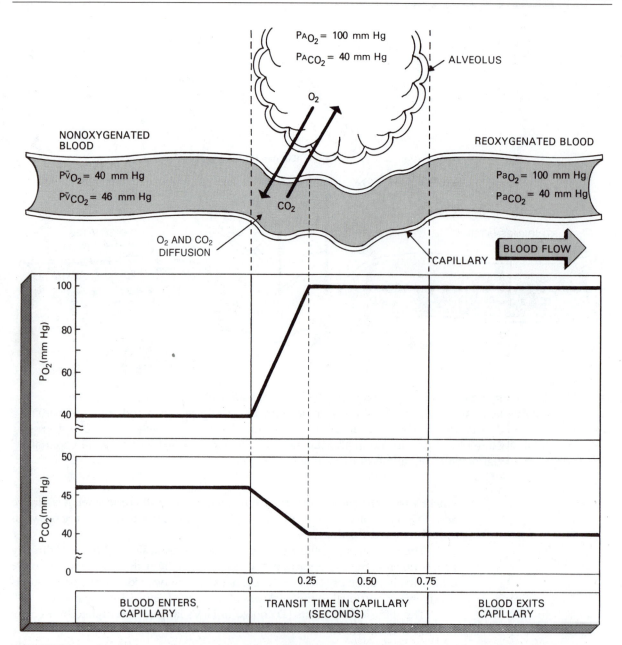

FIGURE 3–4. Under normal resting conditions, blood moves through the alveolar-capillary membrane in about 0.75 second. The oxygen pressure (P_{O_2}) and carbon dioxide pressure (P_{CO_2}) reach equilibrium in about 0.25 second—one third of the time available. $P_{\bar{v}O_2}$ = partial pressure of oxygen in mixed venous blood; $P_{\bar{v}CO_2}$ = partial pressure of carbon dioxide in mixed venous blood; P_{AO_2} = partial pressure of oxygen in alveolar gas; P_{ACO_2} = partial pressure of carbon dioxide in alveolar gas; Pa_{O_2} = partial pressure of oxygen in arterial blood; Pa_{CO_2} = partial pressure of carbon dioxide in arterial blood.

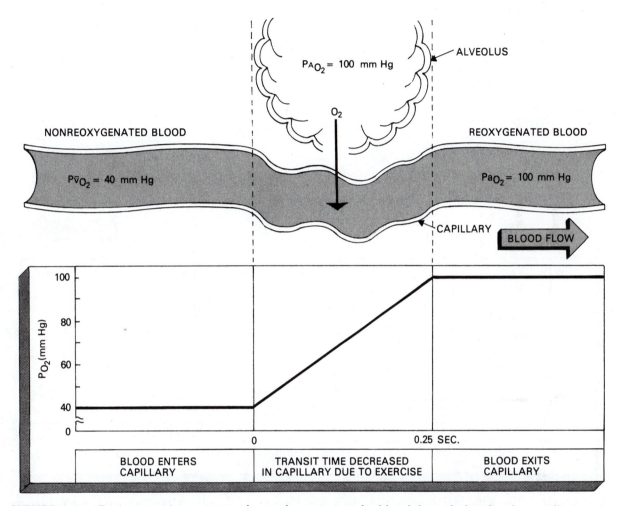

FIGURE 3–5. During exercise or stress, the total transit time for blood through the alveolar-capillary membrane is less than normal (normal = 0.75 sec). In the healthy individual, however, oxygen equilibrium usually occurs. Pv_{O_2} = partial pressure of oxygen in mixed venous blood; PA_{O_2} = partial pressure of oxygen in alveolar gas; Pa_{O_2} = partial pressure of oxygen in arterial blood.

of the liquid. At 37°C and 760 mm Hg pressure, the solubility coefficient of oxygen is 0.0244 ml/mm Hg/ml H_2O. The solubility coefficient of carbon dioxide is 0.592 ml/mm Hg/ml H_2O. The solubility coefficient varies inversely with temperature (i.e., if the temperature rises the solubility coefficient decreases in value).

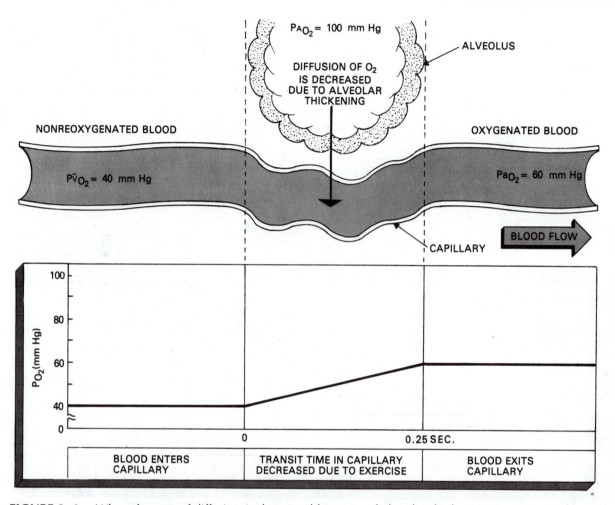

FIGURE 3–6. When the rate of diffusion is decreased because of alveolar thickening, oxygen equilibrium will likely not occur when the total transit time is decreased as a result of exercise or stress. Pv_{O_2} = partial pressure of oxygen in mixed venous blood; Pa_{O_2} = partial pressure of oxygen in alveolar gas; Pa_{O_2} = partial pressure of oxygen in arterial blood.

On the basis of the solubility coefficients of oxygen and carbon dioxide, it can be seen that in a liquid medium (e.g., alveolar-capillary membrane) carbon dioxide is more soluble than oxygen:

$$\frac{\text{Solubility } CO_2}{\text{Solubility } O_2} = \frac{0.592}{0.0244} = \frac{24}{1}$$

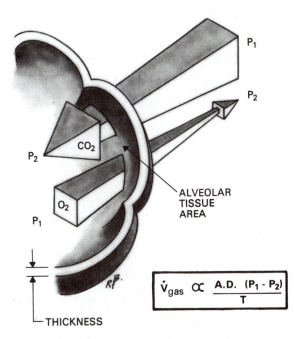

FIGURE 3–7. Fick's law. See text for explanation.

Graham's Law.   Graham's law states that the rate of diffusion of a gas through a liquid is (1) directly proportional to the solubility coefficient of the gas and (2) inversely proportional to the square root of the gram-molecular weight (GMW) of the gas. In comparing the relative rates of diffusion to oxygen (GMW = 32) and carbon dioxide (GMW = 44), it can be seen that, since oxygen is the lighter gas, it moves faster than carbon dioxide:

$$\frac{\text{Diffusion rate for CO}_2}{\text{Diffusion rate for O}_2} = \frac{\sqrt{\text{GMW O}_2}}{\sqrt{\text{GMW CO}_2}} = \frac{\sqrt{32}}{\sqrt{44}}$$

$$= \frac{5.6}{6.6}$$

By combining Graham's and Henry's laws, it can be said that the rates of diffusion of two gases are directly proportional to the ratio of their solubility coefficients, and inversely proportional to the ratio of their gram-molecular weights. For example, when the two laws are used to determine the relative rates of diffusion of carbon dioxide and oxygen, it can be seen that carbon dioxide diffuses about 20 times faster than oxygen.

$$\frac{\text{Diffusion rate for CO}_2}{\text{Diffusion rate for O}_2} = \frac{5.6 \times 0.592}{6.6 \times 0.0244} = \frac{20}{1}$$

To summarize, the diffusion constant (D) for a particular gas is directly proportional to the solubility coefficients (S) of the gas, and inversely proportional to the square root of the gram-molecular weight (GMW) of the gas:

$$D = \frac{S}{\sqrt{GMW}}$$

Mathematically, by substituting the diffusion constants,

$$D = \frac{S}{\sqrt{GMW}}$$

into Fick's law:

$$\dot{V} \, gas \; \alpha \; \frac{A.D. \, (P_1 - P_2)}{T}$$

then Fick's law can be rewritten as:

$$\dot{V} \, gas \; \alpha \; \frac{A.S. \, (P_1 - P_2)}{\sqrt{GMW} \times T}$$

Clinical Application of Fick's Law

Clinically, Fick's law is confirmed by the following general statements:

- The area (A) component of the law is verified in that a decreased alveolar surface area (e.g., caused by alveolar collapse or alveolar fluid) decreases the ability of oxygen to enter the pulmonary capillary blood.
- The $P_1 - P_2$ portion of the law is confirmed in that a decreased alveolar oxygen pressure ($P_{A_{O_2}}$ or P_1) (e.g., caused by high altitudes or alveolar hypoventilation) reduces the diffusion of oxygen into the pulmonary capillary blood.
- The thickness (T) factor is confirmed in that an increased alveolar tissue thickness (e.g., caused by alveolar fibrosis or alveolar edema) reduces the movement of oxygen across the alveolar-capillary membrane.

Fick's law also demonstrates how certain adverse pulmonary conditions may be improved. For example, when a patient's oxygen diffusion rate is decreased because of alveolar thickening, the administration of oxygen therapy to the patient will be beneficial. As the patient's fractional concentration of inspired oxygen ($F_{I_{O_2}}$) increases, the patient's alveolar oxygen pressure (i.e., $P_{A_{O_2}}$ or the P_1) also increases. This causes the movement of oxygen across the alveolar-capillary membrane to increase.

PERFUSION LIMITED GAS

Perfusion limited means that the transfer of gas across the alveolar wall is a function of the amount of blood that flows past the alveoli. Nitrous oxide (N_2O) is an excellent gas to illustrate this concept: When N_2O moves across the alveolar wall and into the blood, it does not chemically combine with hemoglobin. Because of this, the partial pressure of N_2O in the blood plasma rises very quickly. It is estimated that the partial pressure of N_2O will equal that of the alveolar gas when the blood is only about one-tenth of the way through the alveolar-capillary system (Figure 3–8). Once the partial pressures of the N_2O in the blood and in the alveolar gas are equal, the diffusion of N_2O stops. In order for the diffusion of N_2O to resume, additional blood must enter the alveolar-capillary system. The rate of perfusion, therefore, limits the amount of diffusion of N_2O.

DIFFUSION LIMITED GAS

Diffusion limited means that the movement of gas across the alveolar wall is a function of the integrity of the alveolar-capillary membrane itself. Carbon monoxide (CO) is an excellent gas to illustrate this concept: When CO moves across the alveolar wall and into the blood, it rapidly enters the red blood cell (RBC) and tightly bonds to hemoglobin (CO has an affinity for hemoglobin that is about 210 times greater than that of oxygen).

It should be noted that when gases are in chemical combination with hemoglobin, they no longer exert a partial pressure. Thus, since CO has a strong chemical attraction to hemoglobin, most of the CO enters the RBCs, combines with hemoglobin, and no longer exerts a partial pressure in the blood plasma. Because there is no appreciable partial pressure of CO in the blood plasma at any time (i.e., $P_2 - P_1$ stays constant), only the diffusion characteristics of the alveolar-capillary membrane, and not the amount of blood flowing through the capillary, limit the diffusion of CO (Figure 3–9, page 133).

Clinically, this makes CO an excellent gas for evaluating the lung's ability to diffuse gases and is used in what is called the *diffusion capacity of carbon monoxide* ($D_{L_{CO}}$) test. The $D_{L_{CO}}$ test measures the amount of CO that moves across the alveolar-capillary membrane into the blood in a given time. In essence, this test measures the physiologic effectiveness of the alveolar-capillary membrane. The normal diffusion capacity of CO is 25 ml/minute/mm Hg. Figure 3–10 (page 134) shows clinical conditions that may cause problems in diffusion. See Figure 3–6 for an illustration of the diffusion of oxygen during a diffusion limited state.

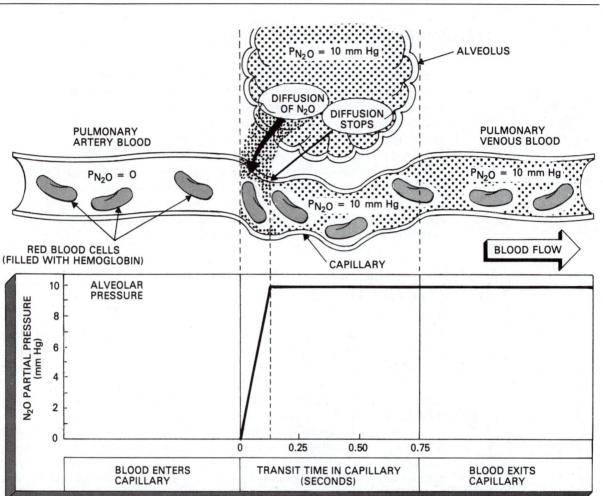

FIGURE 3–8. Nitrous oxide (N_2O) quickly equilibrates with pulmonary blood. When equilibrium occurs, the diffusion of N_2O stops. In order for the diffusion of N_2O to resume, fresh blood (pulmonary artery blood) must enter the alveolar-capillary system. This phenomenon is called *perfusion limited*. P_{N_2O} = partial pressure of nitrous oxide in the blood.

HOW OXYGEN CAN BE EITHER PERFUSION OR DIFFUSION LIMITED

When oxygen diffuses across the alveolar wall and into the blood, it enters the red blood cell and combines with hemoglobin—but not with the same avidity as carbon monoxide. Hemoglobin quickly becomes saturated with oxygen and, once

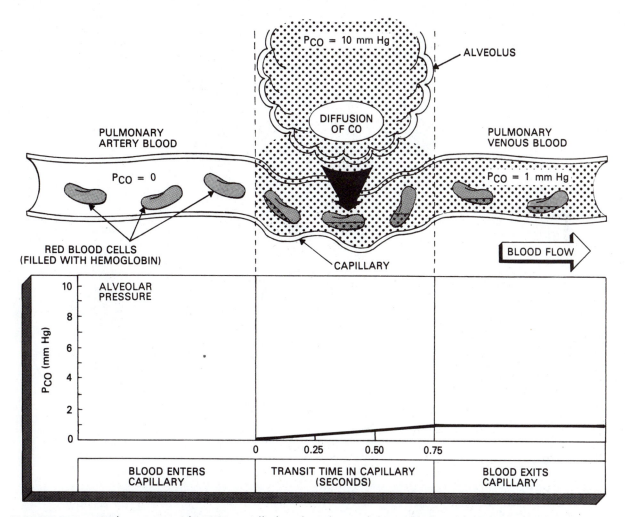

FIGURE 3–9. Carbon monoxide (CO) rapidly bonds to hemoglobin and, thus, does not generate an appreciable partial pressure (P_{CO_2}) in the blood plasma. As a result of this chemical relationship, blood flow (perfusion) does not limit the rate of CO diffusion. However, when the alveolar-capillary membrane is abnormal (e.g., in alveolar fibrosis), the rate of CO diffusion decreases. This phenomenon is called *diffusion limited*. In essence, diffusion limited means that the structure of the alveolar-capillary membrane alone limits the rate of gas diffusion.

this happens, oxygen molecules in the plasma can no longer enter the red blood cell. This, in turn, causes the partial pressure of oxygen in the plasma to increase.

Under normal resting conditions, the partial pressure of oxygen in the capillary blood equals the partial pressure of oxygen in the alveolar gas when the

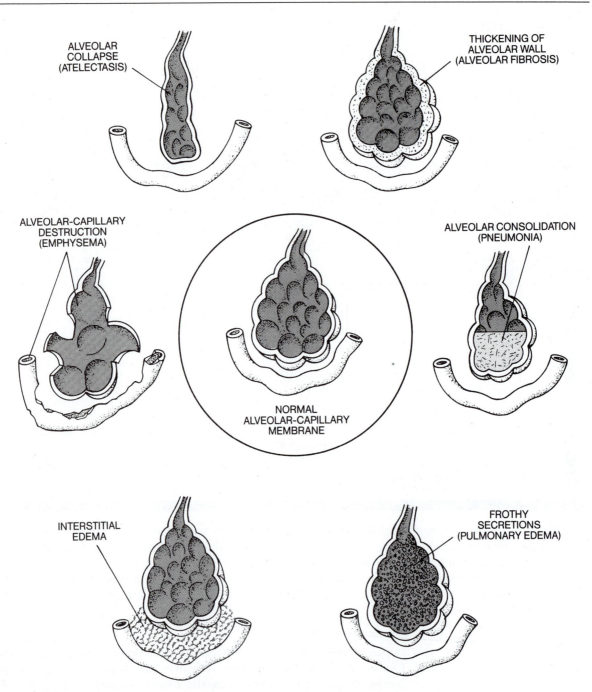

FIGURE 3–10. Clinical conditions that decrease the rate of gas diffusion. These conditions are known as *diffusion limited problems.*

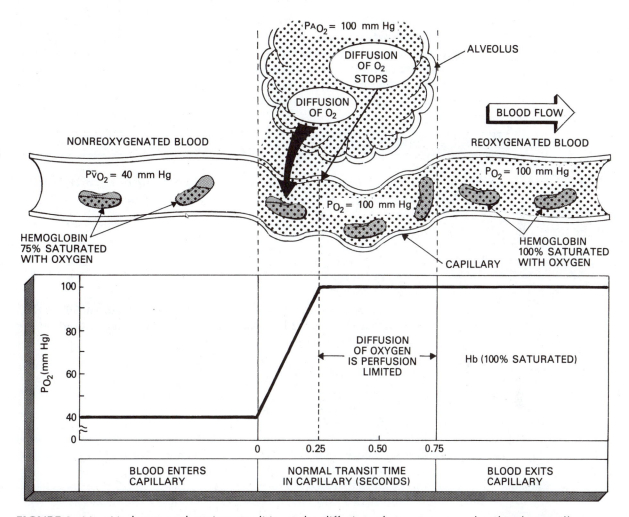

FIGURE 3–11.   Under normal resting conditions, the diffusion of oxygen across the alveolar-capillary membrane stops when blood is about one-third of the way through the capillary. This occurs because the partial pressure of oxygen in the capillary blood (P_{O_2}) equals the partial pressure of oxygen in the alveolus ($P_{A_{O_2}}$). Once oxygen equilibrium occurs between the alveolus and capillary blood, the diffusion of oxygen is *perfusion limited*.

blood is about one-third of the way through the capillary. Beyond this point, the transfer of oxygen is perfusion limited (Figure 3–11). When the patient has either a decreased cardiac output or a decreased hemoglobin level (anemia), the effects of perfusion limitation may become significant.

When the diffusion properties of the lungs are impaired (see Figure 3–10), however, the partial pressure of oxygen in the capillary blood may never equal the partial pressure of the oxygen in the alveolar gas during the normal alveolar-capillary transit time. Thus, under normal circumstances the diffusion of oxygen is perfusion limited, but under certain abnormal pulmonary conditions the transfer of oxygen may become diffusion limited.

SELF-ASSESSMENT QUESTIONS

1. If a container having a volume of 375 ml and a pressure of 15 cm H_2O in it is suddenly reduced to a volume of 150 ml, what would be the pressure in the container?
   a. 17.5 cm H_2O
   b. 28 cm H_2O
   c. 37.5 cm H_2O
   d. 43 cm H_2O
   e. 56.5 cm H_2O

2. If the gas temperature in a closed container that has a pressure of 50 cm H_2O in it is increased from 125 absolute to 235 absolute, what would be the pressure in the container?
   a. 86 cm H_2O
   b. 94 cm H_2O
   c. 102 cm H_2O
   d. 117 cm H_2O
   e. 123 cm H_2O

3. Which of the following gas laws states that in a mixture of gases the total pressure is equal to the sum of the partial pressure of each gas?
   a. Dalton's law
   b. Gay-Lussac's law
   c. Charles' law
   d. Boyle's law
   e. Ideal gas law

4. At sea level, the normal percent of carbon dioxide in the atmosphere is
   a. 5%
   b. 40%
   c. 78%
   d. 0.40%
   e. 0.03%

5. At sea level, the alveolar water vapor pressure is normally about
   a. 0.2 mm Hg

    b. 47 mm Hg

    c. 0.0 mm Hg

    d. 40 mm Hg

    e. one-half the vapor pressure of the atmosphere

6. If a patient is receiving an $F_{I_{O_2}}$ of .60 on a day when the barometric pressure is 725 mm Hg, and if the Pa_{CO_2} is 50 mm Hg, what is the patient's alveolar oxygen tension ($P_{A_{O_2}}$)?

    a. 177 mm Hg

    b. 233 mm Hg

    c. 344 mm Hg

    d. 415 mm Hg

    e. 511 mm Hg

7. The normal transit time for blood through the alveolar-capillary system is about

    a. 0.25 sec

    b. 0.50 sec

    c. 0.75 sec

    d. 1.0 sec

    e. 1.5 secs

8. Under normal resting conditions, the diffusion of oxygen and carbon dioxide is usually completed in about

    I. 0.25 sec

    II. 0.50 sec

    III. 0.75 sec

    IV. 1.0 sec

    V. one-third of the time available

      a. I only

      b. II only

      c. III only

      d. IV and V only

      e. I and V only

9. Which of the following states that the rate of gas diffusion is inversely proportional to the weight of the gas?

    a. Graham's law

    b. Charles' law

    c. Henry's law

    d. Gay-Lussac's law

    e. Boyle's law

10. According to Fick's law, gas diffusion is

    I. directly proportional to the thickness of the tissue

    II. indirectly proportional to the diffusion constants

III. directly proportional to the difference in partial pressure of the gas between the two sides

IV. indirectly proportional to the tissue area

    a. I only

    b. III only

    c. IV only

    d. II and III only

    e. I, III, and IV only

Answers appear in Appendix VII.

CHAPTER 4

PULMONARY FUNCTION MEASUREMENTS

OBJECTIVES

By the end of this chapter, the student should be able to:

1. Define the following *lung volumes:*
   —Tidal volume
   —Inspiratory reserve volume
   —Expiratory reserve volume
   —Residual volume
2. Define the following *lung capacities:*
   —Vital capacity
   —Inspiratory capacity
   —Functional residual capacity
   —Total lung capacity
   —Residual volume/total lung capacity ratio
3. Identify the approximate lung volumes and capacities in milliliters in the average normal male and female between 20 and 30 years of age.
4. Define the following *expiratory flow rate measurements:*
   —Forced vital capacity
   —Forced expiratory volume timed
   —Forced expiratory flow$_{200-1200}$
   —Forced expiratory flow$_{25\%-75\%}$
   —Peak expiratory flow rate
   —Maximum voluntary ventilation
   —Forced expiratory volume$_{1\ sec}$/forced vital capacity ratio
   —Flow-volume curves
5. Identify the following average dynamic flow rate measurements for the healthy male and female between 20 and 30 years of age:
   —Forced expiratory volume timed for periods of 0.5, 1.0, 2.0, and 3.0 seconds
   —Forced expiratory flow$_{200-1200}$

LUNG VOLUMES AND CAPACITIES

The total amount of air that the lungs can accommodate is divided into four separate volumes. Four specific combinations of these lung volumes are used to designate lung capacities (Figure 4–1). The volumes and capacities of the lungs are defined below.

Lung Volumes

Tidal Volume (V_T).   The volume of air that normally moves into and out of the lungs in one quiet breath.

Inspiratory Reserve Volume (IRV).   The maximum volume of air that can be inhaled after a normal tidal volume inhalation.

Expiratory Reserve Volume (ERV).   The maximum volume of air that can be exhaled after a normal tidal volume exhalation.

Residual Volume (RV).   The amount of air remaining in the lungs after a maximal exhalation.

Lung Capacities

Vital Capacity (VC).   The maximum volume of air that can be exhaled after a maximal inspiration (IRV + V_T + ERV). There are two major VC measurements:

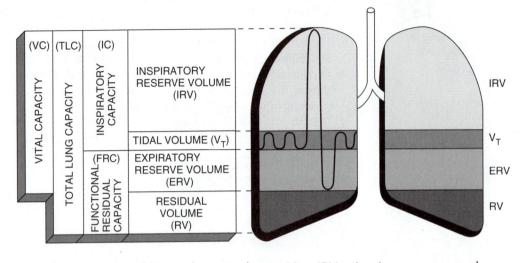

FIGURE 4–1.   Normal lung volumes and capacities. IRV = inspiratory reserve volume;
V_T = tidal volume; RV = residual volume; ERV = expiratory reserve volume;
TLC = total lung capacity; VC = vital capacity; IC = inspiratory capacity;
FRC = functional residual capacity.

slow vital capacity (SVC), in which exhalation is performed slowly; and forced vital capacity (FVC), in which a maximal effort is made to exhale as rapidly as possible.

Inspiratory Capacity (IC).   The volume of air that can be inhaled after a normal exhalation (V_T + IRV).

Functional Residual Capacity (FRC).   The volume of air remaining in the lungs after a normal exhalation (ERV + RV).

Total Lung Capacity (TLC).   The maximum amount of air that the lungs can accommodate (IC + FRC).

Residual Volume/Total Lung Capacity Ratio (RV/TLC × 100).   The percentage of the TLC occupied by the RV.

The amount of air that the lungs can accommodate varies with the age, race, weight, height, and sex of the individual. Table 4–1 lists the normal lung volumes and capacities of the average man and woman between 20 and 30 years of age.

Changes in lung volumes and capacities are seen in trauma and disease. Such changes are commonly classified as either an obstructive lung disorder or a restrictive lung disorder.

In an obstructive lung disorder, the RV, V_T, FRC, and RV/TLC ratio are increased; and the VC, IC, IRV, and ERV are decreased (Figure 4–2). In a restrictive lung disorder, the VC, IC, RV, FRC, V_T, and TLC are all decreased (Figure 4–3, page 145).

TABLE 4–1. Approximate Lung Volumes and Capacities in the Average Normal Subject Between 20 and 30 Years of Age

MEASUREMENT	MALE		FEMALE	
	ml	Approx. % of TLC	ml	Approx. % of TLC
Tidal Volume (V_T)	500	8–10	400–500	8–10
Inspiratory Reserve Volume (IRV)	3100	50	1900	30
Expiratory Reserve Volume (ERV)	1200	20	800	20
Residual Volume (RV)	1200	20	1000	25
Vital Capacity (VC)	4800	80	3200	75
Inspiratory Capacity (IC)	3600	60	2400	60
Functional Residual Capacity (FRC)	2400	40	1800	40
Total Lung Capacity (TLC)	6000	—	4200	—
Residual Volume/Total Lung Capacity Ratio (RV/TLC × 100)	$\dfrac{1200}{6000}$	20	$\dfrac{1000}{4200}$	25

PULMONARY MECHANICS

In addition to measuring volumes and capacities, one can also measure the rate at which gas flows into and out of the lungs. Expiratory flow rate measurements provide data on the integrity of the airways and the severity of airway impairment, as well as indicating whether the patient has a large airway or a small airway problem. Collectively, the tests for measuring expiratory flow rates are referred to as the pulmonary mechanic measurements and are described below.

Forced Vital Capacity (FVC).   The maximum volume of gas that can be exhaled as forcefully and rapidly as possible after a maximal inspiration. Normally FVC equals VC. In obstructive lung disease, however, the FVC is less than the VC (Figure 4–4). The FVC decreases with age.

Forced Expiratory Volume Timed (FEV_T).   The maximum volume of gas that can be exhaled over a specific time period. This measurement is obtained from an FVC.

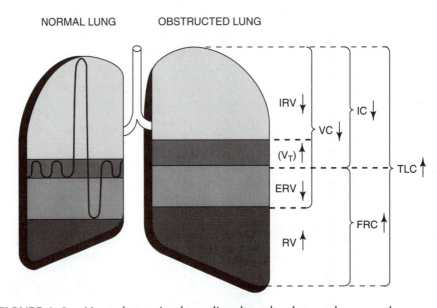

FIGURE 4–2. How obstructive lung disorders alter lung volumes and capacities. IRV = inspiratory reserve volume; V_T = tidal volume; RV = residual volume; ERV = expiratory reserve volume; TLC = total lung capacity; VC = tidal capacity; IC = inspiratory capacity; FRC = functional residual capacity.

The most frequently used time period is 1.0 second; other commonly used periods are 0.5, 2.0, and 3.0 seconds. Normally, the percentage of the total volume exhaled during these time periods is as follows: $FEV_{0.5}$, 60 percent; $FEV_{1.0}$, 83 percent; $FEV_{2.0}$, 94 percent; and $FEV_{3.0}$, 97 percent.

In obstructive disease, the FEV_T decreases (Figure 4–5). The FEV_T normally decreases with age.

Forced Expiratory Flow$_{200-1200}$ ($FEF_{200-1200}$). The average rate of airflow between 200 and 1200 ml of the FVC (Figure 4–6); formerly known as the *maximum expiratory flow rate* (MEFR). The first 200 ml of the FVC is usually exhaled slower than the average flow rate because of (1) the inertia involved in the respiratory maneuver, and (2) the general unreliability of the equipment response time. Because the $FEF_{200-1200}$ measures expiratory flows at high lung volumes (i.e., the initial part, or the *effort dependent portion*,* of the FVC), it is a good index of the integrity of large airway function. The average $FEF_{200-1200}$ for the healthy male between 20 and 30 years of age is about 8 L/sec (480 L/min), and for the

---

*See The Effort-Dependent Portion of a Forced Expiratory Maneuver, later in this chapter.

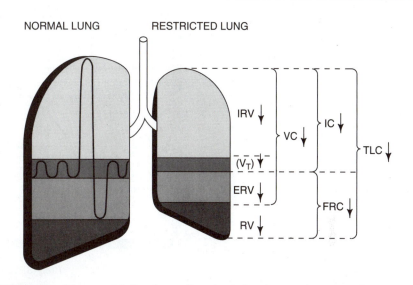

FIGURE 4–3. How restrictive lung disorders alter lung volumes and capacities. IRV = inspiratory reserve volume; V_T = tidal volume; RV = residual volume; ERV = expiratory reserve volume; TLC = total lung capacity; VC = vital capacity; FRC = functional residual capacity.

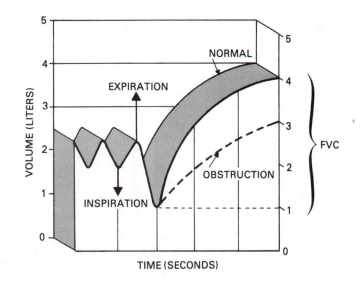

FIGURE 4–4. Forced vital capacity (FVC). A = point of maximal inspiration and the starting point of an FVC.

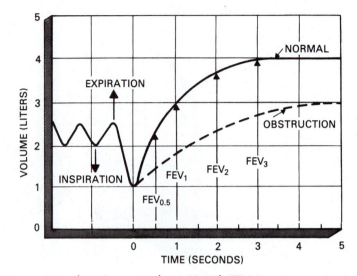

FIGURE 4–5.   Forced expiratory volume timed (FEV_T).

female between 20 and 30 years of age is about 5.5 L/sec (330 L/min). In obstructive lung disease, however, flow rates as low as 1 L/sec (60 L/min) have been reported. The $FEF_{200-1200}$ decreases with age and in obstructive lung disease. Conceptually, the $FEF_{200-1200}$ is similar to measuring, and then averaging, the flow rate from a water faucet when 200 ml and 1200 ml have accumulated in a measuring container (Figure 4–7).

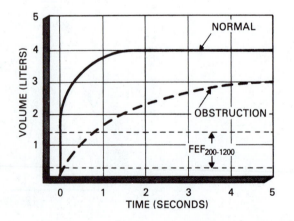

FIGURE 4–6.   Forced expiratory flow$_{200-1200}$ ($FEF_{200-1200}$).

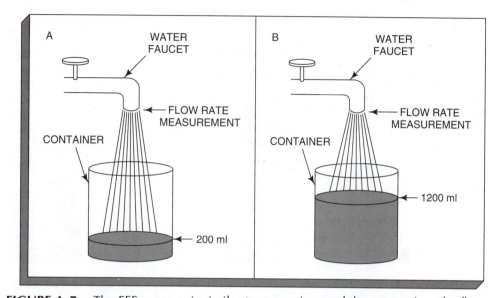

FIGURE 4–7. The $FEF_{200-1200}$ is similar to measuring, and then averaging, the flow rate of water from a faucet at the precise moment when 200 ml and 1200 ml of water have accumulated in a container. Picture the flow rate from the faucet being measured when 200 ml of water have entered the container (A). Again, picture the flow rate from the faucet being measured when 1200 ml of water have entered the container (B). Taking the average of the two flow rates would be similar to the $FEF_{200-1200}$, which measures, and then averages, the flow rate at the precise point when 200 ml and 1200 ml of gas have been exhaled during a FVC maneuver.

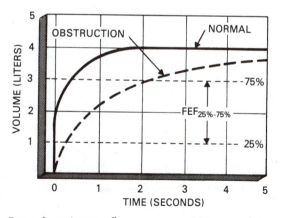

FIGURE 4–8. Forced expiratory flow$_{25\%-75\%}$ ($FEF_{25\%-75\%}$).

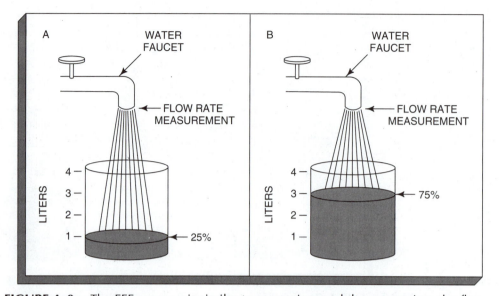

FIGURE 4–9. The FEF$_{25\%-75\%}$ is similar to measuring, and then averaging, the flow rate from a faucet when one liter and three liters of water have accumulated in a four liter container. Picture the flow rate from the faucet being measured when one liter (25%) of water has entered a four-liter container (A). Again, picture the flow rate from the faucet being measured when three liters (75%) of water have entered the container (B). Taking the average of the two flow rates would be similar to the FEF$_{25\%-75\%}$ which measures, and then averages, the flow rate when an individual exhales 25% and 75% of their FVC.

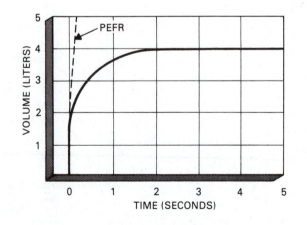

FIGURE 4–10. Peak expiratory flow rate (PEFR).

Forced Expiratory Flow$_{25\%-75\%}$ (FEF$_{25\%-75\%}$). The average flow rate during the middle 50 percent of an FVC measurement (Figure 4–8); also known as the *maximum midexpiratory flow rate* (MMFR). This measurement reflects the status of medium- to small-sized airways. The average FEF$_{25\%-75\%}$ for the normal healthy male between 20 and 30 years old is about 4.5 L/sec (270 L/min), and for the female about 3.5 L/sec (210 L/min). In obstructive lung disease, flow rates as low as 0.3 L/sec (18 L/min) have been reported. The FEF$_{25\%-75\%}$ decreases progressively with age and in obstructive lung disease. Conceptually, the FEF$_{25\%-75\%}$ is similar to measuring, and then averaging, the flow rate from a water faucet when 25% and 75% of a specific volume of water has accumulated in a measuring container (Figure 4–9).

Peak Expiratory Flow Rate (PEFR). The maximum flow rate that can be achieved; also known as *peak flow rate*. The PEFR can be obtained from the FVC (Figure 4–10). The average PEFR for the normal healthy male between 20 and 30 years is about 10 L/sec (600 L/min), and for the female about 7.5 L/sec (450 L/min). The PEFR decreases with age and in obstructive lung disease.

Maximum Voluntary Ventilation (MVV). The largest volume of gas that can be breathed voluntarily in and out of the lungs in 1 minute (the patient actually performs the test for only 12 or 15 seconds); also known as *maximum breathing capacity* (MBC). The MVV is a general test that evaluates the performance of the respiratory muscles, the compliance of the lung and thorax, and the resistance generated by the airways and tissues. The average MVV for the healthy male between 20 and 30 years old is about 170 L/min, and for the female about 110 L/min. In patients with chronic obstructive disease, the MVV is decreased. The MVV decreases with age (Figure 4–11).

Forced Expiratory Volume$_{1\ Sec}$/Forced Vital Capacity Ratio (FEV$_1$/FVC ratio). The ratio of the volume of gas that can be forcefully exhaled in 1 second to the total volume of gas that can be forcefully exhaled after a maximum inspiration. A decreased FEV$_1$/FVC ratio is a broad indicator of airway obstruction, but the absence of a decrease does not exclude the presence of airway obstruction.

Flow-volume Curve. The flow-volume curve is a graphic presentation of a forced vital capacity (FVC) maneuver followed by a forced inspiratory volume (FIV) maneuver. When the FVC and FIV are plotted together, the graphic illustration produced by the two curves is called a **flow-volume loop.** The flow-volume loop compares both the flow rates and volume changes produced at different points of an FVC and FIV maneuver. Depending on the sophistication of the equipment, the

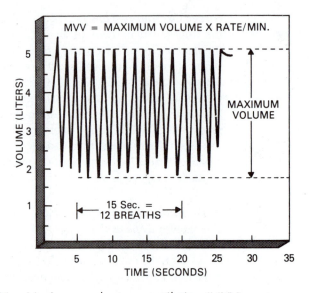

FIGURE 4–11. Maximum voluntary ventilation (MVV).

following measurements can be obtained from the flow-volume loop (Figure 4–12):

- Peak expiratory flow rate (PEFR)
- Peak inspiratory flow rate (PIFR)
- Forced vital capacity (FVC)
- Forced expiratory volume timed (FEV_T)
- Forced expiratory flow$_{25\%-75\%}$ ($FEF_{25\%-75\%}$)
- Forced expiratory flow$_{50\%}$ ($FEF_{50\%}$); also called the $\dot{V}max_{50}$. In the normal subject, the $FEF_{50\%}$ has a straight-line appearance, since the expiratory flow decreases linearly with volume throughout most of the VC range. In subjects with obstructive lung disease, however, flow frequently decreases at low lung volumes, causing the $FEF_{50\%}$ line to appear cuplike or scooped out.

Flow-volume loop measurements graphically illustrate both obstructive (Figure 4–13) and restrictive lung problems (Figure 4–14). Table 4–2 summarizes the average dynamic flow rate values found in the healthy male and female between 20 and 30 years of age.

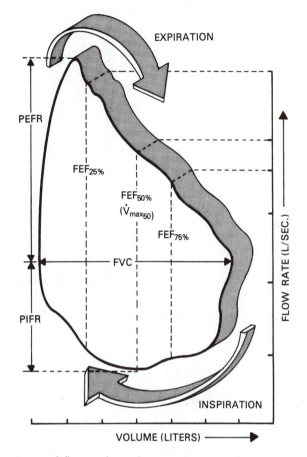

FIGURE 4–12. Normal flow-volume loop. PEFR = peak expiration flow rate; PIFR = peak inspiratory flow rate; FVC = forced vital capacity; $FEF_{25\%-75\%}$ = forced expiratory flow$_{25\%-75\%}$; $FEF_{50\%}$ = forced expiratory flow$_{50\%}$ (also called $Vmax_{50}$).

HOW THE EFFECTS OF DYNAMIC COMPRESSION DECREASE EXPIRATORY FLOW RATES

The Effort-Dependent Portion of a Forced Expiratory Maneuver

Normally, during approximately the first 30 percent of a forced vital capacity maneuver, the maximum peak flow rate is dependent on the amount of muscular

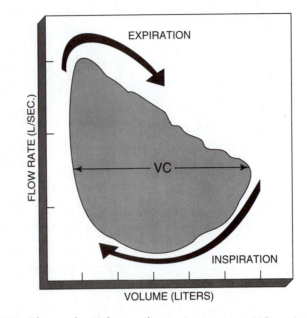

FIGURE 4–13.   Flow-volume loop, obstructive pattern, VC = vital capacity.

effort exerted by the individual. Therefore, the first 30 percent of a forced expiratory maneuver is referred to as **effort-dependent**.

The Effort-Independent Portion of a Forced Expiratory Maneuver

The flow rate during approximately the last 70 percent of a forced vital capacity maneuver is **effort-independent**. That is, once a maximum flow rate has been attained, the flow rate cannot be increased by further muscular effort.

The lung volume at which the patient initiates a forced expiratory maneuver also influences the maximum flow rate. As lung volumes decline, flow also declines. The reduced flow, however, is the maximum flow for that particular volume.

Figure 4–15 illustrates where the effort-dependent and effort-independent portions of a forced expiratory maneuver appear on a flow-volume loop.

Dynamic Compression of the Bronchial Airways

The limitation of the flow rate that occurs during the last 70 percent of a forced vital capacity maneuver is due to the dynamic compression of the walls of the airways. As gas flows through the airways from the alveoli to the atmosphere

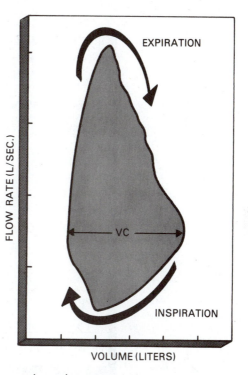

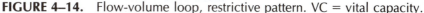

FIGURE 4–14. Flow-volume loop, restrictive pattern. VC = vital capacity.

during passive expiration, the pressure within the airways diminishes to zero (Figure 4–16A).

During a forced expiratory maneuver, however, as the airway pressure decreases from the alveoli to the atmosphere, there is a point at which the pressure within the lumen of the airways equals the pleural pressure surrounding the airways. This point is called the **equal pressure point**.

Downstream (i.e., toward the mouth) from the equal pressure point, the lateral pressure within the airway becomes less than the surrounding pleural pressure. Consequently, the airways are compressed. As muscular effort and pleural pressure increase during a forced expiratory maneuver, the equal pressure point moves upstream (i.e., toward the alveolus). Ultimately, the equal pressure point becomes fixed where the individual's flow rate has achieved maximum (Figure 4–16B). In essence, once dynamic compression occurs during a forced expiratory maneuver, increased muscular effort merely augments airway compression, which in turn increases airway resistance.

TABLE 4–2. Average Dynamic Flow Rate Measurements of the Healthy Male and Female Between 20 and 30 Years of Age

MEASUREMENT	MALE	FEMALE
FEV_T		
$FEV_{0.5}$	60%	60%
$FEV_{1.0}$	83%	83%
$FEV_{2.0}$	94%	94%
$FEV_{3.0}$	97%	97%
$FEF_{200-1200}$	8 L/sec (480 L/min)	5.5 L/sec (330 L/min)
$FEF_{25\%-75\%}$	4.5 L/sec (270 L/min)	3.5 L/sec (210 L/min)
PEFR	10 L/sec (600 L/min)	7.5 L/sec (450 L/min)
MVV	170 L/min	110 L/min

As the structural changes associated with certain respiratory diseases (e.g., chronic obstructive pulmonary diseases) intensify, the patient commonly responds by increasing intrapleural pressure during expiration to overcome the increased airway resistance produced by the disease. By increasing intrapleural pressure during expiration, however, the patient activates the dynamic compression mechanism, which in turn further reduces the diameter of the bronchial airways. This results in an even greater increase in airway resistance.

Flow is normally not limited to effort during inspiration. This is because the airways widen as greater inspiratory efforts are generated. This action enhances gas flow (see Figure 4–12).

Diffusion Capacity of Carbon Monoxide ($D_{L_{CO}}$)

The $D_{L_{CO}}$ study measures the amount of carbon monoxide (a diffusion limited gas*) that moves across the alveolar-capillary membrane. Carbon monox-

---

*See diffusion limited, page 131.

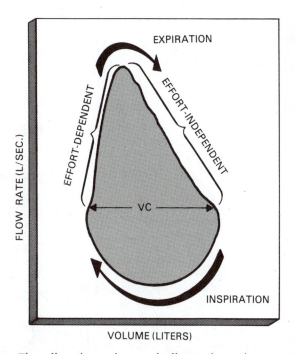

FIGURE 4–15. The effort-dependent and effort-independent portions of a forced expiratory maneuver in a flow-volume loop measurement. VC = vital capacity.

ide (CO) has an affinity for hemoglobin that is about 210 times greater than that of oxygen. Thus, in individuals who have normal amounts of hemoglobin and normal ventilatory function, the only limiting factor to the diffusion of CO is the alveolar-capillary membrane. In essence, the $D_{L_{CO}}$ study measures the physiologic status of the various anatomic structures that compose the alveolar-capillary membrane (see Figure 4–2).

The carbon monoxide single-breath technique is commonly used for this measurement. Under normal conditions, the average $D_{L_{CO}}$ value for the resting male is 25 ml/min/mm Hg (STPD). This value is slightly lower in females, presumably because of their smaller normal lung volumes. The $D_{L_{CO}}$ may increase three-fold in healthy subjects during exercise. The $D_{L_{CO}}$ generally decreases in response to lung disorders that effect the alveolar-capillary membrane. For example, the $D_{L_{CO}}$ is decreased in emphysema because of the alveolar-capillary destruction associate with this lung disease. See Figure 4–10 for other common lung disorders that effect the alveolar-capillary membrane and cause the $D_{L_{CO}}$ to decrease.

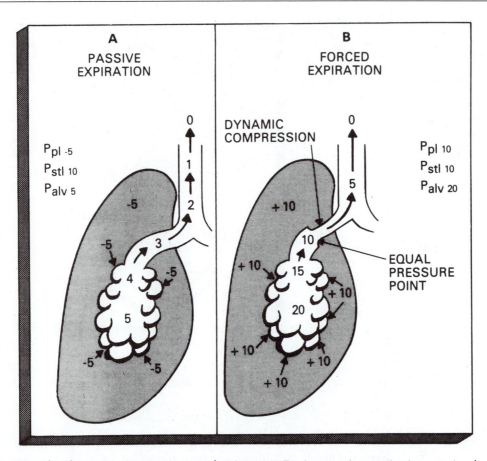

FIGURE 4–16. The dynamic compression mechanism. (*A*) During passive expiration, static elastic recoil pressure of the lungs (P_{stL}) is 10, pleural pressure (P_{pl}) at the beginning of expiration is −5, and alveolar pressure (P_{alv}) is +5. In order for gas to move from the alveolus to the atmosphere during expiration, the pressure must decrease progressively in the airways from +5 to 0. As *A* shows, P_{pl} is always less than the airway pressure. (*B*) During forced expiration, P_{pl} becomes positive (+10 in this illustration). When this P_{pl} is added to the P_{stL} of +10, P_{alv} becomes +20. As the pressure progressively decreases during forced expiration, there must be a point at which the pressures inside and outside the airway wall are equal. This point is the *equal pressure point*. Airway compression occurs downstream (toward the mouth) from this point because the lateral pressure is less than the surrounding wall pressure.

SELF-ASSESSMENT QUESTIONS

1. The volume of air that can be exhaled after a normal tidal volume exhalation is the
    a. IRV
    b. FRC
    c. FVC
    d. ERV
    e. TLC

2. In an obstructive lung disorder, the
    I. FRC is decreased
    II. RV is increased
    III. VC is decreased
    IV. IRV is increased
        a. I and III only
        b. II and III only
        c. II and IV only
        d. II, III, and IV only
        e. I, II, and III only

3. The PEFR in the normal healthy male between 20 and 30 years of age may exceed
        a. 200 L/min
        b. 300 L/min
        c. 400 L/min
        d. 500 L/min
        e. 600 L/min

4. Which of the following can be obtained from a flow-volume loop study?
    I. FVC
    II. PEFR
    III. FEV_T
    IV. $FEF_{25\%-75\%}$
        a. IV only
        b. I and II only
        c. II and III only
        d. I, III, and IV only
        e. I, II, III and IV

5. The MVV in the normal healthy male between 20 and 30 years of age is
        a. 60 L/min
        b. 100 L/min
        c. 170 L/min

   d. 240 L/min
   e. 400 L/min
6. Approximately how much of a forced expiratory maneuver is effort-dependent?
   a. 20%
   b. 30%
   c. 40%
   d. 50%
   e. 60%
7. Which of the following forced expiratory measurements reflects the status of
   medium to small-sized airways?
   a. $FEF_{200-1200}$
   b. PEFR
   c. MVV
   d. $FEF_{25\%-75\%}$
   e. FEV_1/FVC ratio
8. Normally, the percentage of the total volume exhaled during an FEV_1 by a
   20-year-old individual is
   a. 60%
   b. 83%
   c. 94%
   d. 97%
   e. 100%
9. Which of the following forced expiratory measurements is a good index of the
   integrity of large airway function?
   a. FEV_T
   b. $FEF_{200-1200}$
   c. $FEF_{25\%-75\%}$
   d. MVV
   e. FEV_1/FVC
10. The residual volume/total lung capacity ratio in the healthy male between 20
    and 30 years old is
    a. 15%
    b. 20%
    c. 25%
    d. 30%
    e. 35%

11.

CASE
PULMONARY FUNCTION STUDY

A 73-year-old male, with a long history of smoking, demonstrates the following clinical data on a pulmonary function test:

PFT	BELOW NORMAL	NORMAL	ABOVE NORMAL
VC	X		
RV			X
FRC			X
ERV	X		
FEV_T	X		
$FEF_{25\%-75\%}$	X		
PEFR	X		
MVV	X		

Based upon the above information, the patient appears to have:
    a. an obstructive lung disorder
    b. a restrictive lung disorder
    c. both an obstructive and restrictive lung disorder
    d. neither an obstructive or restrictive lung disorder

Answers appear in Appendix VII.

CHAPTER 5

THE CIRCULATORY SYSTEM

OBJECTIVES

By the end of this chapter, the student should be able to:

1. Describe the function of the following specialized cells of the plasma:
   —Erythrocytes
   —Leukocytes
   —Thrombocytes
2. List the chemical components of plasma.
3. Describe the structure and function of the following components of the heart:
   —Inferior and superior venae cavae
   —Right and left atria
   —Right and left ventricles
   —Pulmonary trunk
   —Pulmonary arteries
   —Pulmonary veins
   —Tricuspid valve
   —Bicuspid valve (mitral valve)
   —Pulmonary semilunar valve
   —Aortic semilunar valve
   —Chordae tendineae
   —Papillary muscles
4. Describe how blood flows through the heart.
5. Identify the major blood vessels that nourish the heart.
6. Describe the location and function of the following components of the *conduction system* of the heart:
   —Sinoatrial node
   —Atrioventricular node
   —Bundle of His
   —Right and left bundle branches
   —Purkinje fibers

7. Explain how the following components of the autonomic nervous system coordinate the moment-to-moment *rhythmicity* of the heart:
   —Cardioinhibitor center
   —Cardioaccelerator center
8. Describe the following components of an *electrocardiogram:*
   —P wave
   —QRS complex
   —T wave
9. Identify the *average heart rate* of the normal adult and infant.
10. Describe the following components of the *pulmonary* and *systemic vascular systems:*
    —Arteries
    —Arterioles
    —Capillaries
    —Venules
    —Veins
11. Explain the *neural control* of the vascular systems.
12. Describe the function of the *baroreceptors.*
13. Define the following types of *pressures:*
    —Intravascular pressure
    —Transmural pressure
    —Driving pressure
14. Describe how the following relate to the *cardiac cycle* and *blood pressure:*
    —Ventricular systole
    —Ventricular diastole
15. List the *intraluminal blood pressures* throughout the pulmonary and systemic vascular systems.
16. Describe how blood volume affects blood pressure, and include the following:
    —Stroke volume
    —Heart rate
    —Cardiac output
17. Identify the percentage of blood found throughout the various parts of the pulmonary and systemic systems.
18. Describe the influence of *gravity* on blood flow, and include how it relates to
    —Zone 1
    —Zone 2
    —Zone 3
19. Define the following *determinants of cardiac output:*
    —Ventricular preload

(*continued*)

—Ventricular afterload

—Myocardial contractility

20. Define *vascular resistance*.
21. Describe how the following affect the pulmonary vascular resistance:
    —Active mechanisms
    - Abnormal blood gas values
    - Pharmacologic stimulation
    - Pathologic conditions
    —Passive mechanisms
    - Increased pulmonary arterial pressure
    - Increased left atrial pressure
    - Lung volume and transpulmonary pressure changes
    - Blood volume changes
    - Blood viscosity changes
22. Complete the self-assessment questions at the end of this chapter.

The delivery of oxygen to the cells of the body is a function of blood flow. Thus, when the flow of blood is inadequate, good alveolar ventilation is of little value.

The circulatory system consists of the **blood**, the **heart** (pump), and the **vascular system**.

BLOOD

Blood consists of numerous specialized cells that are suspended in a liquid substance called **plasma**. The cells in the plasma include the **erythrocytes** (red blood cells), **leukocytes** (white blood cells), and **thrombocytes** (or platelets, which are actually cell fragments) (Figure 5–1).

Erythrocytes

The erythrocytes constitute the major portion of the blood cells. In the healthy adult male there are about 5 million red blood cells (RBCs) in each cubic millimeter of blood. The healthy adult female has about 4 million RBCs in each cubic millimeter of blood. The percentage of RBCs in relation to the total blood volume is known as the **hematocrit**. The normal hematocrit is approximately 45

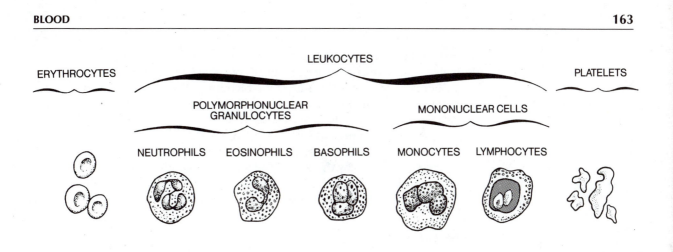

ERYTHROCYTES

LEUKOCYTES

PLATELETS

POLYMORPHONUCLEAR
GRANULOCYTES

MONONUCLEAR CELLS

NEUTROPHILS   EOSINOPHILS   BASOPHILS   MONOCYTES   LYMPHOCYTES

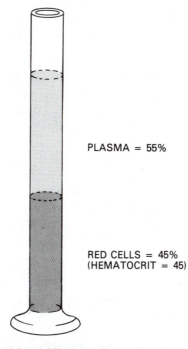

PLASMA = 55%

RED CELLS = 45%
(HEMATOCRIT = 45)

FIGURE 5–2.   When a blood-filled capillary tube is centrifuged, the red blood cells move to the lower portion of the tube. This permits the percentage of red blood cells (hematocrit) to be determined.

percent in the adult male and 42 percent in the adult female (Figure 5–2). In the normal newborn, the hematocrit ranges between 45 and 60 percent.

Microscopically, the RBCs appear as biconcave discs, averaging about 7.5 µ in diameter and 2.5 µ in thickness. They are produced in the red bone marrow in the spongy bone of the cranium, bodies of vertebrae, ribs, sternum, and proximal epiphyses of the humerus and femur. It is estimated that the RBCs are produced at the astonishing rate of 2 million per second. An equal number of worn-out RBCs are destroyed each second by the spleen and liver. The life span of a RBC is about 120 days. The major constituent of the RBCs is **hemoglobin** which is the primary substance responsible for the transport of oxygen and carbon dioxide.

Leukocytes

The primary function of the **leukocytes**, is to protect the body against the invasion of bacteria and other foreign agents that can harm the body. Leukocytes fall into two major groups: (1) the **polymorphonuclear granulocytes**, which include the **neutrophils**, **eosinophils**, and **basophils**; and (2) the **mononuclear** or **nongranulated cells**, which include the **monocytes** and **lymphocytes**. The polymorphonuclear granulocytes are produced in the red bone marrow, and the mononuclear cells develop from lymphoid and myeloid tissue.

The leukocytes are far less numerous than the red blood cells, averaging between 5000 to 9000 cells per cubic millimeter of blood. Because the general function of the leukocytes is to combat inflammation and infection, the clinical diagnosis of an injury or infection often entails what is called a *differential count*, which is the determination of the number of each type of white cell in 100 white blood cells. Table 5–1 shows a normal differential count.

The neutrophils are the most active white cells in response to tissue destruction by bacteria. They are one of several types of cells called phagocytes that ingest and destroy particulate matter. They also release an enzyme called **lysozyme**, which destroys certain bacteria. Thus, a high neutrophil count suggests a bacterial infection.

An elevated eosinophil count indicates an allergic condition, such as an

TABLE 5–1. Normal Differential Count	
POLYMORPHONUCLEAR GRANULOCYTES	**MONONUCLEAR CELLS**
Neutrophils 60–70% Eosinophils 2–4% Basophils 0.5–1%	Lymphocytes 20–25% Monocytes 3–8%

allergic asthmatic episode. Eosinophils are thought to combat the allergen responsible for the allergic reaction. Basophils are also believed to combat allergic reactions.

An elevated number of monocytes indicates a chronic infection (e.g., tuberculosis). Monocytes, which are also phagocytes, take a longer time to reach the site of infection than do neutrophils, but when they do arrive they do so in greater numbers and destroy more bacteria. Lymphocytes are involved in the production of **antibodies**, which are special proteins that inactivate antigens.

Thrombocytes

Thrombocytes, or *blood platelets*, are the smallest of the formed elements in the plasma (see Figure 5–1). The normal platelet count in each cubic millimeter of blood ranges between 250,000 and 500,000. The function of the platelets is to prevent blood loss from a traumatized area of the body involving the smallest blood vessels. They do this by virtue of an activator substance called **platelet factor**, which is a sticky substance that causes blood clotting at the traumatized site. The platelets also contain *serotonin* which, when released, causes smooth muscle constriction and reduced blood flow.

Plasma

When all the cells are removed from the blood, a straw-colored liquid called plasma remains. Plasma constitutes about 55 percent of the total blood volume (see Figure 5–2). Approximately 90 percent of plasma consists of water. The remaining 10 percent is composed of proteins, electrolytes, food substances, respiratory gases, hormones, vitamins, and waste products. Table 5–2 outlines the chemical composition of plasma. Blood serum is plasma without its fibrinogen and several other proteins involved in clotting.

THE HEART

The **heart** is a hollow, four-chambered, muscular organ that consists of the upper right and left **atria** and the lower right and left **ventricles** (Figure 5–3). The atria are separated by a thin muscular wall called the **interatrial septum**; the ventricles are separated by a thick muscular wall called the **interventricular septum**. The heart actually functions as two separate pumps. The right atrium and ventricle act as one pump to propel unoxygenated blood to the lungs. At the same time, the left atrium and ventricle act as another pump to propel oxygenated blood throughout the systemic circulation.

TABLE 5–2. Chemical Composition of Plasma

Water	—93% of plasma weight	**Food Substances**	
		Amino acids	— 40 mg/100 ml
Proteins		Glucose/carbohydrates	—100 mg/100 ml
Albumins	—4.5 g/100 ml	Lipids	—500 mg/100 ml
Globulins	—2.5 g/100 ml	Individual vitamins	—0.0001–2.5 mg/100 ml
Fibrinogen	—0.3 g/100 ml		
		Respiratory Gases	
Electrolytes		O_2	—0.3 ml/100 ml
Cations		CO_2	— 2 ml/100 ml
Na^+	—143 mEq/L	N_2	—0.9 ml/100 ml
K^+	— 4 mEq/L		
Ca_2^+	— 2.5 mEq/L	**Individual Hormones**	—0.000001–0.05 mg/100 ml
Mg_2^+	— 1.5 mEq/L		
Anions		**Waste Products**	
Cl^-	—103 mEq/L	Urea	—34 mg/100 ml
PO_4^{3-}	— 1 mEq/L	Creatinine	— 1 mg/100 ml
SO_4^{2-}	— 0.5 mEq/L	Uric Acid	— 5 mg/100 ml
HCO_3^-	— 27 mEq/L	Bilirubin	—0.2–1.2 mg/100 ml

Blood Flow Through the Heart

As shown in Figure 5–4, the right atrium receives venous blood from the **inferior** and **superior venae cavae**. This blood is low in oxygen and high in carbon dioxide. A one-way valve called the **tricuspid valve** lies between the right atrium and the right ventricle. The tricuspid valve gets its name from its three valve leaflets, or cusps. The tricuspid leaflets are held in place by tendinous cords called **chordae tendineae**. The chordae tendineae are secured to the ventricular wall by the **papillary muscles**. When the ventricles contract, the tricuspid valve closes and blood leaves the right ventricle through the **pulmonary trunk** and enters the lungs by way of the right and left **pulmonary arteries**. The **pulmonary semilunar valve** separates the right ventricle from the pulmonary trunk.

After blood passes through the lungs, it returns to the left atrium by way of the **pulmonary veins**. The returning blood is high in oxygen and low in carbon dioxide. The **bicuspid valve** (also called the *mitral valve*) lies between the left atrium and the left ventricle. The bicuspid valve, which consists of two cusps, prevents blood from returning to the left atrium during ventricular contraction. Similarly to the tricuspid valve, the bicuspid valve is also held in position by chordae tendineae and papillary muscles. The left ventricle pumps blood through

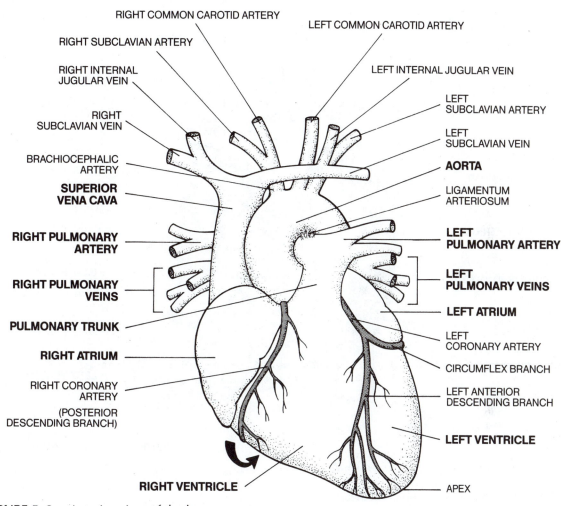

FIGURE 5–3. Anterior view of the heart.

the ascending **aorta**. The **aortic semilunar valve**, which lies at the base of the ascending aorta, closes in response to the increased pressure in the aorta and thus prevents the backflow of blood into the left ventricle (see Figure 5–4).

Blood Supply of the Heart

The blood supply that nourishes the heart originates directly from the aorta by means of two arteries—the **left coronary artery** and the **right coronary artery** (see Figure 5–3).

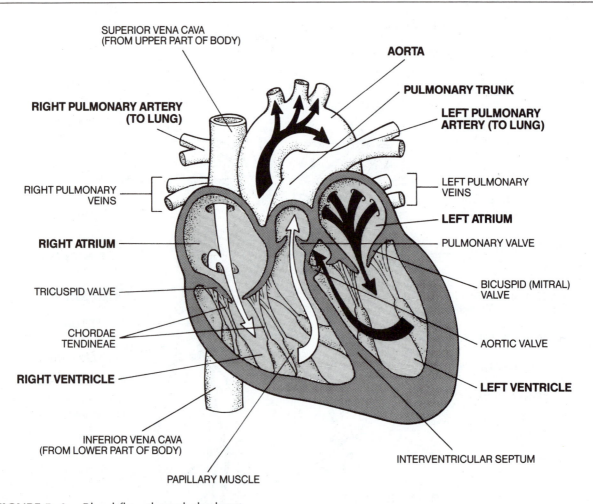

SUPERIOR VENA CAVA
(FROM UPPER PART OF BODY)

AORTA

**RIGHT PULMONARY ARTERY
(TO LUNG)**

PULMONARY TRUNK

**LEFT PULMONARY
ARTERY (TO LUNG)**

RIGHT PULMONARY
VEINS

LEFT PULMONARY
VEINS

RIGHT ATRIUM

LEFT ATRIUM

PULMONARY VALVE

TRICUSPID VALVE

BICUSPID (MITRAL)
VALVE

CHORDAE
TENDINEAE

AORTIC VALVE

RIGHT VENTRICLE

LEFT VENTRICLE

INFERIOR VENA CAVA
(FROM LOWER PART OF BODY)

INTERVENTRICULAR SEPTUM

PAPILLARY MUSCLE

FIGURE 5–4. Blood flow through the heart.

The left coronary artery divides into the **circumflex** and **anterior descending branches**. The circumflex branch, which runs posteriorly, supplies the lateral
wall of the left ventricle and the diaphragmatic surface of the left ventricle. The
anterior descending branch supplies the anterior wall of the left ventricle and
portions of the right ventricle and interventricular septum.

The right coronary artery supplies the right ventricle and the posterior
portion of the septum. The **posterior descending branch** of the right coronary
artery supplies portions of the diaphragmatic surface of the left ventricle.

At rest, the heart receives about 5 percent of the total cardiac output. Most of
the blood delivered to the heart returns to the right atrium via the **coronary sinus**.

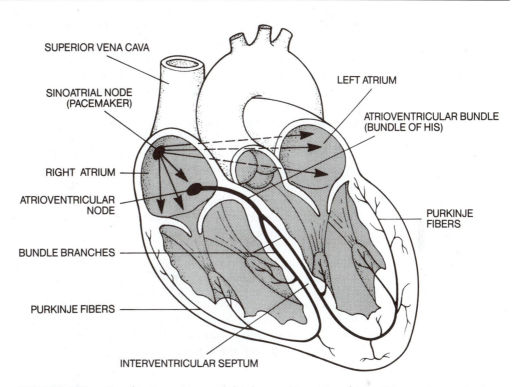

SUPERIOR VENA CAVA

SINOATRIAL NODE
(PACEMAKER)

LEFT ATRIUM

ATRIOVENTRICULAR BUNDLE
(BUNDLE OF HIS)

RIGHT ATRIUM

ATRIOVENTRICULAR
NODE

PURKINJE
FIBERS

BUNDLE BRANCHES

PURKINJE FIBERS

INTERVENTRICULAR SEPTUM

FIGURE 5–5. Conductive system of the heart. SA = sinoatrial; AV = atrioventricular.

Some of the venous blood returns to the ventricular chambers via the **Thebesian veins**. The function of the Thebesian veins, however, is controversial: some investigators feel that, in the left ventricle at least, the Thebesian vein carries oxygenated blood from the ventricular chamber backward into the muscular walls to supply the inner musculature with nutrients.

The Conductive System of the Heart

The cardiac muscle possesses an intrinsic rhythmicity that enables the heart to initiate the heartbeat without extrinsic stimulation. This unique autorhythmicity is a function of the conductive system of the heart. The components of the conductive system are the **sinoatrial node** (SA node), **atrioventricular node** (AV node of AV junction), **bundle of His**, the **right and left bundle branches**, and the **Purkinje fibers** (Figure 5–5).

The SA node, or *pacemaker*, is located in the upper portion of the right atrium. The SA node initiates the cardiac contraction by producing an electrical impulse that travels through the muscle strands of the atria, causing them to contract simultaneously. This action forces the atrial blood into the ventricles. The

AV node, located in the lower portion of the right interatrial septum, receives the electrical impulse and relays it to the ventricles via the bundle of His, the right and left bundle branches, and the Purkinje fibers. Stimulation of the Purkinje fibers causes the ventricles to contract simultaneously.

Although the cardiac muscle has an intrinsic rhythmicity, it is also controlled by the *autonomic nervous system*, which enables the heart to respond to the ever-changing needs of the body. Two areas in the medulla oblongata that are responsible for coordinating the moment-to-moment activity of the heart are called the **cardioinhibitor center** and the **cardioaccelerator center**; collectively, they are known as the **cardiac centers**. When activated, the cardioaccelerator center increases the heart rate and increases the strength of contraction by sending sympathetic impulses to the heart. In contrast, the cardioinhibitor center slows the heart and decreases the strength of contraction by sending parasympathetic (vagal) impulses to the heart.

The Electrocardiogram

The electrical impulses that travel through the conductive system of the heart can be recorded as an **electrocardiogram** (ECG) by means of electrodes placed on the surface of the body. The ECG represents the electrical changes of the heart that result from the depolarization and repolarization of the cardiac muscle (Figure 5–6).

Figure 5–7 illustrates the ECG of a normal cardiac cycle. The P wave represents the depolarization of the atria, the QRS complex represents ventricular depolarization (the P wave repolarizes during the QRS complex and is not seen on the ECG tracing), and the T wave represents ventricular repolarization. The normal adult heart rate is 60 to 100 beats per minute. The normal infant heart rate is 130 to 150 beats per minute.

THE PULMONARY AND SYSTEMIC VASCULAR SYSTEMS

The vascular network of the circulatory system is composed of two major subdivisions: the **systemic system** and the **pulmonary system** (Figure 5–8, page 173). The pulmonary system begins with the pulmonary trunk and ends in the left atrium. The systemic system begins with the aorta and ends in the right atrium. Both systems are composed of arteries, arterioles, capillaries, venules, and veins (see Figure 1–24).

Arteries are vessels that carry blood away from the heart. The arteries are strong, elastic vessels that are well suited for carrying blood under high pressures in the systemic system. The arteries subdivide as they move away from the heart into smaller vessels and, eventually, into vessels called **arterioles**. Arterioles play a

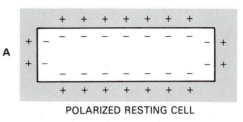

A

POLARIZED RESTING CELL

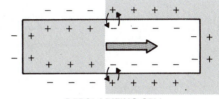

B

DEPOLARIZING CELL

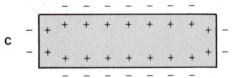

C

DEPOLARIZED CELL

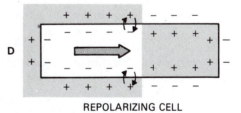

D

REPOLARIZING CELL

FIGURE 5–6. Depolarization and repolarization. A) Polarized resting cell.
The heart muscle is in the resting, or polarized, state: that is, the cell carries an
electrical charge, with the inside negatively charged with potassium and the
outside positively charged with sodium. **B) Depolarizing cell.** When the
muscle cell is stimulated, the cell begins to depolarize: that is, the positively
charged ions flow into the cell, and the negatively charged ions flow out of the
cell. **C) Depolarized cell.** During the period that the cell is depolarized, all the
positively charged ions are on the inside of the cell, and all the negatively
charged ions are on the outside of the cell. **D) Repolarizing cell.** After the
muscle cell has depolarized, it begins to return to the resting state: that is, the
negatively charged ions flow into the cell, and the positively charged ions flow
out of the cell.

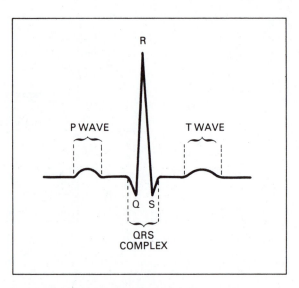

FIGURE 5–7. Normal electrocardiogram (ECG) tracing.

major role in the distribution and regulation of blood pressure and are referred to as the **resistance vessels**.

Gas exchange occurs in the **capillaries**. In the capillaries of the pulmonary system, gas exchange is called **external respiration** (gas exchange between blood and air). In the capillaries of the systemic system, gas exchange is called **internal respiration** (gas exchange between blood and tissues).

The **venules** are tiny veins continuous with the capillaries. The venules empty into the veins, which carry blood back to the heart. The veins differ from the arteries in that they are capable of holding a large amount of blood with very little pressure change. Because of this unique feature, the veins are called **capacitance vessels**. Approximately 60 percent of the body's total blood volume is contained within the venous system.

Neural Control of the Vascular System

The pulmonary arterioles and most of the arterioles in the systemic circulation are controlled by sympathetic impulses. Sympathetic fibers are found in the arteries, arterioles, and, to a lesser degree, in the veins (Figure 5–9). The **vasomotor center**, which is located in the medulla oblongata, governs the number of sympathetic impulses sent to the vascular systems. Under normal circumstances, the vasomotor center transmits a continual stream of sympathetic impulses to the blood vessels, maintaining the vessels in a moderate state of constriction all the time. This state of vascular contraction is called the **vasomotor tone**.

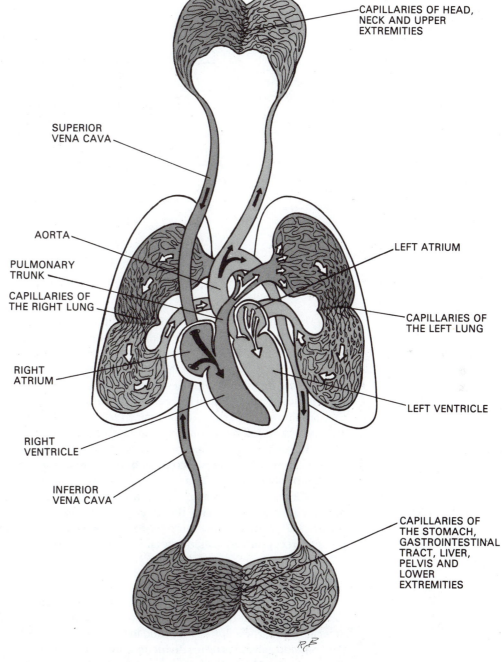

FIGURE 5–8. Pulmonary and systemic circulation. The pulmonary circulation is indicated by open arrows; the systemic circulation is indicated by solid black arrows.

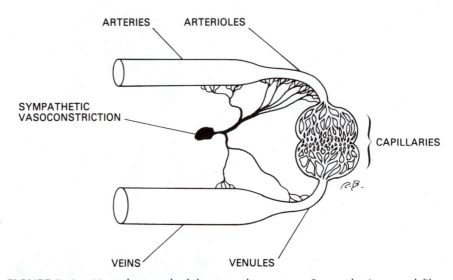

FIGURE 5–9. Neural control of the vascular system. Sympathetic neural fibers to the arterioles are especially abundant.

The vasomotor center coordinates both vasoconstriction and vasodilation by controlling the number of sympathetic impulses that leave the medulla. For example, when the vasomotor center is activated to constrict a particular vascular region (i.e., more than the normal state of constriction), it does so by increasing the number of sympathetic impulses to that vascular area. In contrast, the vasomotor center initiates vasodilation by reducing the number of sympathetic impulses sent to a certain vascular region. (The major vascular beds in the systemic system that are *not* controlled by this mechanism are the arterioles of the heart, brain, and skeletal muscles. Sympathetic impulses to these vessels cause vasodilation.) In addition to the sympathetic control, blood flow through the large veins can be affected by abdominal and intrathoracic pressure changes.

Working together, the vasomotor center and the cardiac centers in the medulla oblongata regulate the arterial blood pressure in response to signals received from special pressure receptors located throughout the body. These pressure receptors are called **arterial baroreceptors**.

The Baroreceptor Reflex

Specialized stretch receptors called **baroreceptors** (also called *pressorecep-tors*) are located in the walls of the carotid arteries and the aorta. In the **carotid arteries**, the baroreceptors are found in the carotid sinuses high in the neck where the common carotid arteries divide into the external and internal carotid arteries (Figure 5–10). The walls of the carotid sinuses are thin and contain a large number

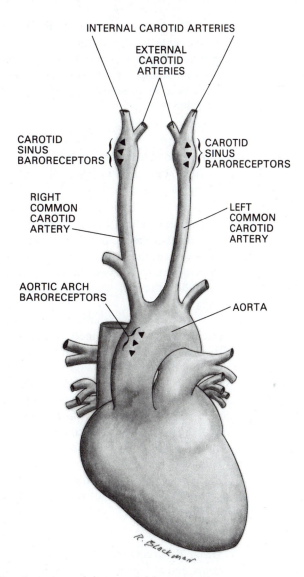

FIGURE 5–10. Location of the arterial baroreceptors.

of branching, vinelike nerve endings that are sensitive to stretch or distortion. The afferent fibers from the carotid sinuses travel with the **glossopharyngeal nerve** (9th cranial) to the medulla. In the aorta, the baroreceptors are located in the **aortic arch** (see Figure 5–10). The afferent fibers from the aortic arch baroreceptors travel with the **vagus nerve** (10th cranial).

The baroreceptors regulate the arterial blood pressure by initiating reflex adjustments to deviations in blood pressure. For example, when the arterial pressure decreases, the neural impulses transmitted from the baroreceptors to the vasomotor and cardiac centers in the medulla also decrease. This causes the medulla to increase its sympathetic activity, which, in turn, causes an increase in the following:

- Heart rate
- Myocardial force of contraction
- Arterial constriction
- Venous constriction

The net result is (1) an increased cardiac output (because of an increased heart rate and stroke volume), (2) an increase in the total peripheral resistance (primarily induced by arterial constriction), and (3) the return of blood pressure toward normal. The vascular constriction occurs primarily in the abdominal region (including the liver, spleen, pancreas, stomach, intestine, kidneys, skin, and skeletal muscles).

In contrast, when the blood pressure increases, the neural impulses from the arterial baroreceptors increase. This causes the medulla to decrease its sympathetic activity, which in turn reduces both the cardiac output and the total peripheral resistance.

Finally, the baroreceptors function as short-term regulators of arterial blood pressure. That is, they respond instantly to any blood pressure change to restore the blood pressure toward normal (to the degree possible in the situation). If, however, the factors responsible for moving the arterial pressure away from normal persist for more than a few days, the arterial baroreceptors will eventually come to "accept" the new pressure as normal. For example, in individuals who have chronically high blood pressure (*hypertension*), the baroreceptors still operate, but at a higher level—in short, their operating point is reset at a higher level.

Other Baroreceptors.   Baroreceptors are also found in the large arteries, large veins, and pulmonary vessels and the cardiac walls themselves. Functionally, most of these receptors are similar to the baroreceptors in the carotid sinuses and aortic arch in that they send an increased rate of neural transmissions to the medulla in response to increased pressure. By means of these additional receptors, the medulla gains a further degree of sensitivity to venous, atrial, and ventricular pressures. For example, a slight decrease in atrial pressure initiates sympathetic activity even before there is a decrease in cardiac output and therefore, a decrease in the arterial blood pressure great enough to be detected by the aortic and carotid baroreceptors.

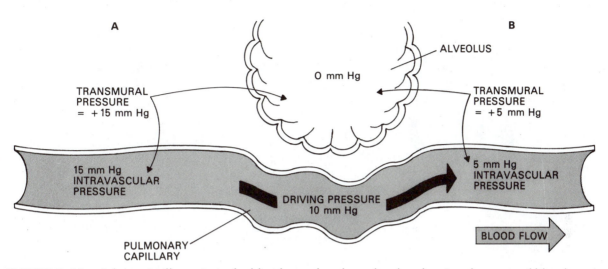

FIGURE 5–11. Schematic illustration of a blood vessel and an alveolus showing the types of blood pressures used to study flood flow. Within the blood vessel, the *intravascular pressure* at point A is 15 mm Hg, and the intravascular pressure at point B is 5 mm Hg. The pressure within the alveolus (which represents the pressure surrounding the blood vessel) is zero. In view of these numbers, the following can be stated: (1) the *transmural pressure* at point A is a positive 15 mm Hg, (2) the *transmural pressure* at point B is a positive 5 mm Hg, and (3) the *driving pressure* between point A and point B is 10 mm Hg.

PRESSURES IN THE PULMONARY AND SYSTEMIC VASCULAR SYSTEMS

Three different types of pressures are used to study the blood flow: (1) **intravascular**, (2) **transmural**, and (3) **driving pressures**.

Intravascular pressure is the actual blood pressure in the lumen of any vessel at any point, relative to the barometric pressure. This pressure is also known as the intraluminal pressure.

Transmural pressure is the difference between the intravascular pressure of a vessel and the pressure surrounding the vessel. The transmural pressure is *positive* when the pressure inside the vessel exceeds the pressure outside the vessel, and *negative* when the pressure inside the vessel is less than the pressure surrounding the vessel.

Driving Pressure is the difference between the pressure at one point in a vessel and the pressure at any other point downstream in the vessel.

Figure 5–11 illustrates the different types of pressures used to study the flow of blood.

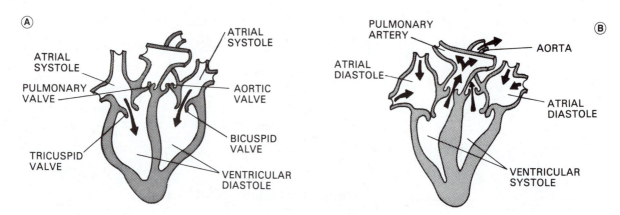

FIGURE 5–12.   Sequence of cardiac contraction. A) Ventricular diastole and atrial systole; B) Ventricular systole and atrial diastole.

THE CARDIAC CYCLE AND ITS EFFECT ON BLOOD PRESSURE

The arterial blood pressure rises and falls in a pattern that corresponds to the phases of the cardiac cycle. When the ventricles contract (ventricular systole), blood is forced into the pulmonary artery and the aorta, and the pressure in these arteries rises sharply. The maximum pressure generated during ventricular contraction is the **systolic pressure**. When the ventricles relax (ventricular diastole), the arterial pressure drops. The lowest pressure that remains in the arteries prior to the next ventricular contraction is the **diastolic pressure** (Figure 5–12). In the systemic system, normal systolic pressure is about 120 mm Hg and normal diastolic pressure is about 80 mm Hg. In the pulmonary system, the normal systolic pressure is about 25 mm Hg and the normal diastolic pressure is about 8 mm Hg (Figure 5–13).

The pulmonary circulation is a low-pressure system. The mean pressure in the pulmonary artery is about 15 mm Hg, and the mean pressure in the left atrium is about 5 mm Hg. Thus, the driving pressure needed to move blood through the lungs is 10 mm Hg. In contrast, the mean intraluminal pressure in the aorta is about 100 mm Hg and the mean right atrial pressure is about 2 mm Hg, making the driving pressure through the systemic system about 98 mm Hg. Compared to the pulmonary circulation, the pressure in the systemic system is about 10 times greater. Figure 5–14 shows the mean intraluminal blood pressures throughout both the pulmonary and systemic vascular systems.

The surge of blood rushing into the arterial system during each ventricular contraction causes the elastic walls of the arteries to expand. When the ventricular contraction stops, the pressure drops almost immediately and the arterial walls

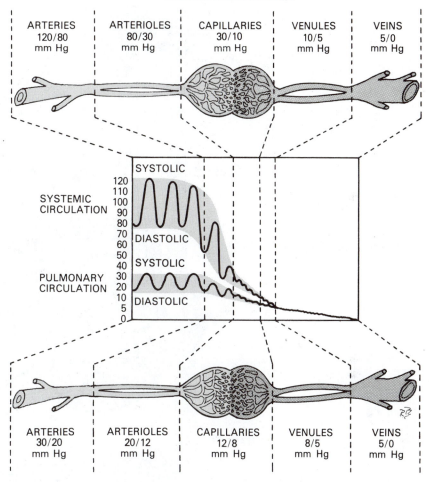

FIGURE 5–13. Summary of diastolic and systolic pressures in various segments of the circulatory system.

recoil. This alternating expansion and recoil of the arterial wall can be felt as a pulse in several systemic arteries that run close to the skin's surface. Figure 5–15 shows the major sites where a pulse can be detected by palpation.

The Blood Volume and Its Effect on Blood Pressure

The volume of blood ejected from the ventricle during each contraction is called the **stroke volume**. Normally, the stroke volume ranges between 40 ml and

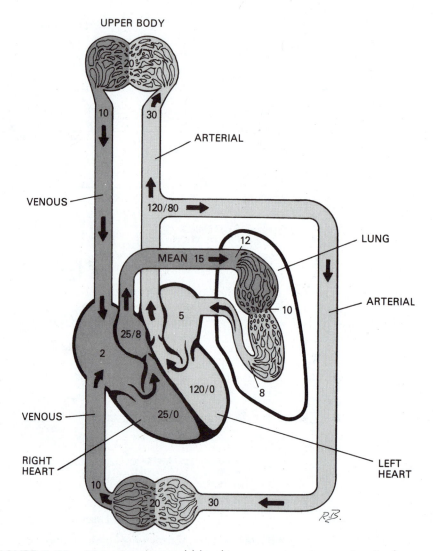

FIGURE 5–14. Mean intraluminal blood pressure at various points in the pulmonary and systemic circulation.

80 ml. The total volume of blood discharged from the ventricles per minute is called **cardiac output**. The cardiac output (CO) is calculated by multiplying the stroke volume (SV) by the heart rate (HR) per minute (CO = SV × HR). Thus, if the stroke volume is 70 ml, and the heart rate is 72 beats per minute, the cardiac output is 5040 ml per minute.

Under normal circumstances, the cardiac output directly influences blood pressure. In other words, *when either the stroke volume or heart rate increases,*

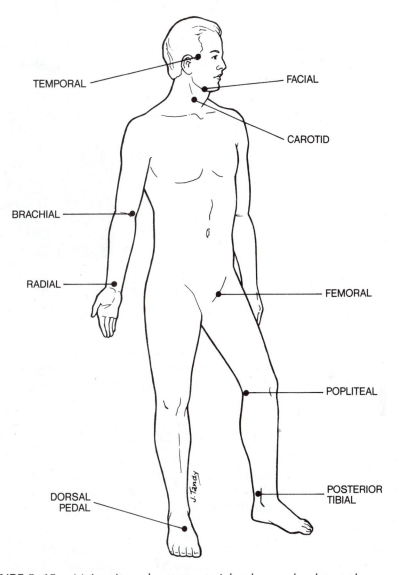

FIGURE 5–15.   Major sites where an arterial pulse can be detected.

the blood pressure increases. Or conversely, when the stroke volume or heart rate decreases, the blood pressure decreases.

Although the total blood volume varies with age, body size, and sex, the normal adult volume is about 5 liters. Of this volume, about 75 percent is in the systemic circulation, 15 percent in the heart, and 10 percent in the pulmonary

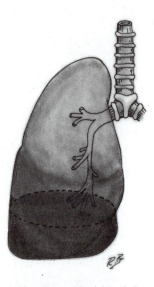

FIGURE 5–16.   Distribution of pulmonary blood flow. In the upright lung, blood flow steadily increases from the apex to the base.

circulation. Overall, about 60 percent of the total blood volume is in the veins, and about 10 percent is in the arteries. Normally, the pulmonary capillary bed contains about 75 ml of blood, although it has the capacity for about 200 ml.

THE DISTRIBUTION OF PULMONARY BLOOD FLOW

In the upright lung, blood flow progressively decreases from the base to the apex (Figure 5–16). This linear distribution of blood is a function of (1) **gravity**, (2) **cardiac output**, and (3) **pulmonary vascular resistance**.

Gravity

Because blood is a relatively heavy substance, it is **gravity-dependent;** i.e., it naturally moves to the portion of the body, or portion of the organ, that is closest to the ground. In the average lung, there is a distance of about 30 centimeters between the base and the apex. The blood that fills the lung from the bottom to the top is analogous to a column of water 30 cm long and, therefore, exerts a pressure of about 30 cm H_2O (22 mm Hg) between the base and apex. Because the pulmonary artery enters each lung about midway between the top and bottom of the lung, the pulmonary artery pressure has to be greater than 15 cm H_2O (11 mm Hg) to overcome the gravitational force and, thereby, supply blood to the lung apex. For this reason, most of the blood flows through (or falls into) the lower half of the lung—the gravity-dependent portion of the lung.

As a result of the gravitational effect on blood flow, the intraluminal pressures of the vessels in the gravity-dependent area (lower lung region) are greater than the intraluminal pressures in the least gravity-dependent area (upper lung region). The high intraluminal pressure of the vessels in the gravity-dependent area causes the vessels to distend. As the vessels widen, the vascular resistance decreases and, thus, permits blood flow to increase. The fact that blood flow is enhanced as the vascular system widens is according to Poiseuille's law for flow ($\dot{V} \simeq Pr^4$).

The position of the body can significantly change the gravity-dependent portion of the lungs. For example, when an individual is in the supine position (lying on the back), the gravity-dependent area is the posterior portion of the lungs; when an individual is in the prone position (lying on the stomach), the gravity-dependent region is the anterior portion of the lungs; when the person is lying on the side, the lower, lateral half of the lung nearest the ground is gravity-dependent; when an individual is suspended upside down, the apices of the lungs become gravity-dependent (Figure 5–17).

Figure 5–18 uses a three-zone model to illustrate the effects of gravity and alveolar pressure on the distribution of pulmonary blood flow:

In **Zone 1** (the least gravity-dependent area), the alveolar pressure is sometimes greater than both the arterial and the venous intraluminal pressures. As a result, the pulmonary capillaries can be compressed and blood is prevented from flowing through this region. Under normal circumstances, this situation does not occur, since the pulmonary arterial pressure (generated by the cardiac output) is usually sufficient to raise the blood to the top of the lungs and to overcome the alveolar pressure. There are, however, a variety of conditions—such as severe hemorrhage, dehydration, and positive pressure ventilation—that can result in the alveolar pressure being higher than the arterial and venous pressures. When the alveoli are ventilated but not perfused, no gas exchange can occur and **alveolar dead space** is said to exist (see Figure 2–28).

In **Zone 2**, the arterial pressure is greater than the alveolar pressure and, therefore, the pulmonary capillaries are perfused. Because the alveolar pressure is greater than the venous pressure, the effective driving pressure for blood flow is determined by the pulmonary arterial pressure minus the alveolar pressure—not the normal arterial-venous pressure difference. Thus, because the alveolar pressure is essentially the same throughout all the lung regions, and because the arterial pressure progressively increases toward the gravity-dependent areas of the lung, the effective driving pressure (arterial pressure minus alveolar pressure) steadily increases down the vertical axis of Zone 2. As a result, from the beginning of the upper portion of Zone 2 (the point at which the arterial pressure equals the alveolar pressure) to the lower portion of Zone 2 (the point at which the venous pressure equals the alveolar pressure) the flow of blood progressively increases.

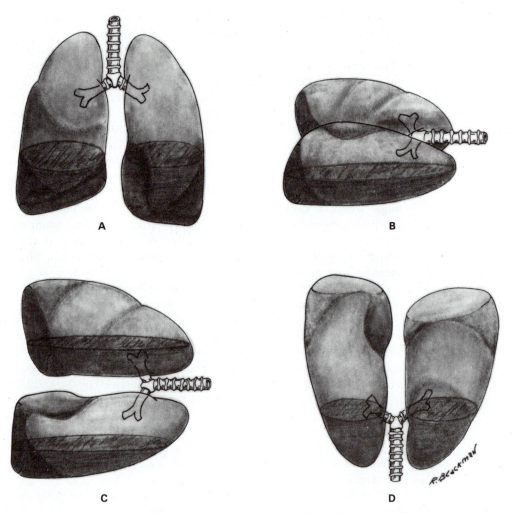

FIGURE 5–17.   Blood flow normally moves into the gravity-dependent areas of the lungs. Thus, body position affects the distribution of the pulmonary blood flow as illustrated in the erect (**A**), supine (**B**), lateral (**C**), and upside-down (**D**) positions.

In **Zone 3** (gravity-dependent area), both the arterial and the venous pressures are greater than the alveolar pressure, and therefore blood flow through this region is constant. Because the arterial pressure and venous pressure both increase equally downward in Zone 3, the arterial-venous pressure difference and, therefore, blood flow is essentially the same throughout all of Zone 3.

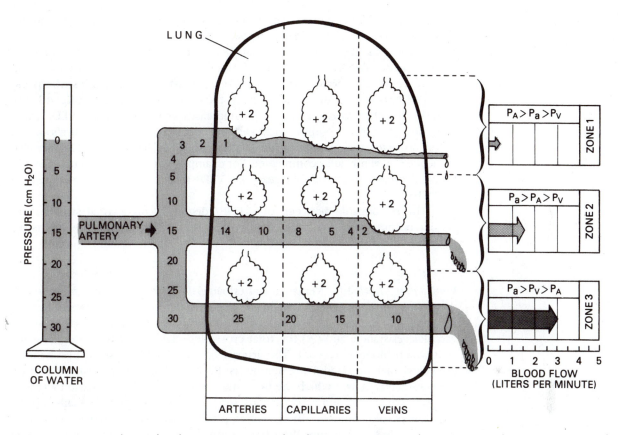

FIGURE 5–18. Relationship between gravity, alveolar pressure (PA), pulmonary arterial pressure (Pa), and pulmonary venous pressure (Pv) in different lung zones. Note: The +2 cm H_2O pressure in the alveoli (e.g., during expiration) was arbitrarily selected for this illustration.

Determinants of Cardiac Output

As described earlier, the cardiac output is equal to the stroke volume times the heart rate. The stroke volume is determined by (1) ventricular preload, (2) ventricular afterload, and (3) myocardial contractility.

Ventricular Preload. Ventricular preload refers to the degree that the myocardial fiber is stretched prior to contraction (*end-diastole*). Within limits, the more the myocardial fiber is stretched during diastole (*preload*), the more strongly it will contract during systole, and therefore the greater the myocardial contractility will be. This mechanism enables the heart to convert an increased venous return into an increased stroke volume. Beyond a certain point, however, the cardiac output does not improve as the preload increases.

Because the degree of myocardial fiber stretch (*preload*) is a function of the pressure generated by the volume of blood returning to the ventricle during diastole, ventricular preload is reflected in the **ventricular end-diastolic pressure (VEDP)**—which, in essence, reflects the ventricular **end-diastolic volume (VEDV)**. In other words, as the VEDV increases or decreases, the VEDP (and, therefore, the cardiac output) increases or decreases, respectively. It should be noted, however, that, similar to lung compliance (C_L), VEDP and VEDV are also influenced by ventricular compliance. For example, when the ventricular compliance is decreased as a result of disease, the VEDP increases significantly more than the VEDV.

The relationship between the VEDP (degree of myocardial stretch) and cardiac output (stroke volume) is known as the **Frank-Starling relationship** (Figure 5–19).

Ventricular Afterload.   Ventricular afterload is defined as the force against which the ventricles must work to pump blood. It is determined by several factors, including (1) the volume and viscosity of the blood ejected, (2) the peripheral vascular resistance, and (3) the total cross-sectional area of the vascular space into which blood is ejected. The arterial systolic blood pressure best reflects the ventricular afterload. For example, as the arterial systolic pressure increases, the resistance (against which the heart must work to eject blood) also increases. Clinically, this condition is particularly serious in the patient with a failing heart and low stroke volume. By reducing the peripheral resistance (*afterload reduction*) in such patients, the stroke volume increases with little or no change in the blood pressure. This is because blood pressure (BP) is a function of the cardiac output (CO) times the systemic vascular resistance (SVR) (BP = CO × SVR).

Myocardial Contractility.   Myocardial contractility may be regarded as the force generated by the myocardium when the ventricular muscle fibers shorten. In general, when the contractility of the heart increases or decreases, the cardiac output increases or decreases, respectively.

There is no single measurement that defines contractility in the clinical setting. Changes in contractility, however, can be inferred through clinical assessment (e.g., pulse, blood pressure, skin temperature) and serial hemodynamic measurements (discussed in Chapter Six). An increase in myocardial contractility is referred to as **positive inotropism**. A decrease in myocardial contractility is referred to as **negative inotropism**.

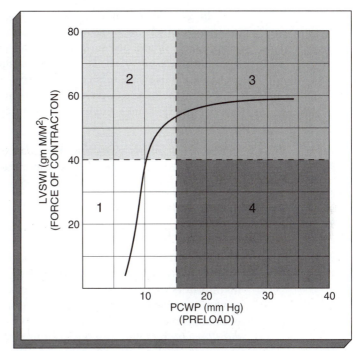

FIGURE 5–19. Frank-Starling curve. The Frank-Starling curve shows that the more the myocardial fiber is stretched as a result of the blood pressure that develops as blood returns to the chambers of the heart during diastole, the more the heart muscle will contract during systole. In addition, it will contract with greater force. The stretch produced within the myocardium at end-diastole is called *preload*. Clinically, it would be best to determine the preload of the left ventricle by measuring the end-diastolic pressure of the left ventricle or left atrium. However, since it is impractical to measure this at the patient's bedside, the best preload approximation of the left heart is the *pulmonary capillary wedge pressure* (PCWP). As shown in this illustration, the relationship of the PCWP (preload) to the *left ventricular stroke work index* (LVSWI) (force of contraction) may appear in four quadrants: (1) hypovolemia, (2) optimal function, (3) hypervolemia, and (4) cardiac failure.

Vascular Resistance

Circulatory resistance is derived by dividing the mean blood pressure (BP) by the cardiac output (CO):

$$Resistance = \frac{BP}{CO}$$

In general, when the vascular resistance increases, the blood pressure increases (which, in turn, increases the ventricular afterload). Because of this relationship, blood pressure monitoring can be used to reflect pulmonary or systemic resistance. That is, when resistance increases or decreases, the blood pressure will likely increase or decrease.

In the pulmonary system, there are several known mechanisms that change the vascular resistance. Such mechanisms are classified as either *active* or *passive mechanisms*.

Active Mechanisms Affecting Vascular Resistance. Active mechanisms that affect vascular resistance include abnormal blood gases, pharmacologic stimulation, and pathologic conditions that have a direct effect on the vascular system.

Abnormal Blood Gases

- Decreased PO_2 (Hypoxia)

The pulmonary vascular system constricts in response to a decreased alveolar oxygen pressure. The exact mechanism of this phenomenon is unclear. Some investigators suggest that alveolar hypoxia causes the lung parenchyma to release a substance that produces vasoconstriction. It is known, however, that the partial pressure of oxygen in the *alveoli* ($P_{A_{O_2}}$)—not the partial pressure of oxygen of the *capillary blood* (Pc_{O_2})—controls this response. The effect of hypoxic vasoconstriction is to direct blood away from the hypoxic lung regions to lung areas that have a higher partial pressure of oxygen.

Clinically, when the number of hypoxic regions becomes significant (e.g., the advanced stages of emphysema or chronic bronchitis), generalized pulmonary vasoconstriction can develop. This can cause a substantial increase in the pulmonary vascular resistance and in the work of the right heart. This in turn leads to right ventricular hypertrophy, or *cor pulmonale*.

- Increased P_{CO_2} (Hypercapnia)

Pulmonary vascular resistance increases in response to an acute increase in the P_{CO_2} level. It is believed, however, that the vasoconstriction that occurs is most likely due to the increased H^+ concentration (*respiratory acidosis*) that develops from a sudden increase in the P_{CO_2} level, rather than to the P_{CO_2} itself. This is supported by the fact that pulmonary vasoconstriction does not occur when hypercapnia is accompanied by a normal pH (*compensated respiratory acidosis*).

- Decreased pH (Acidemia)

Pulmonary vasoconstriction develops in response to decreased pH (increased H^+ concentration) of either metabolic or respiratory origin.

Pharmacologic Stimulation. The pulmonary vessels constrict in response to various pharmacologic agents, including

- Epinephrine (Adrenalin)
- Norepinephrine (Levophed, Levarterenol).
- Dobutamine (Dobutrex)
- Dopamine (Intropin)
- Phenylephrine (Neo-Synephrine)

Constricted pulmonary vessels relax in response to the following agents:

- Oxygen
- Isoproterenol (Isuprel)
- Aminophylline
- Calcium blocking agents

Pathologic Conditions.   Pulmonary vascular resistance increases in response to a number of pathologic conditions. Some of the more common ones are:

- Vessel blockage or obstruction—e.g., caused by a thrombus or an embolus (blood clot, fat cell, air bubble, or tumor mass)
- Vessel wall diseases—e.g., sclerosis, polyarteritis, or scleroderma
- Vessel destruction or obliteration—e.g., emphysema or pulmonary interstitial fibrosis
- Vessel compression—e.g., pneumothorax, hemothorax, or tumor mass

Pathologic disturbances in the pulmonary vasculary system can develop in the arteries, arterioles, capillaries, venules, or veins. When increased vascular resistance originates in the venules or veins, the transmural pressure increases and, in severe cases, causes the capillary fluid to spill into the alveoli. **This is called pulmonary edema.** Left ventricular failure will cause the same pathologic disturbances. When the resistance originates in the arteries or arterioles, the pulmonary artery pressure will increase but the pulmonary capillary pressure will be normal or low. Regardless of the origin of the pathologic disturbance, a severe and persistent pulmonary vascular resistance is ultimately followed by an elevated right ventricular pressure, right ventricular strain, right ventricular hypertrophy, and right heart failure.

Passive Mechanisms Affecting Vascular Resistance.   The term *passive mechanism* refers to a secondary change in pulmonary vascular resistance that occurs in response to another mechanical change. In other words, when a mechanical factor in the respiratory system changes, a passive increase or decrease in the caliber of the pulmonary blood vessels also occurs. Some of the more common passive mechanisms are:

Pulmonary Arterial Pressure Changes.   As pulmonary arterial pressure increases (either by increasing the height of the perfusion reservoir or by increasing blood

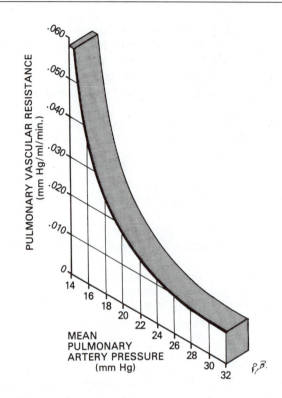

FIGURE 5–20. Increased mean pulmonary arterial pressure decreases pulmonary vascular resistance.

flow), the pulmonary vascular resistance decreases (Figure 5–20). This is assuming that lung volume and left atrial pressure remain constant. The pulmonary vascular resistance decreases because of the increase in intraluminal distending pressure, which increases the total cross-sectional areas of the pulmonary vascular system through the mechanisms of **recruitment** and **distension**.

As shown in Figure 5–21, *recruitment* entails the opening of vessels that were closed or not being utilized for blood flow before the vascular pressure increased. *Distention,* on the other hand, entails the stretching or widening of vessels that were open, but not to their full capacity. Both of these mechanisms increase the total cross-sectional area of the vascular system, which, in turn, reduces the vascular resistance. These mechanisms, however, have their limits.

Left Atrial Pressure Changes.   As the left atrial pressure increases, while the lung volume and pulmonary arterial pressure are held constant, pulmonary vascular resistance decreases.

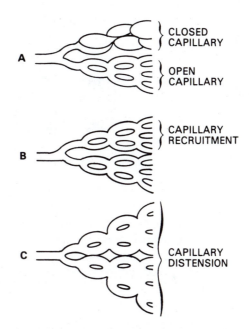

FIGURE 5–21. Schematic drawing of the mechanisms that may be activated to decrease pulmonary vascular resistance when the mean pulmonary artery pressure increases. (*A*) A group of pulmonary capillaries, one-half of which are not perfused. (*B*) The previously unperfused capillaries shown in *A* are recruited (i.e., opened) in response to the increased pulmonary artery pressure. (*C*) The increased blood pressure has distended the capillaries that are already open.

Lung Volume Changes. The effect of changes in lung volume on pulmonary vascular resistance varies according to the location of the vessel. Two major groups of vessels must be considered: (1) **alveolar vessels**—those vessels that surround the alveoli (*pulmonary capillaries*)—and (2) **extra-alveolar vessels**—the larger arteries and veins.

Alveolar Vessels. Because the pulmonary capillary vessels are so thin, intrapleural pressure changes directly affect the anatomy of the capillaries. During normal inspiration, the alveolar vessels progressively stretch and flatten. During expiration, the alveolar vessels shorten and widen. Thus, as the lungs are inflated, the resistance offered by the alveolar vessels progressively increases (Figure 5–22). During the inspiratory phase of mechanical ventilation (*positive pressure phase*), moreover, the resistance generated by the alveolar vessels may become excessively high and, as a result, restrict the flow of pulmonary blood. The pressure difference between the alveoli and the inside of the pulmonary capillaries is called the *transmural pressure* (see Figure 5–11).

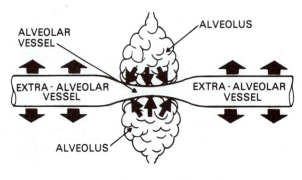

DURING INSPIRATION

FIGURE 5–22. Schematic illustration of pulmonary vessels during inspiration. The *alveolar vessels* (pulmonary capillaries) are exposed to the intrapleural pressure change and are stretched and flattened. The *extra-alveolar vessels* expand as the intrapleural pressure becomes more negative during inspiration.

Extra-alveolar Vessels.   The extra-alveolar vessels (the large arterioles and veins) are also exposed to the intrapleural pressure. However, they behave differently from the pulmonary capillaries (alveolar vessels) when subjected to volume and pressure changes. That is, as the lung volume increases in response to a more negative intrapleural pressure during inspiration, the transmural pressure increases (i.e., the pressure within the vessels becomes more positive) and the extra-alveolar vessels distend (see Figure 5–22). A second factor that dilates the extra-alveolar vessels at higher lung volumes is the radial traction generated by the connective tissue and by the alveolar septa that hold the larger vessels in place throughout the lung.

Another type of extra-alveolar vessel is the so-called "corner vessel," located at the junction of the alveolar septa. As the lung volume increases, the corner vessels are also pulled open (greater radius) by the radial traction force created by the expansion of the alveoli (Figure 5–23).

To summarize, at low lung volumes (low distending pressures), the extra-alveolar vessels narrow and cause the vascular resistance to increase. The alveolar vessels, however, widen and cause the vascular resistance to decrease. In contrast, at high lung volumes (high distending pressures), the extra-alveolar vessels dilate and cause the vascular resistance to decrease. The alveolar vessels, however, flatten and cause the vascular resistance to increase.

Finally, because the alveolar and extra-alveolar vessels are all part of the same vascular system, the resistance generated by the two groups of vessels is additive at any lung volume. The effect of changes in lung volume on the total pulmonary vascular resistance demonstrates a U-shaped curve (Figure 5–24).

PULMONARY VASCULAR RESISTANCE

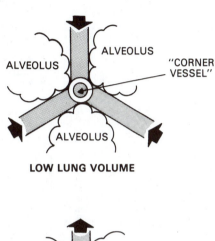

LOW LUNG VOLUME

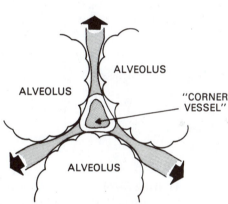

HIGH LUNG VOLUME

FIGURE 5–23.   Schematic drawing of the extra-alveolar "corner vessels" found at the junction of the alveolar septa. Expansion of the alveoli generates radial traction on the corner vessels, causing them to dilate. The alveolar vessels are compressed and flattened at high lung volumes.

Thus, the pulmonary vascular resistance (PVR) is lowest near the functional residual capacity (FRC) and increases in response to both high and low lung volumes.

Blood Volume Changes.   As blood volume increases, the recruitment and distention of pulmonary vessels will ensue, and pulmonary vascular resistance will tend to decrease (see Figure 5–21).

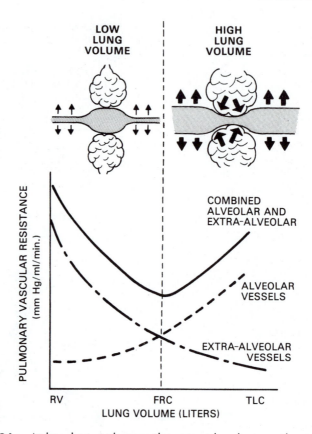

FIGURE 5–24. At low lung volumes, the extra-alveolar vessels generate a greater resistance to pulmonary blood flow; at high lung volumes, the alveolar vessels generate a greater resistance to pulmonary blood flow. When added together, the resistances of the extra-alveolar and alveolar vessels demonstrate a U-shaped curve. Pulmonary vascular resistance (PVR) is lowest near the functional residual capacity (FRC) and increases at both high and low lung volumes. RV = residual volume; TLC = total lung capacity.

Blood Viscosity Changes. The viscosity of blood is derived from the hematocrit, the integrity of red blood cells, and the composition of plasma. As blood viscosity increases, the pulmonary vascular resistance increases. Table 5–3 summarizes the active and passive mechanisms of vascular resistance.

TABLE 5–3. Summary of *Active* and *Passive* Mechanisms on Vascular Resistance

	↑RESISTANCE (VASCULAR CONSTRICTION)	↓RESISTANCE (VASCULAR DILATION)
ACTIVE MECHANISMS		
Abnormal Blood Gases		
↓ PO_2	X	
↑ PCO_2	X	
↓ pH	X	
Pharmacologic Stimulation		
Epinephrine (Adrenalin)	X	
Norepinephrine (Levophed)	X	
Dobutamine (Dobutrex)	X	
Dopamine (Intropin)	X	
Phenylephrine (Neo-Synephrine)	X	
Oxygen		X
Isoproterenol (Isuprel)		X
Aminophylline		X
Calcium Blocking Agents		X
PASSIVE MECHANISMS		
Pathologic Conditions		
Vessel Blockage/Obstruction	X	
Vessel Wall Disease	X	
Vessel Destruction	X	
Vessel Compression	X	
↑ Pulmonary Arterial Pressure		X
↑ Left Atrial Pressure		X
↑ Lung Volume (Extreme)	X	
↓ Lung Volume (Extreme)	X	
↑ Blood Volume		X
↑ Blood Viscosity	X	

SELF-ASSESSMENT QUESTIONS

1. Which of the following are polymorphonuclear granulocytes?
   I. Neutrophils
   II. Monocytes
   III. Eosinophils
   IV. Lymphocytes
   V. Basophils
      a. I only
      b. II only
      c. V only
      d. II and IV only
      e. I, III, and V only

2. In the normal male, the hematocrit is about
      a. 25%
      b. 35%
      c. 45%
      d. 65%
      e. 75%

3. Which of the following agents cause pulmonary vascular constriction?
   I. Isoproterenol
   II. Epinephrine
   III. Oxygen
   IV. Dopamine
      a. I only
      b. III only
      c. II and IV only
      d. I, II, and IV only
      e. I, II, III, and IV

4. If the pressure in the pulmonary artery is 34 mm Hg, and the pressure in the left atrium is 9 mm Hg, what is the driving pressure?
      a. 9 mm Hg
      b. 17 mm Hg
      c. 25 mm Hg
      d. 34 mm Hg
      e. 43 mm Hg

5. The tricuspid valve lies between the
      a. right atrium and the right ventricle
      b. left ventricle and the aorta
      c. right ventricle and the pulmonary artery
      d. left atrium and the left ventricle
      e. right ventricle and the semilunar valve

6. The QRS complex represents which of the following?
   a. Atrial depolarization only
   b. Ventricular repolarization only
   c. Atrial repolarization only
   d. Ventricular depolarization only
   e. Both atrial and ventricular repolarization

7. The mean intraluminal pressure in the pulmonary capillaries is
   a. 5 mm Hg
   b. 10 mm Hg
   c. 15 mm Hg
   d. 20 mm Hg
   e. 25 mm Hg

8. An increase in which of the following suggests a bacterial infection?
   a. Lymphocytes
   b. Neutrophils
   c. Monocytes
   d. Eosinophils
   e. Basophils

9. The force the ventricles must work against to pump blood is called
   a. myocardial contractility
   b. ventricular afterload
   c. negative inotropism
   d. ventricular preload
   e. positive inotropism

10. Compared to the systemic circulation, the pressure in the pulmonary circulation is about
    a. 1/10 the pressure
    b. 1/4 the pressure
    c. 1/3 the pressure
    d. 1/2 the pressure
    e. the same pressure

11. The difference between the pressure in the lumen of a vessel and that of the pressure surrounding the vessel is called the
    a. driving pressure
    b. transmural pressure
    c. diastolic pressure
    d. intravascular pressure
    e. transpulmonary pressure

12. Which of the following cause(s) pulmonary vasoconstriction?
    I. Hypercapnia
    II. Hypoxia
    III. Acidemia
    IV. Increased H^+ concentration

     a. I only
     b. III only
     c. II and IV only
     d. II, III, and IV only
     e. I, II, III, and IV

13. The cardioinhibitor center of the medulla slows the heart by sending neural impulses by way of the

    I. 10th cranial nerve
   II. parasympathetic nervous system
  III. sympathetic nervous system
  IV. vagus nerve
     a. I only
     b. IV only
     c. III only
     d. I and IV only
     e. I, II, and IV only

14. Which of the following cause passive changes in the pulmonary vascular resistance?

    I. pH changes
   II. Transpulmonary pressure changes
  III. P_{CO_2} changes
  IV. Blood viscosity changes
     a. II only
     b. III only
     c. I and III only
     d. II and IV only
     e. I, III, and IV only

15. Which of the following cause blood clotting at a traumatized site?

     a. Thrombocytes
     b. Basophils
     c. Monocytes
     d. Eosinophils
     e. Neutrophils

Answers appear in Appendix VII.

CHAPTER 6

HEMODYNAMIC MEASUREMENTS

OBJECTIVES

By the end of this chapter, the student should be able to:

1. List the abbreviations and normal ranges of the following hemodynamic values *directly* measured by means of the pulmonary artery catheter:
   —Central venous pressure
   —Right atrial pressure
   —Mean pulmonary artery pressure
   —Pulmonary capillary wedge pressure
   —Cardiac output
2. List the abbreviations and normal ranges of the following *computed* hemodynamic values:
   —Stroke volume
   —Stroke volume index
   —Cardiac index
   —Right ventricular stroke work index
   —Left ventricular stroke work index
   —Pulmonary vascular resistance
   —Systemic vascular resistance
3. List factors that increase and decrease the following:
   —Stroke volume
   —Stroke volume index
   —Cardiac output
   —Cardiac index
   —Right ventricular stroke work index
   —Left ventricular stroke work index
4. List the factors that increase and decrease the *pulmonary vascular resistance*.
5. List the factors that increase and decrease the *systemic vascular resistance*.
6. Complete the self-assessment questions at the end of this chapter.

HEMODYNAMIC MEASUREMENTS DIRECTLY OBTAINED BY MEANS OF THE PULMONARY ARTERY CATHETER

The term **hemodynamics** is defined as the study of the forces that influence the circulation of blood. With the advent of the pulmonary artery catheter (Figure 6–1), the hemodynamic status of the critically ill patient can be accurately determined at the bedside.* The pulmonary artery catheter has enabled the respiratory care practitioner to measure several hemodynamic parameters directly. These direct measurements, in turn, can be used to compute other important hemodynamic values. Table 6–1 lists the major hemodynamic values that can be directly measured.

HEMODYNAMIC VALUES COMPUTED FROM DIRECT MEASUREMENTS

Table 6–2 lists the major hemodynamic values that can be calculated from the direct measurements listed in Table 6–1. Today, such calculations are obtained either from a programmed calculator or by using the specific hemodynamic formula and a simple hand-held calculator. It should be noted, moreover, that since the hemodynamic parameters vary with the size of an individual, some hemodynamic values are "indexed" by body surface area (BSA). Clinically, the BSA is obtained from a height–weight nomogram (see Appendix IV). The normal adult BSA is 1.5 to 2 m^2.

Stroke Volume

The stroke volume (SV) is the volume of blood ejected by the ventricles with each contraction. The preload, afterload, and myocardial contractility are the major determinants of stroke volume. Stroke volume is derived by dividing the cardiac output (CO) by the heart rate (HR).

$$SV = \frac{CO}{HR}$$

*See Appendix V for a representative example of a cardiopulmonary profile sheet used to monitor the hemodynamic status of the critically ill patient.

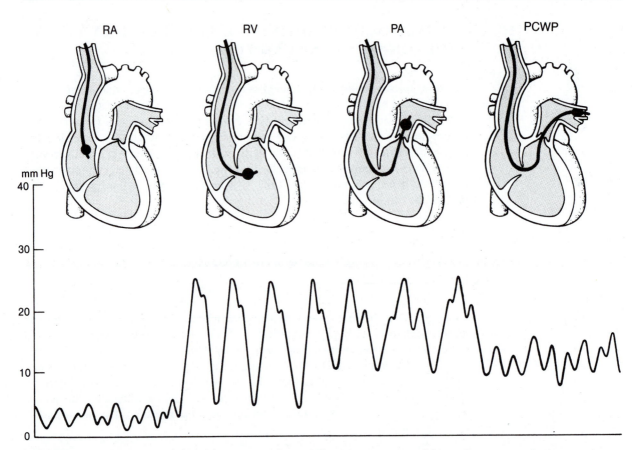

FIGURE 6–1. Insertion of the pulmonary catheter. The insertion site of the pulmonary catheter may be the basilic, brachial, femoral, subclavian, or internal jugular veins. The latter two are the most common insertion sites. As the catheter advances, pressure readings and waveforms are monitored to determine the catheter's position as it moves through the right atrium (RA), right ventricle (RV), pulmonary artery (PA), and finally into a pulmonary capillary "wedge" pressure (PCWP) position. Immediately after a PCWP reading, the balloon is deflated to allow blood to flow past the tip of the catheter. When the balloon is deflated, the catheter continuously monitors the pulmonary artery pressure.

For example, if an individual has a cardiac output of 4.5 L/min (4500 ml/min) and a heart rate of 75 beats/min, the stroke volume would be calculated as follows:

$$SV = \frac{CO}{HR}$$

$$= \frac{4500 \text{ ml/min}}{75 \text{ beats/min}}$$

$$= 60 \text{ ml/beat}$$

TABLE 6–1. Hemodynamic Values Directly Obtained by Means of the Pulmonary Artery Catheter

HEMODYNAMIC VALUE	ABBREVIATION	NORMAL RANGE
Central venous pressure	CVP	1–7 mm Hg
Right atrial pressure	RAP	1–7 mm Hg
Mean pulmonary artery pressure	$\overline{PA}$	15 mm Hg
Pulmonary capillary wedge pressure (also called pulmonary artery wedge; pulmonary artery occlusion)	PCWP PAW PAO	8–12 mm Hg
Cardiac output	CO	4–6 L/min

TABLE 6–2. Computed Hemodynamic Values

HEMODYNAMIC VARIABLE	ABBREVIATION	NORMAL RANGE
Stroke volume	SV	40–80 ml
Stroke volume index	SVI	40 ± 7 ml/beat/m^2
Cardiac index	CI	3.0 ± 0.5 L/min/m^2
Right ventricular stroke work index	RVSWI	7–12 g m/m^2
Left ventricular stroke work index	LVSWI	40–60 g m/m^2
Pulmonary vascular resistance	PVR	50–150 dynes $\times$ sec $\times$ cm^{-5}
Systemic vascular resistance	SVR	800–1500 dynes $\times$ sec $\times$ cm^{-5}

Table 6–3 lists factors that increase and decrease the stroke volume.

Stroke Volume Index

The stroke volume index (SVI) (also known as stroke index) is derived by dividing the stroke volume (SV) by the body surface area (BSA).

$$SVI = \frac{SV}{BSA}$$

TABLE 6–3. Factors Increasing and Decreasing Stroke Volume (SV), Stroke Volume Index (SVI), Cardiac Output (CO), Cardiac Index (CI), Right Ventricular Stroke Work Index (RVSWI), and Left Ventricular Stroke Work Index (LVSWI)

INCREASES	DECREASES
Drugs (Increased Contractility)	**Drugs (Decreased Contractility)**
Dobutamine (Dobutrex)	Propranolol (Inderal)
Epinephrine	Timolol (Brocadren)
Dopamine (Intropin)	Metoprolol (Lopressor)
Isoproterenol (Isuprel)	Atenolol (Tenormin)
Digitalis	Nadolol (Corgard)
Inocor (Amrinone)	
	Abnormal Conditions
Abnormal Conditions	Septic shock (late stages)
Septic shock (early stages)	Congestive heart failure
Hyperthermia	Hypovolemia
Hypervolemia	Pulmonary emboli
Decreased vascular resistance	Increased vascular resistance
	Myocardial infarction
	Hyperinflation of Lungs
	Mechanical ventilation
	Continuous Positive Airway Pressure (CPAP)
	Positive End-Expiratory Pressure (PEEP)

For example, if a patient has a stroke volume of 60 ml and a body surface area of 2 m^2, the stroke volume index would be determined as follows:

$$SVI = \frac{SV}{BSA}$$

$$= \frac{60 \text{ ml/beat}}{2 \text{ m}^2}$$

$$= 30 \text{ ml/beat/m}^2$$

Assuming that the heart rate remains the same, as the stroke volume index increases or decreases, the cardiac index also increases or decreases. The stroke volume index reflects the (1) contractility of the heart, (2) overall blood volume status, and (3) amount of venous return.

Table 6–3 lists factors that increase and decrease the stroke volume index.

Cardiac Index

The cardiac index (CI) is calculated by dividing the cardiac output (CO) by the body's surface area (BSA).

$$CI = \frac{CO}{BSA}$$

For example, if a patient has a cardiac output of 5 liters per minute and a body surface area of 2 m^2, the cardiac index is computed as follows:

$$CI = \frac{CO}{BSA}$$

$$= \frac{5 \text{ L/min}}{2 \text{ m}^2}$$

$$= 2.5 \text{ L/min/m}^2$$

See Table 6–3 for a list of factors that increase and decrease the cardiac index.

Right Ventricular Stroke Work Index

The right ventricular stroke work index (RVSWI) measures the amount of work required by the right ventricle to pump blood. The RVSWI is a reflection of the contractility of the right ventricle. In the presence of normal right ventricular contractility, increases in afterload (e.g., caused by pulmonary vascular constriction) cause the RVSWI to increase, until a pleateau is reached. When the contractility of the right ventricle is dimished by disease states, however, the RVSWI does not appropriately increase. The RVSWI is derived from the following formula:

$$RVSWI = SVI \times (\overline{PA} - CVP) \times 0.0136 \text{ g/ml}$$

where SVI is stroke volume index, $\overline{PA}$ is mean pulmonary artery pressure, CVP is central venous pressure, and the density of mercury factor 0.0136 g/ml is needed to convert the equation to the proper units of measurement—i.e., gram meters/m^2 (g m/m^2).

For example, if a patient has an SVI of 35 ml, a $\overline{PA}$ of 20 mm Hg, and a CVP of 5 mm Hg, the patient's RVSWI is calculated as follows:

$$RVSWI = SVI \times (\overline{PA} - CVP) \times 0.0136 \text{ g/ml}$$

$$= 35 \text{ ml/beat/m}^2 \times (20 \text{ mm Hg} - 5 \text{ mm Hg}) \times 0.0136 \text{ g/ml}$$

$$= 35 \text{ ml/beat/m}^2 \times 15 \text{ mm Hg} \times 0.0136 \text{ g/ml}$$

$$= 7.14 \text{ g m/m}^2$$

Factors that increase and decrease the right ventricular stroke work index are listed in Table 6–3.

Left Ventricular Stroke Work Index

The left ventricular stroke work index (LVSWI) measures the amount of work required by the left ventricle to pump blood. The LVSWI is a reflection of the contractility of the left ventricle. In the presence of normal left ventricular contractility, increases in afterload (e.g., caused by systemic vascular constriction) cause the LVSWI to increase until a plateau is reached. When the contractility of the left ventricle is diminished by disease states, however, the LVSWI does not increase appropriately. The following formula is used for determining this hemodynamic variable:

$$LVSWI = SVI \times (MAP - PCWP) \times 0.0136 \text{ g/ml}$$

where SVI is stroke volume index, MAP is mean arterial pressure, PCWP is pulmonary capillary wedge pressure, and the density of mercury factor 0.0136 g/ml is needed to convert the equation to the proper units of measurement—i.e., gram meters/m^2 (g m/m^2).

For example, if a patient has an SVI of 30 ml, an MAP of 100 mm Hg, and a PCWP of 5 mm Hg, then:

$$LVSWI = SVI \times (MAP - PCWP) \times 0.0136 \text{ g/ml}$$

$$= 30 \text{ ml/beat/m}^2 \times (100 \text{ mm Hg } - 5 \text{ mm Hg}) \times 0.0136 \text{ g/ml}$$

$$= 30 \text{ ml/beat/m}^2 \times (95 \text{ mm Hg}) \times 0.0136 \text{ g/ml}$$

$$= 38.76 \text{ g m/m}^2$$

Table 6–3 lists factors that increase and decrease the left ventricular stroke work index.

Vascular Resistance

As blood flows through the pulmonary and the systemic vascular system there is resistance to flow. The pulmonary system is a *low resistance* system. The systemic vascular system is a *high resistance* system.

Pulmonary Vascular Resistance (PVR).   The PVR measurement reflects the afterload of the right ventricle. It is calculated by the following formula:

$$PVR = \frac{\overline{PA} - PCWP}{CO} \times 80$$

where $\overline{PA}$ is the mean pulmonary artery pressure, PCWP is the pulmonary capillary wedge pressure, CO is the cardiac output, and 80 is a conversion factor for adjusting to the correct units of measurement (dyne $\times$ sec $\times$ cm^{-5}).

TABLE 6–4. Factors that Increase Pulmonary Vascular Resistance (PVR)

CHEMICAL STIMULI

Decreased alveolar oxygenation
  (alveolar hypoxia)
Decreased pH (acidemia)
Increased P_{CO_2} (hypercapnia)

PHARMACOLOGIC AGENTS

Epinephrine
Norepinephrine (Levophed, Levarterenol)
Dobutamine (Dobutrex)
Dopamine (Intropin)
Phenylephrine (Neo-synephrine)

HYPERINFLATION OF LUNGS

Mechanical ventilation
  Continuous Positive Airway Pressure (CPAP)
  Positive End-Expiratory Pressure (PEEP)

PATHOLOGIC FACTORS

Vascular blockage
  Pulmonary emboli
  Air bubble
  Tumor mass

Vascular wall disease
  Sclerosis
  Endarteritis
  Polyarteritis
  Scleroderma

Vascular Destruction
  Emphysema
  Pulmonary interstitial fibrosis

Vascular Compression
  Pneumothorax
  Hemothorax
  Tumor mass

HUMORAL SUBSTANCES

Histamine
Angiotensin
Fibrinopeptides
Prostaglandin $F_{2\alpha}$
Serotonin

For example, to determine the PVR of a patient who has a $\overline{\text{PA}}$ of 15 mm Hg, a PCWP of 5 mm Hg, and a CO of 5 L/min:

$$PVR = \frac{\overline{\text{PA}} - \text{PCWP}}{\text{CO}} \times 80$$

$$= \frac{15 \text{ mm Hg} - 5 \text{ mm Hg}}{5 \text{ L/min}} \times 80$$

$$= \frac{10 \text{ mm Hg}}{5 \text{ L/min}} \times 80$$

$$= 160 \text{ dynes} \times \sec \times cm^{-5}$$

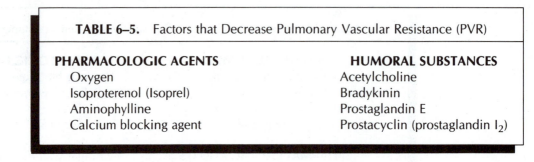

TABLE 6–5. Factors that Decrease Pulmonary Vascular Resistance (PVR)

PHARMACOLOGIC AGENTS	HUMORAL SUBSTANCES
Oxygen	Acetylcholine
Isoproterenol (Isoprel)	Bradykinin
Aminophylline	Prostaglandin E
Calcium blocking agent	Prostacyclin (prostaglandin I_2)

Table 6–4 (page 207) lists factors that increase the pulmonary vascular resistance. Factors that decrease the pulmonary vascular resistance are listed in Table 6–5.

Systemic or Peripheral Vascular Resistance (SVR).   The SVR measurement reflects the afterload of the left ventricle. It is calculated by the following formula:

$$SVR = \frac{MAP - CVP}{CO} \times 80$$

TABLE 6–6. Factors that Increase and Decrease Systemic Vascular Resistance (SVR)

INCREASES	DECREASES
Vasoconstricting Agents	**Vasodilating Agents**
Dopamine (Intropin)	Nitroglycerin
Norepinephrine (Levarterenol, Levophed)	Nitroprusside (Nipride)
Epinephrine	Morphine
Phenylephrine (Neo-synephrine)	Inocor (Amrinone)
	Hydralazine (Apresoline)
Abnormal Conditions	Methyldopa (Aldomet)
Hypovolemia	Diazoxide (Hyperstat)
Septic shock (late stages)	
$\downarrow P_{CO_2}$	**Abnormal Conditions**
	Septic shock (early stages)
	$\uparrow P_{CO_2}$

where MAP is the mean arterial pressure, CVP is the central venous pressure, CO is the cardiac output, and 80 is a conversion factor for adjusting to the correct units of measurement ($dyne \times sec \times cm^{-5}$). (Note: The right atrial pressure (RAP) can be used in place of the CVP value.)

For example, if a patient has an MAP of 80 mm Hg, a CVP of 5 mm Hg, and a CO of 5 L/min, then:

$$SVR = \frac{MAP - CVP}{CO} \times 80$$

$$= \frac{80 \text{ mm Hg} - 5 \text{ mm Hg}}{5 \text{ L/min}} \times 80$$

$$= \frac{75 \text{ mm Hg} \times 80}{5 \text{ L/min}}$$

$$= 1200 \text{ dynes} \times sec \times cm^{-5}$$

Table 6–6 (page 8) lists factors that increase and decrease the systemic vascular resistance.

SELF-ASSESSMENT QUESTIONS

Directions: On the line next to the hemodynamic parameters in Column A, match the normal range from Column B. Items in Column B can be used once, more than once, or not at all.

COLUMN A	COLUMN B
Hemodynamic Parameters	*Normal Range*

1. _____ Mean pulmonary artery pressure

2. _____ Pulmonary vascular resistance

3. _____ Cardiac output

4. _____ Left ventricular stroke work index

5. _____ Central venous pressure

6. _____ Stroke volume index

7. _____ Pulmonary capillary wedge pressure

a. 4–6 L/min
b. 800–1500 $dynes \times sec \times cm^{-5}$
c. 40–80 ml
d. −1 to 7 mm Hg
e. 50–150 $dynes \times sec \times cm^{-5}$
f. 15 mm Hg
g. 40 ± 7 ml/beat/m^2
h. 80 mm Hg
i. 3 ± 0.5 L/min/m^2
j. 8–12 mm Hg

continued

8. _____ Systemic vascular   k. 40–60 g m/m^2
                  resistance   l. 7–12 g m/m^2
9. _____ Right atrial pressure
10. _____ Cardiac index

Multiple Choice

1. Which of the following increases an individual's cardiac output?
    I. Epinephrine
    II. Hypovolemia
    III. Mechanical ventilation
    IV. Hypothermia
        a. I only
        b. II only
        c. III only
        d. I and IV only
        e. I, II, and IV only

2. Pulmonary vascular resistance increases in response to:
    I. Acidemia
    II. Oxygen
    III. Mechanical ventilation
    IV. Epinephrine
        a. I only
        b. II only
        c. III only
        d. I and III only
        e. I, III, and IV only

3. An individual's systemic vascular resistance increases in response to:
    I. Morphrine
    II. Hypovolemia
    III. An increased P_{CO_2}
    IV. Epinephrine
        a. I only
        b. II only
        c. III only
        d. II and IV only
        e. I, III, and IV only

4. Which of the following decreases an individual's stroke volume index?
    I. Dobutamine
    II. Mechanical ventilation
    III. Propranolol
    IV. Congestive heart failure
        a. I only

    b. II only

    c. IV only

    d. I and III only

    e. II, III, and IV only

5. An individual's pulmonary vascular resistance decreases in response to:

    I. Bradykinin

    II. Emphysema

    III. Norepinephrine

    IV. Hypercapnia

        a. I only

        b. II only

        c. III only

        d. II and III only

        e. II, III, and IV only

Answers appear in Appendix VII.

CHAPTER 7

OXYGEN TRANSPORT

OBJECTIVES

By the end of this chapter, the student should be able to:

1. Calculate the quantity of oxygen that *dissolves in the plasma* of the blood.
2. Describe the major features of *hemoglobin*, including:
   —Heme portion
   - Iron
   —Globin portion
   - Four amino acid chains
     ○ Two alpha chains
     ○ Two beta chains
   —Ferrous state vs. ferric state
   —Normal hemoglobin concentrations in the adult male and female and in the infant
3. Calculate the quantity of oxygen that *combines with hemoglobin*.
4. Calculate the *total amount* of oxygen in the *blood*.
5. Identify the abbreviations for the following:
   —Oxygen content of arterial blood
   —Oxygen content of mixed venous blood
   —Oxygen content of capillary blood
6. Describe how the following relate to the *oxygen dissociation curve*:
   —Oxygen pressure
   —Percentage of hemoglobin bound to oxygen
   —Oxygen content
7. Describe the clinical significance of the
   —flat portion of the oxygen dissociation curve
   —steep portion of the oxygen dissociation curve
   —P_{50}
8. Identify the factors that shift the oxygen dissociation curve to the right.
9. Identify the factors that shift the oxygen dissociation curve to the left.
10. Explain the clinical significance of a right or left shift of the oxygen dissociation curve in regard to the
    —loading of oxygen in the lungs
    —unloading of oxygen at the tissues

11. Calculate the following oxygen transport studies:
    —Total oxygen delivery
    —Arterial-venous oxygen content difference
    —Oxygen consumption
    —Oxygen extraction ratio
    —Mixed venous oxygen saturation
    —Pulmonary shunting
12. Identify the factors that increase and decrease the *oxygen transport* studies.
13. Differentiate between the following forms of *pulmonary shunting*:
    —Anatomic shunt
    —Capillary shunt
    —Shunt-like effect
14. Explain the meaning of *venous admixture*.
15. Calculate the *shunt equation*.
16. Describe the clinical significance of intrapulmonary shunting.
17. Define the following four, main types of tissue hypoxia:
    —Hypoxic hypoxia
    —Anemic hypoxia
    —Circulatory hypoxia
    —Histotoxic hypoxia
18. Explain the meaning of
    —cyanosis
    —polycythemia
19. Complete the self-assessment questions at the end of this chapter.

An understanding of oxygen transport is essential to the study of pulmonary physiology and to the clinical interpretation of arterial and venous blood gases. Table 7–1 lists the normal blood gas values.* To fully understand this subject, the student must understand (1) how oxygen is transported from the lungs to the tissues, (2) the oxygen dissociation curve and its clinical significance, (3) how various oxygen transport studies are used to identify the patient's cardiac and ventilatory status, and (4) the major forms of tissue hypoxia.

---

*See Appendix V for a representative example of a cardiopulmonary profile sheet used to monitor the blood gas values of the critically ill patient.

TABLE 7–1. Normal Blood Gas Value Ranges

BLOOD GAS VALUE	ARTERIAL	VENOUS
pH	7.35–7.45	7.30–7.40
P_{CO_2}	35–45 mm Hg (Pa_{CO_2})	42–48 mm Hg ($P\bar{v}_{CO_2}$)
HCO_3^-	22–28 mEq/L	24–30 mEq/L
P_{O_2}	80–100 mm Hg (Pa_{O_2})*	35–45 mm Hg ($P\bar{v}_{O_2}$)

Technically, only the oxygen (P_{O_2}) and carbon dioxide (P_{CO_2}) pressure readings are "true" blood gas values. The pH indicates the balance between the bases and acids in the blood. The bicarbonate (HCO_3^-) reading is an indirect measurement that is calculated from the pH and P_{CO_2} levels.

*For each year over 60 years, subtract 1 mm Hg from 80 mm Hg for the lower arterial Pa_{O_2} limit.

OXYGEN TRANSPORT

The transport of oxygen between the lungs and the cells of the body is a function of the blood and the heart. Oxygen is carried in the blood in two forms: (1) as dissolved oxygen in the blood plasma, and (2) chemically bound to the hemoglobin (Hb) that is encased in the erythrocytes, or red blood cells (RBCs).

Oxygen Dissolved in the Blood Plasma

As oxygen diffuses from the alveoli into the pulmonary capillary blood, it dissolves in the plasma of the blood. The term **dissolve** means that when a gas like oxygen enters the plasma, it maintains its precise molecular structure (in this case, O_2) and moves freely throughout the plasma in its normal gaseous state. Clinically, it is this portion of the oxygen that is measured to assess the patient's partial pressure of oxygen (P_{O_2}) (see Table 7–1).

The quantity of oxygen that dissolves in the plasma is a function of Henry's law, which states that the amount of gas that dissolves in a liquid (in this case, plasma) at a given temperature is proportional to the partial pressure of the gas. At normal body temperature, about 0.003 ml of oxygen will dissolve in 100 ml of blood for every 1 mm Hg of P_{O_2}. Thus, in the healthy individual with an arterial oxygen partial pressure (Pa_{O_2}) of 100 mm Hg, approximately 0.3 ml of oxygen is dissolved in every 100 ml of plasma (0.003 × 100 mm Hg = 0.3 ml). This is written as 0.3 volumes percent (vol%). Vol% represents the amount of O_2 in milliliters that is in 100 ml of blood (vol% = ml O_2/100 ml bd). For example, 10 vol% of O_2 means that there are 10 ml of O_2 in 100 ml of blood. In terms of total oxygen transport, a relatively small percentage of oxygen is transported in the form of dissolved oxygen.

Oxygen Bound with Hemoglobin

Hemoglobin.   Most of the oxygen that diffuses into the pulmonary capillary blood rapidly moves into the RBCs and chemically attaches to the hemoglobin. Each RBC contains approximately 280 million hemoglobin molecules, highly specialized to transport oxygen and carbon dioxide.

Normal adult hemoglobin, which is designated Hb A, consists of (1) four heme groups, which are the pigmented, iron-containing non-protein portions of the hemoglobin molecule, and (2) four amino acid chains (polypeptide chains) that collectively constitute globin (a protein) (Figure 7–1).

At the center of each heme group, the iron molecule can combine with one oxygen molecule in an easily reversible reaction to form oxyhemoglobin:

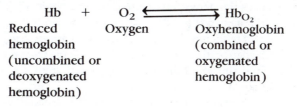

Hb   + O_2 ⇌ Hb_{O_2}
Reduced   Oxygen   Oxyhemoglobin
hemoglobin   (combined or
(uncombined or   oxygenated
deoxygenated   hemoglobin)
hemoglobin)

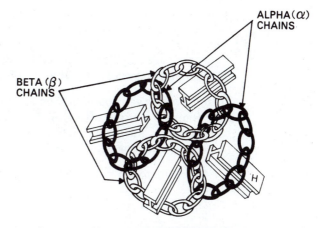

FIGURE 7–1.   Schematic illustration of a hemoglobin molecule. The globin (protein) portion consists of two identical alpha (α) chains and two beta (β) chains. The four heme (iron-containing) portions are in the center of each globin molecule.

Since there are four heme/iron groups in each Hb molecule, a total of four oxygen molecules can combine with each Hb molecule. When four oxygen molecules are bound to one Hb molecule, the Hb is said to be 100 percent saturated with oxygen; a Hb molecule with three oxygen molecules is 75 percent saturated; and so forth. Hemoglobin bound with oxygen (Hb_{O_2}) is called **oxyhemoglobin**. Hemoglobin not bound with oxygen (Hb) is called **reduced hemoglobin** or **deoxyhemoglobin**. The amount of oxygen bound to Hb is directly related to the partial pressure of oxygen.

The globin portion of each Hb molecule consists of two identical alpha (α) chains, each with 141 amino acids, and two identical beta (β) chains, each with 146 amino acids ($\alpha_2\beta_2$). Normal fetal hemoglobin (Hb F) has two alpha (α) chains and two gamma (γ) chains ($\alpha_2\gamma_2$). This increases hemoglobin's attraction to oxygen and facilitates transfer of maternal oxygen across the placenta. Fetal hemoglobin is gradually replaced with Hb A over the first year of postnatal life.

When the precise number, sequence, or spatial arrangement of the globin amino acid chains is altered, the hemoglobin will be abnormal. For example, sickle cell hemoglobin (Hb S) has a different amino acid substituted into the β chain. This causes the deoxygenated hemoglobin molecule (hemoglobin not bound to oxygen) to change the RBC shape from biconcave to a crescent or "sickle" form that have a tendency to provide thrombi. Various drugs and chemicals, such as nitrites, can change the iron molecule in the heme from the *ferrous state* to the *ferric state*, eliminating the ability of hemoglobin to transport oxygen. This type of hemoglobin is known as *methemoglobin*.

The normal hemoglobin value for the adult male is 14 to 16 g/100 ml of blood. In other words, if all the hemoglobin were to be extracted from all the RBCs in 100 milliliters of blood, the hemoglobin would actually weigh between 14 and 16 grams. Clinically, the weight measurement of hemoglobin, in reference to 100 ml of blood, is referred to as either the *gram percent of hemoglobin* (g% Hb) or *grams per deciliter* (g/dl). The average adult female hemoglobin value is 12 to 15 g%. The average infant hemoglobin value is 14 to 20 g%. Hemoglobin constitutes about 33 percent of the RBC weight.

Quantity of Oyxgen Bound to Hemoglobin.   Each g% of Hb is capable of carrying approximately 1.34 ml* of oxygen. Thus, if the hemoglobin level is 15 g%, and if the hemoglobin is fully saturated, about 20.1 vol% of oxygen will be bound to the hemoglobin. The figure 20.1 is calculated using the following formula:

$$O_2 \text{ bound to Hb} = 1.34 \text{ ml } O_2 \times 15 \text{ g\% Hb}$$

$$= 20.1 \text{ vol\% } O_2$$

---

*The literature also reports the values 1.36, 1.38, and 1.39. The figure 1.34 is the commonly used factor and is used in this textbook.

At a normal arterial oxygen pressure (Pa_{O_2}) of 100 mm Hg, however, the hemoglobin saturation (Sa_{O_2}) is only about 97 percent because of these normal physiologic shunts:

- Thebesian venous drainage into the left atrium
- Bronchial venous drainage into the pulmonary veins
- Alveoli that are underventilated in proportion to pulmonary blood flow

Thus, the amount of arterial oxygen in the above equation must be adjusted to 97 percent. The equation is written as follows:

$$
\begin{array}{r}
20.1 \text{ vol\% } O_2 \\
\times \quad .97 \\
\hline
19.5 \text{ vol\% } O_2
\end{array}
$$

Total Oxygen Content

To determine the total amount of oxygen in 100 ml of blood, the dissolved oxygen and the oxygen bound to hemoglobin must be added together. The following case example summarizes the calculations required to compute an individual's total oxygen content.

CASE STUDY: ANEMIC PATIENT

A 27-year-old woman with a long history of anemia (decreased hemoglobin concentration) is showing signs of respiratory distress. Her respiratory rate is 36 breaths per minute, her heart rate is 130 beats per minute, and her blood pressure is 155/90. Her hemoglobin concentration is 6 g%, and her Pa_{O_2} is 80 mm Hg (Sa_{O_2} 90%).

Based upon this information, the patient's total oxygen content is computed as follows:

1. Dissolved O_2:

$$
\begin{array}{r}
80 \text{ } Pa_{O_2} \\
\times \quad 0.003 \text{ (dissolved } O_2 \text{ factor)} \\
\hline
0.24 \text{ vol\% } O_2
\end{array}
$$

2. Oxygen bound to hemoglobin:

$$
\begin{array}{r}
6 \text{ g\% Hb} \\
\times \text{ } 1.34 \text{ } (O_2 \text{ bound to Hb factor)} \\
\hline
8.04 \text{ vol\% } O_2 \text{ (at } Sa_{O_2} \text{ of 100\%)}
\end{array}
$$

$$\begin{array}{r} 8.04 \text{ vol\% } O_2 \\ \times \quad .90 \text{ Sa}_{O_2} \\ \hline 7.236 \text{ vol\% } O_2 \end{array}$$

3. Total Oxygen Content:

$$\begin{array}{r} 7.236 \text{ vol\% } O_2 \text{ (bound to hemoglobin)} \\ + \; 0.24 \quad \text{vol\% } O_2 \text{ (dissolved } O_2) \\ \hline 7.476 \text{ vol\% } O_2 \text{ (total amount of } O_2/100 \text{ ml of blood)} \end{array}$$

Note that the patient's total arterial oxygen content is less than 50 percent of normal. Her hemoglobin concentration, which is the primary mechanism for transporting oxygen, is very low. Once this problem is corrected, the clinical manifestations of respiratory distress should no longer be present.

The total oxygen content of the arterial blood (Ca_{O_2}), mixed venous blood (Cv_{O_2}), and pulmonary capillary blood (Cc_{O_2}) is calculated as follows:

Ca_{O_2}: Oxygen content of arterial blood
$(Hb \times 1.34 \times Sa_{O_2}) + (Pa_{O_2} \times 0.003)$

Cv_{O_2}: Oxygen content of mixed venous blood
$(Hb \times 1.34 \times Sv_{O_2}) + (Pv_{O_2} \times 0.003)$

Cc_{O_2}: Oxygen content of pulmonary capillary blood
$(Hb \times 1.34)* + (P_{A_{O_2}}\dagger \times 0.003)$

It will be shown later in this chapter how various mathematical manipulations of the Ca_{O_2}, Cv_{O_2}, and Cc_{O_2} values are used in different oxygen transport studies to reflect important factors concerning the patient's cardiac and ventilatory status.

OXYGEN DISSOCIATION CURVE

As shown in Figure 7–2, the oxygen dissociation curve is part of a nomogram that graphically illustrates the *percentage of hemoglobin* (left-hand side of the graph) that is chemically bound to oxygen at each *oxygen pressure* (bottom portion of the graph). On the right-hand side of the graph, a second scale is included that gives the precise *oxygen content* that is carried by the hemoglobin at each oxygen pressure.

---

*It is assumed that the hemoglobin saturation with oxygen in the pulmonary capillary blood is 100 percent or 1.0.
†See Ideal Alveolar Gas Equation, Chapter Three.

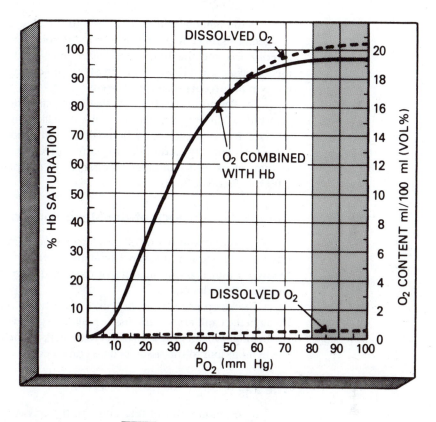

FIGURE 7–2.   Oxygen dissociation curve.

The curve is S-shaped with a steep slope between 10 and 60 mm Hg and a flat portion between 70 and 100 mm Hg. The steep portion of the curve shows that oxygen rapidly combines with hemoglobin as the P_{O_2} increases. Beyond this point (60 mm Hg), a further increase in the P_{O_2} produces only a slight increase in oxygen/hemoglobin bonding. In fact, because the hemoglobin is already 90 percent saturated at a P_{O_2} of 60 mm Hg, an increase in the P_{O_2} from 60 to 100 mm Hg elevates the total saturation of the hemoglobin by only 7 percent (see Figure 7–2).

Clinical Significance of the Flat Portion of the Curve

The P_{O_2} can fall from 100 to 60 mm Hg and the hemoglobin will still be 90 percent saturated with oxygen. Thus, the upper curve plateau illustrates that hemoglobin has an excellent safety zone for the loading of oxygen in the lungs.

As the hemoglobin moves through the alveolar-capillary system to pick up oxygen, a significant partial pressure difference continues to exist between the alveolar gas and the blood even after most of the oxygen is transferred. This mechanism enhances the diffusion of oxygen during the transit time the hemoglobin is in the alveolar-capillary system.

The flat portion also means that increasing the P_{O_2} beyond 100 mm Hg adds very little additional oxygen to the blood. In fact, once the P_{O_2} increases enough to saturate 100 percent of the hemoglobin with oxygen, the hemoglobin will no longer accept any additional oxygen molecules. However, a small additional amount of oxygen continues to dissolve in the plasma as the P_{O_2} rises ($P_{O_2} \times 0.003$ = dissolved O_2).

Clinical Significance of the Steep Portion of the Curve

P_{O_2} reductions below 60 mm Hg produce a rapid decrease in the amount of oxygen bound to hemoglobin. Clinically, therefore, when the P_{O_2} continues to fall below 60 mm Hg, the quantity of oxygen delivered to the tissue cells may be significantly reduced.

The steep portion of the curve also shows that as the hemoglobin moves through the capillaries of the tissue cells, a large amount of oxygen is released from the hemoglobin for only a small decrease in P_{O_2}. Thus, the diffusion of oxygen from the hemoglobin to the tissue cells is enhanced.

The P_{50}

A common point of reference on the oxygen dissociation curve is the P_{50} (Figure 7–3). The P_{50} represents the partial pressure at which the hemoglobin is 50 percent saturated with oxygen—i.e., when there are two oxygen molecules on each hemoglobin molecule. Normally, the P_{50} is about 27 mm Hg. Clinically, however, there are a variety of abnormal conditions that can shift the oxygen dissociation curve to either the right or left. When this happens the P_{50} changes. For example, when the curve shifts to the right, the affinity of hemoglobin for oxygen decreases, causing the hemoglobin to be less saturated at a given P_{O_2}. Thus, *when the curve shifts to the right, the P_{50} increases.* On the other hand, when the curve moves to the left, the affinity of hemoglobin for oxygen increases, causing the hemoglobin to be more saturated at a given P_{O_2}. Thus, *when the curve shifts to the left, the P_{50} decreases* (see Figure 7–3).

Factors That Shift the Oxygen Dissociation Curve

pH. As the blood hydrogen-ion concentration increases (decreased pH), the oxygen dissociation curve shifts to the right. This mechanism enhances the unloading of oxygen at the cellular level, since the pH decreases in this area as carbon dioxide (the acidic end-product of cellular metabolism) moves into the

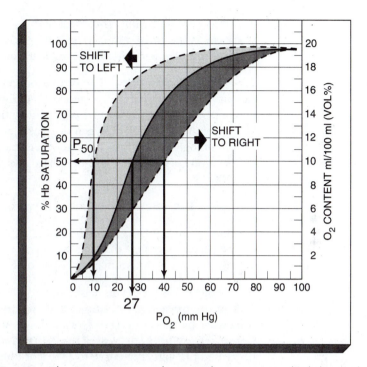

FIGURE 7–3. The P_{50} represents the partial pressure at which hemoglobin is 50 percent saturated with oxygen. When the oxygen dissociation curve shifts to the right, the P_{50} increases. When the oxygen dissociation curve shifts to the left, the P_{50} decreases.

blood. In contrast, as the blood hydrogen-ion concentration decreases, the curve shifts to the left. This mechanism facilitates the loading of oxygen onto hemoglobin as blood passes through the lungs, since the pH increases as carbon dioxide moves out of the blood and into the alveoli.

Temperature. As the body temperature increases, the curve moves to the right. Thus, actively metabolizing tissue (e.g., exercise), which has an elevated temperature, enhances the release of oxygen as blood flows through the muscle capillaries. Conversely, as the body temperature decreases, the curve shifts to the left. This mechanism partly explains why an individual's lips, ears, and fingers appear blue while swimming in very cold water. That is, their Pa_{O_2} is normal, but oxygen is not readily released from the hemoglobin at the tissue sites.

Carbon Dioxide. As the P_{CO_2} level increases (increased H^+ concentration), the oxyhemoglobin saturation decreases, shifting the oxyhemoglobin dissociation curve to the right, whereas decreasing P_{CO_2} levels (decreased H^+ concentrations) shift the curve to the left. The effect of P_{CO_2} and pH on the oxyhemoglobin curve is known as the **Bohr effect**. The Bohr effect is most active in the capillaries of working muscles, particularly the myocardium.

2,3-Diphosphoglycerate.   The red blood cells (RBCs) contain a large quantity (about 15 mol/g Hb) of the substance 2,3-diphosphoglycerate (2,3-DPG). 2,3-DPG is a metabolic intermediary that is formed by the RBCs during anerobic glycolysis. Hemoglobin's affinity for oxygen decreases as the 2,3-DPG level increases. Thus, the physiologic effect of an elevated concentration of 2,3-DPG is to shift the oxygen dissociation curve to the right. Clinically, a variety of conditions affect the level of 2,3-DPG.

Hypoxia.   Regardless of the etiology, hypoxia increases the 2,3-DPG level.

Anemia.   The 2,3-DPG level increases as the hemoglobin concentration decreases. It is suggested that this mechanism may explain why individuals with anemia frequently do not manifest signs or symptoms associated with hypoxia.

pH Changes.   As the pH increases, the 2,3-DPG concentration increases. Thus, the shift of the oxygen dissociation curve to the left by the increased pH is offset somewhat by the increased 2,3-DPG level, which shifts the curve to the right. Conversely, as the pH decreases, the 2,3-DPG concentration decreases. Thus, as the decreased pH shifts the curve to the right, the decreased 2,3-DPG level works to shift the curve to the left.

Stored Blood.   Blood stored for as little as one week has been shown to have very low concentrations of 2,3-DPG. Thus, when patients receive stored blood, the oxygen unloading at their tissue sites may be reduced because of the decreased 2,3-DPG level.

Fetal Hemoglobin.   Fetal hemoglobin (Hb F) is chemically different from adult hemoglobin (Hb A). Hb F has a greater affinity for oxygen and therefore shifts the oxygen dissociation curve to the left (reducing the P_{50}). During fetal development, the higher affinity of Hb F enhances the transfer of oxygen from maternal blood to fetal blood. After birth, Hb F progressively disappears and is completely absent after about one year.

Carbon Monoxide Hemoglobin.   Carbon monoxide (CO) has about 210 times the affinity of oxygen for hemoglobin. Because of this, a small amount of CO can tie up a large amount of hemoglobin (COHb) and, as a result, prevent oxygen molecules from bonding to hemoglobin. This mechanism can seriously reduce the amount of oxygen transferred to the tissue cells. In addition, when COHb is present the affinity of hemoglobin for oxygen increases and shifts the oxygen dissociation curve to the left. Thus, the oxygen molecules that do manage to combine with hemoglobin are unable to unload easily at the tissues.

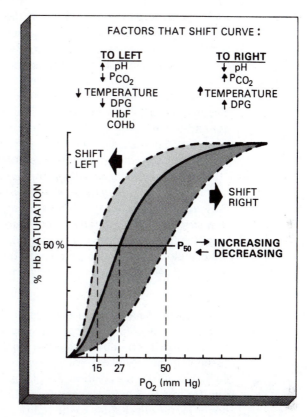

FIGURE 7–4. Factors that shift the oxygen dissociation curve to the right and left.

Figure 7–4 summarizes factors that shift the oxygen dissociation curve to the right and left and, additionally, how the P_{50} is affected by these shifts.

Clinical Significance of Shifts in the O_2 Dissociation Curve

When an individual's blood Pa_{O_2} is within normal limits (80–100 mm Hg), a shift of the oxygen dissociation curve to the right or left does not significantly affect the hemoglobin's ability to transport oxygen to the peripheral tissues. This is because shifts in this pressure range (80–100 mm Hg) occur on the flat portion of the curve. However, when an individual's blood Pa_{O_2} falls below the normal range, a shift to the right or left can have a remarkable effect on the hemoglobin's ability to pick up and release oxygen. This is because shifts below the normal pressure range occur on the steep portion of the curve. For example, consider the loading and unloading of oxygen during the following clinical conditions:

Right Shifts—Loading of Oxygen in the Lungs. Picture the loading of oxygen onto hemoglobin as blood passes through the alveolar-capillary system at a time when the alveolar oxygen tension ($P_{A_{O_2}}$) is moderately low—say, 60 mm Hg (caused, for example, by an acute asthmatic episode). Normally, when the $P_{A_{O_2}}$ is 60 mm Hg, the P_{O_2} of the pulmonary capillary blood ($P_{c_{O_2}}$) is also about 60 mm Hg. Thus, the hemoglobin is about 90 percent saturated with oxygen as it leaves the alveoli (Figure 7–5). If, however, the oxygen dissociation curve shifts to the right, as indicated in Figure 7–6 (caused by a pH of about 7.1), the hemoglobin will only be about 75 percent saturated with oxygen as it leaves the alveoli—in spite of the fact that the patient's plasma P_{O_2} is still 60 mm Hg.

In view of this gas transport phenomenon, therefore, it should be stressed that the total oxygen delivery may be much lower than indicated by a particular Pa_{O_2} when the patient has some disease process that causes the oxygen dissociation curve to shift to the right (see Figure 7–4). It should also be noted that when a right shift is accompanied by either a decreased cardiac output or a reduced level of hemoglobin, the patient's ability to transport oxygen will be jeopardized even more.

Right Shifts—Unloading of Oxygen at the Tissues. Although the total oxygen delivery may decrease in the above situation, the plasma P_{O_2} at the tissue sites does not have to fall as much to unload oxygen from the hemoglobin. For example, if the tissue cells metabolize 5 vol% oxygen at a time when the oxygen dissociation curve is in its normal position, the plasma P_{O_2} must fall from 60 mm Hg to about 35 mm Hg to free 5 vol% oxygen from the hemoglobin (Figure 7–7, page 227). If, however, the curve shifts to the right in response to a pH of 7.1, the plasma P_{O_2} at the tissue sites would only have to fall from 60 mm Hg to about 40 mm Hg to unload 5 vol% oxygen from the hemoglobin (Figure 7–8, page 228).

Left Shifts—Loading of Oxygen in the Lungs. If the oxygen dissociation curve shifts to the left, as indicated in Figure 7–9, page 229 (caused by a pH of about 7.6), at a time when the $P_{A_{O_2}}$ is 60 mm Hg, the hemoglobin will be about 95 percent saturated with oxygen as it leaves the alveoli, even though the patient's plasma P_{O_2} is only 60 mm Hg.

Left Shifts—Unloading of Oxygen at the Tissues. Although the total oxygen delivery increases in the above situation, the plasma P_{O_2} at the tissue sites must decrease more than normal in order for oxygen to dissociate from the hemoglobin. For example, if the tissue cells require 5 vol% oxygen at a time when the oxygen dissociation curve is in its normal position, the plasma P_{O_2} will fall from 60 mm Hg to about 35 mm Hg to free 5 vol% of oxygen from the hemoglobin (see Figure 7–7). If, however, the curve shifts to the left because of a pH of 7.6, the plasma P_{O_2}

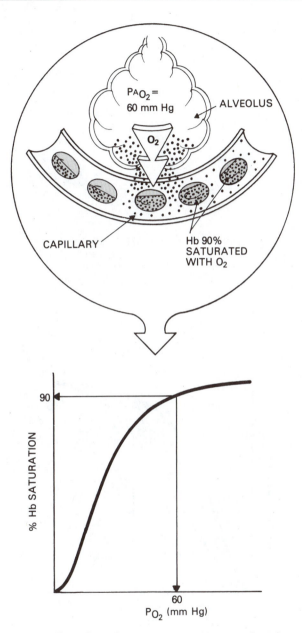

FIGURE 7–5.   Normally, when the $P_{A_{O_2}}$ is 60 mm Hg, the plasma P_{O_2} of the alveolar-capillary blood is also about 60 mm Hg and the hemoglobin is about 90 percent saturated with oxygen as it leaves the alveoli.

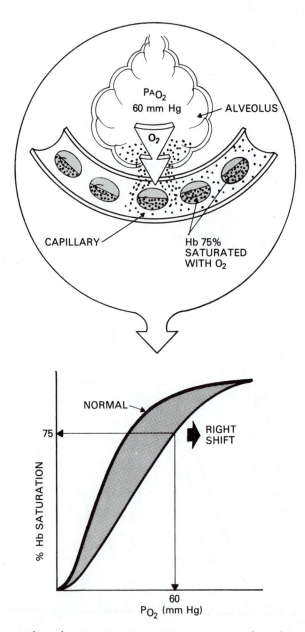

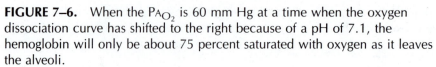

FIGURE 7–6. When the $P_{A_{O_2}}$ is 60 mm Hg at a time when the oxygen dissociation curve has shifted to the right because of a pH of 7.1, the hemoglobin will only be about 75 percent saturated with oxygen as it leaves the alveoli.

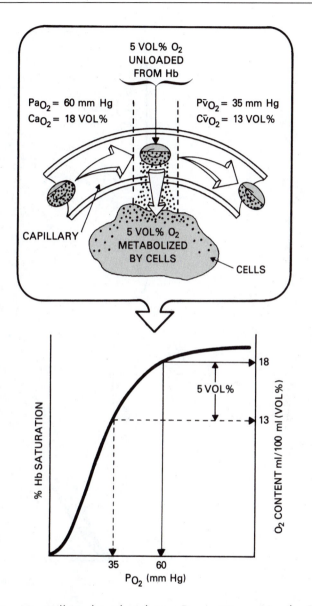

FIGURE 7–7. Normally, when the plasma P_{O_2} is 60 mm Hg, the P_{O_2} must fall from 60 mm Hg to about 35 mm Hg to free 5 vol% oxygen from the hemoglobin for tissue metabolism.

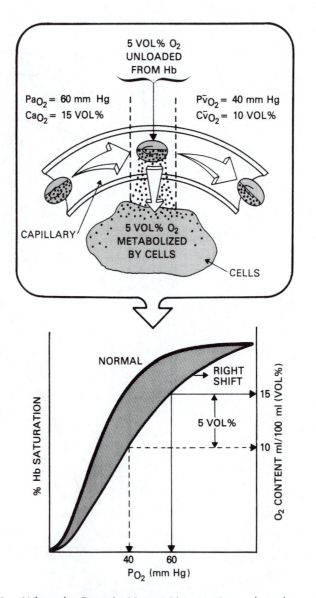

FIGURE 7–8. When the $P_{A_{O_2}}$ is 60 mm Hg at a time when the oxygen dissociation curve has shifted to the right because of a pH of 7.1, the plasma P_{O_2} at the tissue sites would only have to fall from 60 mm Hg to about 40 mm Hg to unload 5 vol% oxygen from the hemoglobin.

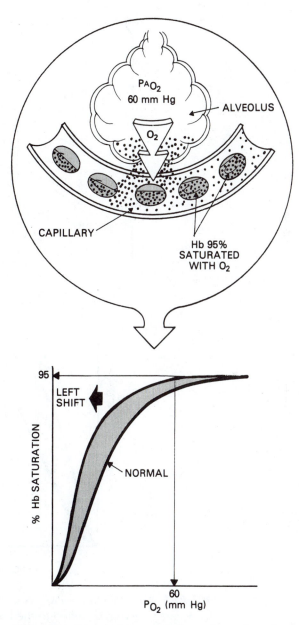

FIGURE 7–9. When the $P_{A_{O_2}}$ is 60 mm Hg at a time when the oxygen dissociation curve has shifted to the left because of a pH of 7.6, the hemoglobin will be about 95 percent saturated with oxygen as it leaves the alveoli.

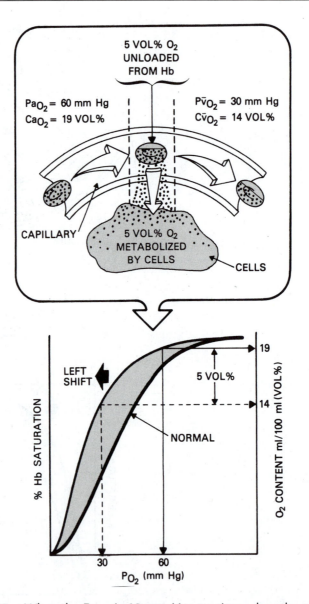

FIGURE 7–10. When the $P_{A_{O_2}}$ is 60 mm Hg at a time when the oxygen dissociation curve has shifted to the left because of a pH of 7.6, the plasma P_{O_2} at the tissue sites would have to fall from 60 mm Hg to about 30 mm Hg to unload 5 vol% oxygen from the hemoglobin.

at the tissue sites would have to fall from 60 mm Hg to about 30 mm Hg in order to unload 5 vol% oxygen from the hemoglobin (Figure 7–10).

OXYGEN TRANSPORT STUDIES

Various mathematical manipulations of the Ca_{O_2}, $C\bar{v}_{O_2}$, and Cc_{O_2} values can serve as excellent indicators of an individual's cardiac and ventilatory status. Clinically, the most common oxygen transport studies performed are (1) total oxygen delivery, (2) arterial-venous oxygen content difference, (3) oxygen consumption, (4) oxygen extraction ratio, (5) mixed venous oxygen saturation, and (6) pulmonary shunting.*

Total Oxygen Delivery

The total amount of oxygen delivered or transported to the peripheral tissues is dependent on (1) the body's ability to oxygenate blood, (2) the hemoglobin concentration, and (3) the cardiac output (Q). **Total oxygen delivery** (D_{O_2}) is calculated as follows:

$$D_{O_2} = \dot{Q}T \times (Ca_{O_2} \times 10)$$

where $\dot{Q}_T$ is total cardiac output (L/min); Ca_{O_2} is the oxygen content of arterial blood (ml oxygen/100 ml blood); and the factor 10 is needed to convert the Ca_{O_2} to ml O_2/L blood.

For example, if an individual has a cardiac output of 5 L/min and a Ca_{O_2} of 20 vol%, the total amount of oxygen delivered to the peripheral tissues will be about 1000 ml O_2 per minute:

$$D_{O_2} = \dot{Q}_T \times (Ca_{O_2} \times 10)$$
$$= 5 \text{ L} \times (20 \text{ vol\%} \times 10)$$
$$= 1000 \text{ ml } O_2/\text{minute}$$

Oxygen delivery decreases when there is a decline in (1) blood oxygenation, (2) hemoglobin concentration, or (3) cardiac output. When possible, an individual's hemoglobin concentration or cardiac output will often increase in an effort to compensate for a reduced oxygen delivery.

---

*See Appendix V for a representative example of a cardiopulmonary profile sheet used to monitor the oxygen transport status of the critically ill patient.

Arterial-venous Oxygen Content Difference

The **arterial-venous oxygen content difference**, $C(a - \bar{v})_{O_2}$, is the difference between the Ca_{O_2} and the $C\bar{v}_{O_2}$ ($Ca_{O_2} - C\bar{v}_{O_2}$). Clinically, the mixed venous blood needed to compute the $C\bar{v}_{O_2}$ is obtained from the patient's pulmonary artery (see Figure 6–1).

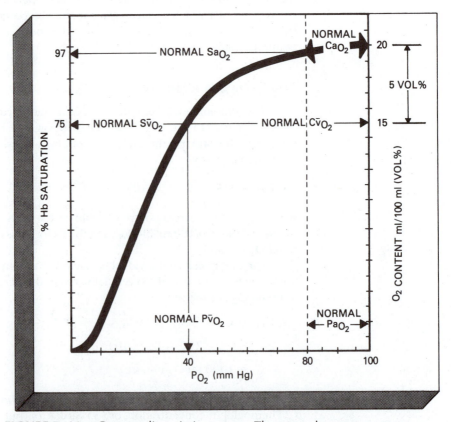

FIGURE 7–11. Oxygen dissociation curve. The normal oxygen content difference between arterial and venous blood is about 5 vol%. Note that both the right side and the left side of the graph illustrate that approximately 25 percent of the available oxygen is used for tissue metabolism, and therefore the hemoglobin returning to the lungs is normally about 75 percent saturated with oxygen.

Normally, the Ca_{O_2} is about 20 vol% and the $C\bar{v}_{O_2}$ is 15 vol% (Figure 7–11). Thus, the normal $C(a - \bar{v})_{O_2}$ is about 5 vol%:

$$C(a - \bar{v})_{O_2} = Ca_{O_2} - C\bar{v}_{O_2}$$

$$= 20 \text{ vol\%} - 15 \text{ vol\%}$$

$$= 5 \text{ vol\%}$$

In other words, 5 ml of oxygen are extracted from each 100 ml of blood for tissue metabolism (50 ml O_2/L). Since the average individual has a cardiac output of about 5 liters per minute, and a $C(a - \bar{v})_{O_2}$ of about 5 vol%, approximately 250 ml of oxygen are extracted from the blood during the course of one minute (50 ml O_2/L × 5 L/min).

Clinically, the $C(a - \bar{v})_{O_2}$ can provide useful information regarding the patient's cardiopulmonary status, since oxygen changes in mixed venous blood can occur earlier than oxygen changes in arterial blood gas. Table 7–2 lists factors that can cause the $C(a - \bar{v})_{O_2}$ to increase. Factors that can cause the $C(a - \bar{v})_{O_2}$ to decrease are listed in Table 7–3.

Oxygen Consumption

The amount of oxygen extracted by the peripheral tissues during the period of one minute is called **oxygen consumption**, or *oxygen uptake* ($\dot{V}_{O_2}$). An individual's oxygen consumption is calculated by using this formula:

$$\dot{V}_{O_2} = \dot{Q}_T [C(a - \bar{v})_{O_2} \times 10]$$

where $\dot{Q}_T$ is the total cardiac output (L/min); $C(a - \bar{v})_{O_2}$ is the arterial-venous oxygen content difference ($Ca_{O_2} - C\bar{v}_{O_2}$); and the factor 10 is needed to convert the $C(a - \bar{v})_{O_2}$ to ml O_2/L.

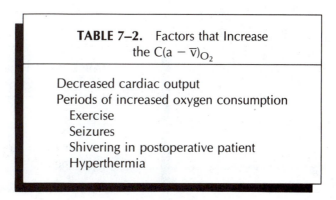

TABLE 7–2. Factors that Increase the $C(a - \bar{v})_{O_2}$

Decreased cardiac output
Periods of increased oxygen consumption
    Exercise
    Seizures
    Shivering in postoperative patient
    Hyperthermia

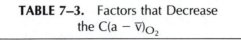

TABLE 7–3. Factors that Decrease
the $C(a - \bar{v})_{O_2}$

Increased cardiac output
Skeletal relaxation (e.g., induced by drugs)
Peripheral shunting (e.g., sepsis, trauma)
Certain poisons (e.g., cyanide prevents cellular
  metabolism)
Hypothermia

For example, if an individual has a cardiac output of 5 L/min, and a $C(a - \bar{v})_{O_2}$ of 5 vol%, the total amount of oxygen metabolized by the tissues in one minute will be 250 ml:

$$\dot{V}_{O_2} = \dot{Q}_T\,[C(a - \bar{v})_{O_2} \times 10]$$

$$= 5 \text{ L/min} \times 5 \text{ vol\%} \times 10$$

$$= 250 \text{ ml O}_2/\text{min}$$

Clinically, the oxygen consumption is commonly indexed by the patient's body surface area (BSA) (see Appendix IV), since the amount of oxygen extracted by the peripheral cells varies with the height and weight of an individual. The patient's oxygen consumption index is derived by dividing the $\dot{V}_{O_2}$ by the BSA. The average oxygen consumption index ranges between 125 to 165 ml O_2/m^2.

Factors that cause an increase in oxygen consumption are listed in Table 7–4. Table 7–5 lists factors that cause a decrease in oxygen consumption.

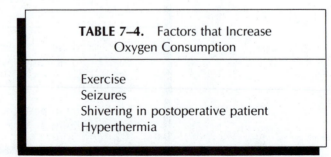

TABLE 7–4. Factors that Increase
Oxygen Consumption

Exercise
Seizures
Shivering in postoperative patient
Hyperthermia

TABLE 7–5. Factors that Decrease Oxygen Consumption
Skeletal relaxation (e.g., induced by drugs)
Peripheral shunting (e.g., sepsis, trauma)
Certain poisons (e.g., cyanide prevents cellular metabolism)
Hypothermia

Oxygen Extraction Ratio

The **oxygen extraction ratio** (O_2ER) is the amount of oxygen extracted by the peripheral tissues divided by the amount of oxygen delivered to the peripheral cells. The O_2ER is also known as the *oxygen coefficient ratio* or the *oxygen utilization ratio*.

The O_2ER is easily calculated by dividing the $C(a - \bar{v})_{O_2}$ by the Ca_{O_2}. In considering the normal Ca_{O_2} of 20 vol%, and the normal $C\bar{v}_{O_2}$ of 15 vol% (see Figure 7–11), the O_2ER ratio of the healthy individual is about 25 percent:

$$O_2ER = \frac{Ca_{O_2} - C\bar{v}_{O_2}}{Ca_{O_2}}$$

$$= \frac{20 \text{ vol\%} - 15 \text{ vol\%}}{20 \text{ vol\%}}$$

$$= \frac{5 \text{ vol\%}}{20 \text{ vol\%}}$$

$$= .25$$

Under normal circumstances, therefore, an individual's hemoglobin returns to the alveoli approximately 75 percent saturated with oxygen (see Figure 7–11). In an individual with a total oxygen delivery of 1000 ml/minute, an extraction ratio of 25 percent would mean that during the course of one minute, 250 ml of oxygen are metabolized by the tissues and 750 ml of oxygen are returned to the lungs.

Factors that can cause the O_2ER to increase are listed in Table 7–6. Table 7–7 lists factors that can cause the O_2ER to decrease.

The O_2ER provides an important view of an individual's oxygen transport

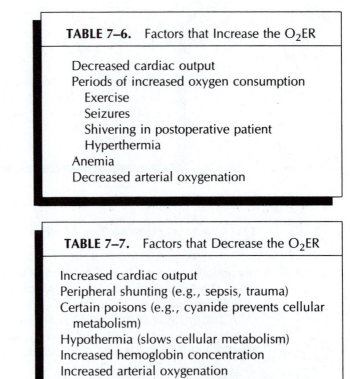

TABLE 7–6.   Factors that Increase the O_2ER

Decreased cardiac output
Periods of increased oxygen consumption
    Exercise
    Seizures
    Shivering in postoperative patient
    Hyperthermia
Anemia
Decreased arterial oxygenation

TABLE 7–7.   Factors that Decrease the O_2ER

Increased cardiac output
Peripheral shunting (e.g., sepsis, trauma)
Certain poisons (e.g., cyanide prevents cellular
    metabolism)
Hypothermia (slows cellular metabolism)
Increased hemoglobin concentration
Increased arterial oxygenation

status that is not readily available from other oxygen transport measurements. For example, in an individual with:

$$\begin{array}{ll} Ca_{O_2}: & 20 \text{ vol\%} \\ -\ C\bar{v}_{O_2}: & 15 \text{ vol\%} \\ \hline C(a-\bar{v})_{O_2} = & 5 \text{ vol\%} \end{array}$$

the $C(a-v)_{O_2}$ is 5 vol% and the O_2ER is 25 percent (normal). In an individual, however, with:

$$\begin{array}{ll} Ca_{O_2}: & 10 \text{ vol\%} \\ -\ C\bar{v}_{O_2}: & 5 \text{ vol\%} \\ \hline C(a-\bar{v})_{O_2} = & 5 \text{ vol\%} \end{array}$$

the $C(a-\bar{v})_{O_2}$ is still 5 vol% (assuming O_2 consumption remains constant), but the O_2ER is now 50 percent—clinically, a potentially dangerous oxygen transport status.

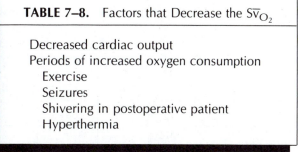

TABLE 7–8. Factors that Decrease the $S\overline{v}_{O_2}$

Decreased cardiac output
Periods of increased oxygen consumption
    Exercise
    Seizures
    Shivering in postoperative patient
    Hyperthermia

NOTE: A decreased $S\overline{v}_{O_2}$ indicates that the $C(a - \overline{v})_{O_2}$, $\dot{V}_{O_2}$, and O_2ER are increasing.

Mixed Venous Oxygen Saturation

In the presence of a normal arterial oxygen saturation level (Sa_{O_2}) and hemoglobin concentration, the continuous monitoring of mixed venous oxygen saturation ($S\overline{v}_{O_2}$) is often used in the clinical setting as an early indicator of changes in the patient's $C(a - \overline{v})_{O_2}$, $\dot{V}_{O_2}$, and O_2ER. Normally, the $S\overline{v}_{O_2}$ is about 75 percent (see Figure 7–11). Clinically, an $S\overline{v}_{O_2}$ of about 65 percent is acceptable.

Factors that can cause the $S\overline{v}_{O_2}$ to decrease are listed in Table 7–8. Table 7–9 lists factors that can cause the $S\overline{v}_{O_2}$ to increase.

Continuous $S\overline{v}_{O_2}$ monitoring can signal changes in the patient's $C(a - \overline{v})_{O_2}$, $\dot{V}_{O_2}$, and O_2ER earlier than routine arterial blood gas monitoring, since the Pa_{O_2} and Sa_{O_2} levels are often normal during early $C(a - \overline{v})_{O_2}$, $\dot{V}_{O_2}$, and O_2ER changes. Table 7–10 summarizes how various clinical factors will likely alter an individual's total oxygen delivery. $\dot{V}_{O_2}$, $C(a - \overline{v})_{O_2}$, O_2ER, and $S\overline{v}_{O_2}$.

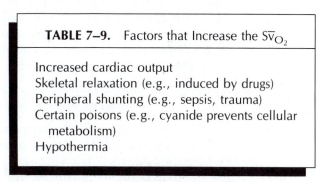

TABLE 7–9. Factors that Increase the $S\overline{v}_{O_2}$

Increased cardiac output
Skeletal relaxation (e.g., induced by drugs)
Peripheral shunting (e.g., sepsis, trauma)
Certain poisons (e.g., cyanide prevents cellular
    metabolism)
Hypothermia

NOTE: An increased $S\overline{v}_{O_2}$ indicates that the $C(a - \overline{v})_{O_2}$, $\dot{V}_{O_2}$, and O_2ER are decreasing.

TABLE 7–10. Clinical Factors Affecting Various Oxygen Transport Study Values

CLINICAL FACTORS	OXYGEN TRANSPORT STUDIES				
	D_{O_2} (1000 ml O_2/min)	$\dot{V}_{O_2}$ (250 ml O_2/min)	$C(a - \bar{v})_{O_2}$ (5 vol%)	O_2ER (25%)	$S\bar{v}_{O_2}$ (75%)
↑O_2 Consumption	Same	↑	↑	↑	↓
↓O_2 Consumption	Same	↓	↓	↓	↑
↓Cardiac Output	↓	Same	↑	↑	↓
↑Cardiac Output	↑	Same	↓	↓	↑
↓Pa_{O_2}	↓	Same	Same	↑	↓
↑Pa_{O_2}	↑	Same	Same	↓	↑
↓Hb	↓	Same	Same	↑	↓
↑Hb	↑	Same	Same	↓	↑
Peripheral Shunting	Same	↓	↓	↓	↑

↑: increase; ↓: decrease.

Mechanisms of Pulmonary Shunting

Pulmonary shunting is defined as that portion of the cardiac output that enters the left side of the heart without exchanging gases with alveolar gases (*true shunt*) or as blood that does exchange gases with alveolar gases but does not obtain a P_{O_2} that equals that of a normal alveolus (*shunt-like effect*). Because the physiologic effect of pulmonary shunting is **hypoxemia** (decreased arterial oxygen tensions), it is important to understand clinical conditions that produce (1) true shunt, and (2) shunt-like effect.

True Shunt. Clinical conditions that cause true shunt can be grouped under two major categories: **anatomic shunts** and **capillary shunts**.

Anatomic Shunts. An anatomic shunt exists when blood flows from the right side of the heart to the left side without coming in contact with an alveolus for gas exchange (see Figures 7–12A and 7–12B). Normally this is calculated to be about 2 to 5 percent of the cardiac output. This normal shunted blood comes from the bronchial, pleural, and Thebesian veins, which are systemic veins that empty into the pulmonary venous system. The following are common abnormalities that cause anatomic shunting.

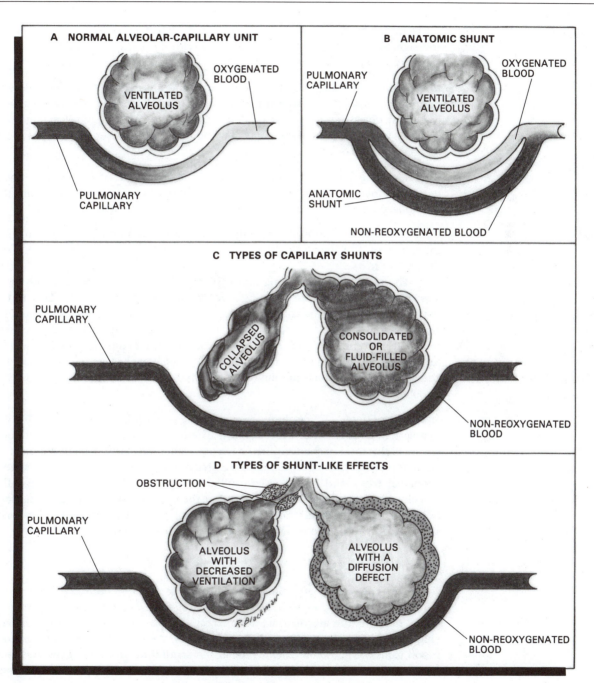

FIGURE 7–12. Pulmonary shunting. *A*) Normal alveolar-capillary unit; *B*) anatomic shunt; *C*) types of capillary shunts; *D*) types of shunt-like effects.

Congenital Heart Disease.   Certain congenital defects permit blood to flow from the right side of the heart to the left side without going through the alveolar-capillary system for gas exchange (e.g., defect of the ventricular septum).

Intrapulmonary Fistula.   In this type of anatomic shunting, a right-to-left flow of pulmonary blood does not pass through the alveolar-capillary system. It may be caused by chest trauma or disease. For example, a penetrating chest wound that damages both the arteries and veins of the lung can leave an arterial-venous shunt as a result of the healing process.

Vascular Lung Tumors.   Some lung tumors can become very vascular. Some permit pulmonary arterial blood to move through the tumor mass and into the pulmonary veins without passing through the alveolar-capillary system.

Capillary Shunts.   Capillary shunting is commonly caused by (1) alveolar collapse or atelectasis, (2) alveolar fluid accumulation, or (3) alveolar consolidation (see Figure 7–12*C*).

The sum of the anatomic and capillary shunts is referred to as **true**, or **absolute shunt**. Absolute shunting is *refractory* to oxygen therapy. That is, the hypoxemia produced by this form of pulmonary shunting cannot be treated by simply increasing the concentration of inspired oxygen, since (1) the alveoli are unable to accommodate any form of ventilation, and (2) the blood that passes by functioning alveoli cannot carry more oxygen once it has become fully saturated—except for a very small amount that dissolves in the plasma ($P_{O_2} \times 0.003 =$ dissolved O_2).

Shunt-Like Effect.   When pulmonary capillary perfusion is in excess of alveolar ventilation, a **shunt-like effect** is said to exist (see Figure 7–12*D*). Common causes of this form of shunting are (1) hypoventilation, (2) uneven distribution of ventilation (e.g., bronchospasm or excessive mucus accumulation in the tracheo-bronchial tree), and (3) alveolar-capillary diffusion defects (even though the alveolus may be ventilated in this condition, the blood passing by the alveolus does not have time to equilibrate with the alveolar oxygen tension). Pulmonary shunting due to the above conditions is readily corrected by oxygen therapy.

Venous Admixture

The end result of pulmonary shunting is **venous admixture**. Venous admixture is the mixing of shunted, *non-reoxygenated blood* with *reoxygenated blood* distal to the alveoli (i.e., downstream in the pulmonary venous system) (Figure 7–13). When venous admixture occurs, the shunted, non-reoxygenated blood gains oxygen molecules while, at the same time, the reoxygenated blood loses oxygen molecules. This process continues until (1) the P_{O_2} throughout all the plasma of the newly mixed blood is in equilibrium and (2) all the hemoglobin molecules carry the same number of oxygen molecules. The end result is a blood

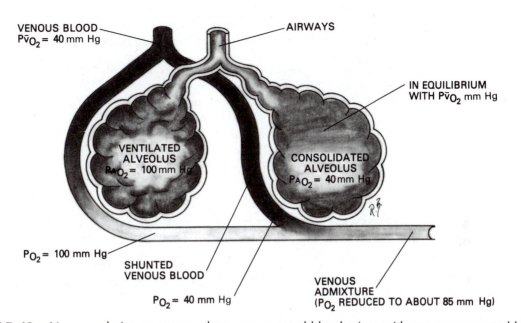

FIGURE 7–13. Venous admixture occurs when reoxygenated blood mixes with non-reoxygenated blood distal to the alveoli.

mixture that has a higher P_{O_2} and oxygen content value than the original shunted, non-reoxygenated blood, but a lower P_{O_2} and oxygen content than the original reoxygenated blood. Clinically, it is this blood mixture that is evaluated downstream (e.g., from the radial artery) to determine an individual's arterial blood gas measurements (see Table 7–1).

Shunt Equation

Because pulmonary shunting and venous admixture are common complications in respiratory disorders, knowledge of the degree of shunting is often desirable when developing patient care plans. The amount of intrapulmonary shunting can be calculated by using the **classic shunt equation**, which is written as follows:

$$\frac{\dot{Q}s}{\dot{Q}T} = \frac{Cc_{O_2} - Ca_{O_2}}{Cc_{O_2} - C\bar{v}_{O_2}}$$

where $\dot{Q}s$ is cardiac output that is shunted, $\dot{Q}T$ is total cardiac output, Cc_{O_2} is oxygen content of capillary blood, Ca_{O_2} is oxygen content of arterial blood, and $C\bar{v}_{O_2}$ is oxygen content of mixed venous blood.

In order to obtain the data necessary to calculate the degree of pulmonary shunting, the following clinical information must be gathered:

- P_B (barometric pressure)
- Pa_{O_2} (partial pressure of arterial oxygen)
- Pa_{CO_2} (partial pressure of arterial carbon dioxide)
- Pv_{O_2} (partial pressure of mixed venous oxygen)
- Hb (hemoglobin concentration)
- PA_{O_2} (partial pressure of alveolar oxygen)*
- $F_{I_{O_2}}$ (fractional concentration of inspired oxygen)

CASE STUDY: MOTORCYCLE ACCIDENT VICTIM

A 38-year-old man is on a volume-cycled mechanical ventilator on a day when the barometric pressure is 750 mm Hg. The patient is receiving an $F_{I_{O_2}}$ of .70. The following clinical data are obtained:

Hb: 13 g%
Pa_{O_2}:   50 mm Hg (Sa_{O_2} = 85%)
Pa_{CO_2}:   43 mm Hg
Pv_{O_2}:   37 mm Hg (Sv_{O_2} = 65%)

With this information, the patient's PA_{O_2}, Cc_{O_2}, Ca_{O_2}, and Cv_{O_2} can now be calculated. (Remember: P_{H_2O} represents alveolar water vapor pressure and is always considered 47 mm Hg.)

1. PA_{O_2} = $(P_B - P_{H_2O})F_{I_{O_2}} - Pa_{CO_2}(1.25)$
   = $(750 - 47).70 - 43(1.25)$
   = $(703).70 - 53.75$
   = $492.1 - 53.75$
   = 438.35 mm Hg
2. Cc_{O_2} = $(Hb \times 1.34)† + (PA_{O_2}* \times 0.003)$
   = $(13 \times 1.34) + (438.35 \times 0.003)$
   = $17.42 + 1.315$
   = 18.735 (vol% O_2)

---

†It is assumed that the hemoglobin saturation with oxygen in the pulmonary capillary blood is 100 percent or 1.0.
*See Ideal Alveolar Gas Equation, Chapter Three.

3. $Ca_{O_2} = (Hb \times 1.34 \times Sa_{O_2}) + (Pa_{O_2} \times 0.003)$
$= (13 \times 1.34 \times .85) + (50 \times 0.003)$
$= 14.807 + 0.15$
$= 14.957 (vol\% \ O_2)$

4. $C\bar{v}_{O_2} = (Hb \times 1.34 \times S\bar{v}_{O_2}) + (P\bar{v}_{O_2} \times 0.003)$
$= (13 \times 1.34 \times .65) + (37 \times 0.003)$
$= 11.323 + 0.111$
$= 11.434 (vol\% \ O_2)$

Based upon the above calculations, the patient's degree of pulmonary shunting can now be calculated:

$$\frac{\dot{Q}s}{\dot{Q}_T} = \frac{Cc_{O_2} - Ca_{O_2}}{Cc_{O_2} - C\bar{v}_{O_2}}$$

$$= \frac{18.735 - 14.957}{18.735 - 11.434}$$

$$= \frac{3.778}{7.301}$$

$$= .517$$

Thus, in this case 51.7 percent of the patient's pulmonary blood flow is perfusing lung tissue that is not being ventilated.

Today, most critical care units have programmed the oxygen transport calculations into inexpensive personal computers. What was once a time-consuming, error-prone task is now quickly and accurately performed.

The Clinical Significance of Pulmonary Shunting

Pulmonary shunting below 10 percent reflects normal lung status.

A shunt between 10 and 20 percent is indicative of an intrapulmonary abnormality, but is seldom of clinical significance.

Pulmonary shunting between 20 and 30 percent denotes significant intrapulmonary disease, and may be life-threatening in patients with limited cardiovascular or central nervous system function.

When the pulmonary shunting is greater than 30 percent, a potentially life-threatening situation exists and aggressive cardiopulmonary supportive measures are almost always necessary.

Calculating the degree of pulmonary shunting is not reliable in patients who demonstrate (1) a questionable perfusion status, (2) a decreased myocardial reserve, or (3) an unstable oxygen consumption demand. This is because these conditions directly affect a patient's Ca_{O_2} and $C\bar{v}_{O_2}$ values—two major components of the shunt equation.

TISSUE HYPOXIA

Tissue hypoxia means that the amount of oxygen available for cellular metabolism is inadequate. There are four main types of hypoxia: (1) **hypoxic hypoxia**, (2) **anemic hypoxia**, (3) **circulatory hypoxia**, and (4) **histotoxic hypoxia**. When hypoxia exists, alternate anaerobic mechanisms are activated in the tissues that produce dangerous metabolites (such as lactate and hydrogen ions) as waste products. These ions form a nonvolatile acid known as lactic acid and cause the blood pH to decrease.

Hypoxic Hypoxia

Hypoxic hypoxia (also called hypoxemic hypoxia) refers to the condition in which the Pa_{O_2} and Ca_{O_2} are abnormally low. Clinically, this form of hypoxia is better known as *hypoxemia* (low oxygen concentration in the blood). This form of hypoxia can develop from **pulmonary shunting** and from the following conditions:

Low Aveolar P_{O_2} (i.e., decreased PA_{O_2}). Because the arterial P_{O_2} (Pa_{O_2}) is determined by the alveolar P_{O_2} (PA_{O_2}), conditions that decrease the PA_{O_2} will lead to reductions in the Pa_{O_2} and Ca_{O_2} levels. A low PA_{O_2} can develop from such conditions as (1) hypoventilation from any cause (e.g., chronic obstructive pulmonary disease, drug overdose, or neuromuscular diseases that affect the respiratory muscles, such as myasthenia gravis), (2) ascent to high altitudes, and (3) the breathing of gas mixtures that contain less than 21 percent oxygen (e.g., suffocation).

Diffusion Impairment. In the presence of certain pulmonary diseases, the time available for oxygen equilibrium across the alveolar-capillary membrane may not be adequate. Such conditions include interstitial fibrosis, alveolar consolidation, and interstitital or alveolar edema (see Figure 3–6).

Ventilation/Perfusion ($\dot{V}/\dot{Q}$ Ratio) Mismatch. When the pulmonary capillary blood flow is in excess of the alveolar ventilation, a decreased $\dot{V}/\dot{Q}$ ratio is said to exist. This condition can cause a shunt-like effect, which in turn causes the Pa_{O_2} and Ca_{O_2} to decrease (the effects of different ventilation/perfusion relationships are discussed in greater detail in Chapter Nine). While the presence of hypoxemia strongly suggests the possibility of tissue hypoxia, it does not necessarily indicate the absolute existence of cellular hypoxia. The reduced level of oxygen in the arterial blood may be offset by an increased cardiac output.

Anemic Hypoxia

In this type of hypoxia, the oxygen tension in the arterial blood is normal, but the oxygen-carrying capacity of the blood is inadequate. This form of hypoxia can develop from (1) a low amount of hemoglobin in the blood or (2) a deficiency in the ability of hemoglobin to carry oxygen, as occurs in carbon monoxide poisoning or methemoglobinemia.

Anemic hypoxia develops in carbon monoxide poisoning because the affinity of carbon monoxide for hemoglobin is about 210 times greater than that of oxygen. As carbon monoxide combines with hemoglobin, the ability of hemoglobin to carry oxygen diminishes and tissue hypoxia may ensue. In methemoglobinemia, iron atoms in the hemoglobin are oxidized to the ferric state which in turn eliminates the hemoglobin's ability to carry oxygen. Increased cardiac output is the main compensatory mechanism for anemic hypoxia.

Circulatory Hypoxia

In circulatory hypoxia, the arterial blood that reaches the tissue cells may have a normal oxygen tension and content, but the amount of blood—and therefore the amount of oxygen—is not adequate to meet tissue needs. The two main causes of circulating hypoxia are (1) stagnant hypoxia and (2) arterial-venous shunting.

Stagnant hypoxia can occur when the peripheral capillary blood flow is slow or stagnant (*pooling*). This condition can be caused by a decreased cardiac output, vascular insufficiency, or neurochemical abnormalities. When blood flow through the tissue capillaries is sluggish, the time needed for oxygen exchange increases while, at the same time, the oxygen supply decreases. Because tissue metabolism continues at a steady rate, the oxygen pressure gradient between the blood and the tissue cells can become insufficient, causing tissue hypoxia. Stagnant hypoxia is primarily associated with cardiovascular disorders and often occurs in the absence of arterial hypoxemia. It is commonly associated with a decreased $S\bar{v}_{O_2}$.

When arterial blood completely bypasses the tissue cells and moves into the venous system, an *arterial-venous shunt* is said to exist. This condition can also cause tissue hypoxia, since arterial blood is prevented from delivering oxygen to the tissue cells. Localized arterial or venous obstruction can cause a similar form of tissue hypoxia, since the flow of blood in or out of the tissue capillaries is impeded. A circulatory hypoxia can also develop when the tissues' need for oxygen exceeds the available oxygen supply from the blood.

Histotoxic Hypoxia

Histotoxic hypoxia develops in any condition that impairs the ability of tissue cells to utilize oxygen. Cyanide poisoning produces this form of hypoxia. Clinically, the Pa_{O_2} and Ca_{O_2} in the blood are normal, but the tissue cells are extremely hypoxic. The $P\bar{v}_{O_2}$, $C\bar{v}_{O_2}$, and $S\bar{v}_{O_2}$ are elevated because oxygen is not utilized.

CYANOSIS

When hypoxemia is severe, signs of cyanosis may develop. Cyanosis is the term used to describe the blue-gray or purplish discoloration seen on the mucous membranes, fingertips, and toes whenever the blood in these areas contains at least 5 g% of reduced hemoglobin per dl (100 ml). When the normal 14 to 15 g% of hemoglobin is fully saturated, the Pa_{O_2} will be about 97 to 100 mm Hg and there will be about 20 vol% of oxygen in the blood. In a cyanotic patient with one-third (5 g%) of the hemoglobin reduced, the Pa_{O_2} will be about 30 mm Hg and there will be about 13 vol% of oxygen in the blood (Figure 7–14). In the patient with polycythemia, however, cyanosis may be present at a Pa_{O_2} well above 30 mm Hg, since the amount of reduced hemoglobin is often greater than 5 g% in these patients—even when their total oxygen transport is within normal limits (about 20 vol% of O_2).

The detection and interpretation of cyanosis is difficult and there is wide individual variation between observers. The recognition of cyanosis depends on

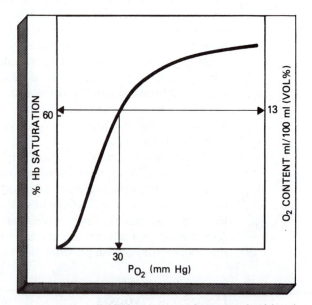

FIGURE 7–14. Cyanosis will likely appear whenever the blood contains at least 5 g% (g/dl) of reduced hemoglobin. In the normal individual with 15 g% hemoglobin, a Pa_{O_2} of about 30 mm Hg will produce 5 g% of reduced hemoglobin. Overall, however, the hemoglobin is still about 60 percent saturated with oxygen.

the acuity of the observer, on the lighting conditions in the examining room, and the pigmentation of the patient. Cyanosis of the nail beds is also influenced by the temperature, since vasoconstriction induced by cold may slow circulation to the point where the blood becomes bluish in the surface capillaries even though the arterial blood in the major vessels is not oxygen-poor.

POLYCYTHEMIA

When pulmonary disorders produce chronic hypoxemia, the hormone **erythropoietin** responds by stimulating the bone marrow to increase red blood cell (RBC) production. RBC production is known as **erythropoiesis**. An increased level of RBCs is called **polycythemia**. The polycythemia that results from hypoxemia is an adaptive mechanism designed to increase the oxygen-carrying capacity of the blood.

Unfortunately, the advantage of the increased oxygen-carrying capacity in polycythemia is offset by the increased viscosity of the blood when the hematocrit reaches about 55 to 60 percent. Because of the increased viscosity of the blood, a greater driving pressure is needed to maintain a given flow. The work of the right and left ventricles must increase in order to generate the pressure needed to overcome the increased viscosity. This can ultimately lead to left ventricular hypertrophy and failure and to right ventricular hypertrophy, or *cor pulmonale*.

SELF-ASSESSMENT QUESTIONS

1. If a patient has a 14 g% Hb level, and a Pa_{O_2} of 55 mm Hg (85 percent saturated with oxygen), approximately how much oxygen is transported to the peripheral tissues in each 100 ml of blood?
    a. 16 vol%
    b. 17 vol%
    c. 18 vol%
    d. 19 vol%
    e. 20 vol%

2. When the blood pH decreases, the oxygen dissociation curve shifts to the
    a. right and the P_{50} decreases
    b. left and the P_{50} increases
    c. right and the P_{50} increases
    d. left and the P_{50} decreases
    e. right and the P_{50} remains the same

3. When shunted, non-reoxygenated blood mixes with reoxygenated blood distal to the alveoli (*venous admixture*), the

I. P_{O_2} of the non-reoxygenated blood increases

II. Ca_{O_2} of the reoxygenated blood decreases

III. P_{O_2} of the reoxygenated blood increases

IV. Ca_{O_2} of the non-reoxygenated blood decreases

    a. I only

    b. IV only

    c. I and II only

    d. III and IV only

    e. II and III only

4. The lowest acceptable Pa_{O_2} for a 75-year-old patient is about

    a. 60 mm Hg

    b. 65 mm Hg

    c. 70 mm Hg

    d. 75 mm Hg

    e. 80 mm Hg

5. The normal calculated anatomic shunt is about

    a. 0.5–1%

    b. 2–5%

    c. 6–9%

    d. 10–12%

    e. 13–20%

6. In which of the following types of hypoxia is the oxygen pressure of the arterial blood (Pa_{O_2}) usually normal?

I. Hypoxic hypoxia

II. Anemic hypoxia

III. Circulatory hypoxia

IV. Histotoxic hypoxia

    a. I only

    b. II only

    c. III only

    d. III and IV only

    e. II, III, and IV only

7. If a patient normally has a 12 g% Hb, cyanosis will likely appear when

    a. 11 g% Hb is saturated with oxygen

    b. 10 g% Hb is saturated with oxygen

    c. 9 g% Hb is saturated with oxygen

    d. 8 g% Hb is saturated with oxygen

    e. 7 g% Hb is saturated with oxygen

8. The advantages of polycythemia begin to be offset by the increased blood viscosity when the hematocrit reaches about

    a. 30–40%

    b. 40–50%

    c. 55–60%

      d. 60–70%

      e. 70–80%

9. Assuming everything else remains the same, when an individual's cardiac output decreases, the

    I. $C(a - \bar{v})_{O_2}$ increases

    II. O_2ER decreases

    III. $\dot{V}_{O_2}$ increases

    IV. $S\bar{v}_{O_2}$ decreases

      a. I only

      b. IV only

      c. II and III only

      d. I and IV only

      e. I, II, and IV only

10. Under normal conditions, the O_2ER is about

      a. 5%

      b. 10%

      c. 15%

      d. 20%

      e. 25%

11. Case Study: Automobile Accident Victim

A 37-year-old woman is on a volume-cycled mechanical ventilator on a day when the barometric pressure is 745 mm Hg. The patient is receiving an $F_{I_{O_2}}$ of .50. The following clinical data are obtained:

    Hb: 11 g% Hb

    Pa_{O_2}: 60 mm Hg (Sa_{O_2} = 90%)

    $P\bar{v}_{O_2}$: 35 mm Hg ($S\bar{v}_{O_2}$ = 65%)

    Pa_{CO_2}: 38 mm Hg

    Cardiac Output: 6 L/minute

Based on the above information, calculate the patient's

    a. total oxygen delivery

      Answer: _____

    b. arterial-venous oxygen content difference

      Answer: _____

    c. intrapulmonary shunting

      Answer: _____

    d. oxygen consumption

      Answer: _____

    e. oxygen extraction ratio

      Answer: _____

Answers appear in Appendix VII.

CHAPTER 8

CARBON DIOXIDE TRANSPORT AND ACID-BASE BALANCE

OBJECTIVES

By the end of this chapter, the student should be able to:

1. List the three ways in which carbon dioxide is transported in the *plasma*.
2. List the three ways in which carbon dioxide is transported in the *red blood cells*.
3. Describe how carbon dioxide is converted to HCO_3^- at the tissue sites and then transported in the plasma to the lungs.
4. Explain how carbon dioxide is eliminated at the lungs.
5. Describe how the *carbon dioxide dissociation curve* differs from the *oxygen dissociation* curve.
6. Explain how the *Haldane effect* relates to the carbon dioxide dissociation curve.
7. Define the meaning of
   —Electrolytes
   —Buffer
   —Strong acid
   —Weak acid
   —Weak base
   —Strong base
   —Dissociation constant
   —pH
8. List the three major mechanisms that maintain the narrow pH range.
9. Describe the components of the *Henderson-Hasselbalch equation*.
10. Explain how the P_{CO_2}, HCO_3^-, and pH levels change in the following respiratory acid-base imbalances:
    —Acute ventilatory failure
    —Chronic ventilatory failure and renal compensation
    —Acute alveolar hyperventilation
    —Chronic alveolar hyperventilation and renal compensation

11. Describe how the P_{CO_2}, HCO_3^-, and pH levels change in the following metabolic acid-base imbalances:
   —Metabolic acidosis
      • Lactic acidosis
      • Keto-acidosis
      • Renal failure
   —Chronic metabolic acidosis and respiratory compensation
   —Metabolic alkalosis
      • Hypokalemia
      • Hypochloremia
      • Gastric suction or vomiting
      • Excessive administration of steroids
      • Excessive administration of sodium bicarbonate
   —Chronic metabolic alkalosis and respiratory compensation
12. Complete the self-assessment questions at the end of this chapter.

In addition to understanding oxygen transport, an understanding of carbon dioxide (CO_2) transport is also essential to the study of pulmonary physiology and to the clinical interpretation of arterial blood gases (see Table 7–1). To fully comprehend this subject, a basic understanding of (1) how carbon dioxide is transported from the tissues to the lungs, (2) acid-base balance, (3) the P_{CO_2}/HCO_3^-/pH relationship in respiratory acid-base imbalances, and (4) the P_{CO_2}/HCO_3^-/pH relationship in metabolic acid-base imbalances is necessary.

CARBON DIOXIDE TRANSPORT

At rest, the metabolizing tissue cells consume about 250 ml of oxygen and produce about 200 ml of carbon dioxide each minute. The newly formed carbon dioxide is transported from the tissue cells to the lungs by six different mechanisms—three mechanisms in the plasma and three mechanisms in the red blood cells (RBCs) (Figure 8–1).

In Plasma

• Carbamino Compound (bound to protein)

Although relatively insignificant, about 1 percent of the CO_2 that dissolves in the plasma chemically combines with free amino groups of protein molecules and forms a carbamino compound (see Figure 8–1).

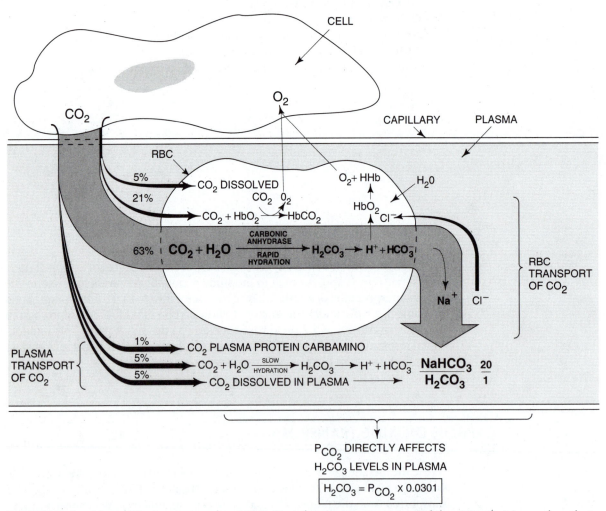

FIGURE 8–1.   How CO_2 is converted to HCO_3^- at the tissue sites. Most of the CO_2 that is produced at the tissue cells is carried to the lungs in the form of HCO_3^-. CA = carbonic anhydrase.

• Bicarbonate

Approximately 5 percent of the CO_2 that dissolves in the plasma ionizes as bicarbonate (HCO_3^-). Initially, CO_2 combines with water in a process called *hydrolysis*. The hydrolysis of CO_2 and water forms carbonic acid (H_2CO_3), which in turn rapidly ionizes into HCO_3^- and H^+ ions.

$$CO_2 + H_2O \rightleftharpoons H_2CO_3 \rightleftharpoons HCO_3^- + H^+$$

The resulting H^+ ions are buffered by the plasma proteins. The rate of this hydrolysis reaction in the plasma is very slow and, therefore, the amount of HCO_3^- and H^+ ions that form by this mechanism is small.

• Dissolved CO_2

Dissolved carbon dioxide in the plasma accounts for about 5 percent of the total CO_2 released at the lungs. Clinically, it is this portion of the carbon dioxide transport system in the venous blood that is measured to assess the patient's partial pressure of carbon dioxide (P_{CO_2}) (see Table 7–1).

It should also be noted that the concentration of H_2CO_3 that forms in the plasma is about 1/1000 that of the physically dissolved carbon dioxide (P_{CO_2}) and, therefore, is proportional to the partial pressure of the CO_2. The H_2CO_3 concentration can be determined by multiplying the partial pressure of carbon dioxide by the factor 0.03. For example, a P_{CO_2} of 40 mm Hg generates a H_2CO_3 concentration of 1.2 mEq/L ($0.03 \times 40 = 1.2$) (see Figure 8–1).

In Red Blood Cells

• Dissolved CO_2

Dissolved carbon dioxide in the intracellular fluid of the red blood cells accounts for about 5 percent of the total CO_2 released at the lungs (see Figure 8–1).

• Carbamino-Hb (combined with hemoglobin)

About 21 percent of the carbon dioxide combines with the red blood cell hemoglobin to form a compound called carbamino-Hb. The O_2 that is released from this reaction is available for tissue metabolism (see Figure 8–1).

• Bicarbonate

Most of the carbon dioxide (about two thirds, or 63 percent) is transported from the tissue cells to the lungs in the form of bicarbonate (HCO_3^-). The major portion of the dissolved CO_2 that enters the red blood cells (RBCs) is converted to HCO_3^- by the following reactions (see Figure 8–1):

1. The bulk of dissolved CO_2 that enters the RBC undergoes hydrolysis according to the following reaction:

$$CO_2 + H_2O \overset{CA}{\rightleftharpoons} H_2CO_3 \rightleftharpoons H^+ + HCO_3^-$$

This reaction, which is normally a very slow process in the plasma, is greatly enhanced in the RBC by the enzyme carbonic anhydrase (CA).

2. The resulting H^+ ions are buffered by the reduced hemoglobin.

3. The rapid hydrolysis of CO_2 causes the RBC to become saturated with HCO_3^-. To maintain a concentration equilibrium between the RBC and plasma, the excess HCO_3^- diffuses out of the RBC.

4. Once in the plasma, the HCO_3^- combines with sodium (Na^+), which is normally in the plasma in the form of sodium/chloride (NaCl). The HCO_3^- is then transported to the lungs as $NaHCO_3$ in the plasma of the venous blood.

5. As HCO_3^- moves out of the RBC, the Cl^- (which has been liberated from the NaCl compound) moves into the RBC to maintain electric neutrality. This movement is known as the **chloride shift,** or the **Hamburger phenomenon,** or as an **anionic shift to equilibrium.** During the chloride shift, some water moves into the RBC to preserve the osmotic equilibrium. This action causes the RBC to slightly swell in the venous blood.

6. In the plasma, the ratio of HCO_3^- and H_2CO_3 is normally maintained at 20 : 1. This 20 : 1 ratio keeps the blood pH level within the normal range of 7.35 to 7.45. The pH of the blood becomes more alkaline as the ratio increases and less alkaline as the ratio decreases.

CARBON DIOXIDE ELIMINATION AT THE LUNGS

As shown in Figure 8–2, as the venous blood enters the alveolar capillaries, the chemical reactions occurring at the tissue level are reversed. These chemical processes continue until the CO_2 pressure is equal throughout the entire system. Table 8–1 summarizes the percentage and quantity of the total carbon dioxide that is transported from the tissue cells to the lungs by the six carbon dioxide mechanisms each minute.

CARBON DIOXIDE DISSOCIATION CURVE

Similar to the oxygen dissociation curve, the loading and unloading of carbon dioxide in the blood can be illustrated in graphic form (Figure 8–3). Unlike the S-shaped oxygen dissociation curve, however, the carbon dioxide curve is almost linear. This means that in comparison to the oxygen dissociation curve there is a more direct relationship between the partial pressure of carbon dioxide (P_{CO_2}) and the amount of carbon dioxide (CO_2 content) in the blood. For example, when the P_{CO_2} increases from 40 to 46 mm Hg between the arterial and venous blood,

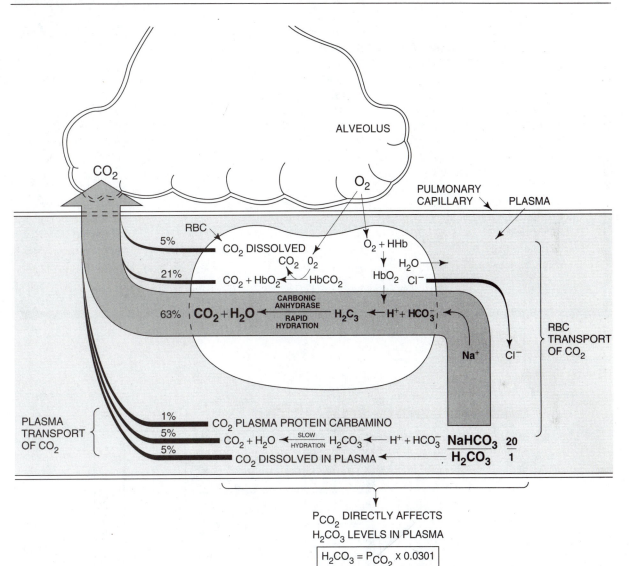

FIGURE 8–2. How HCO_3^- is transformed back into CO_2 and eliminated into the alveoli. CA = carbonic anhydrase.

the CO_2 content increases by about 5 vol% (Figure 8–4). The same partial pressure change of oxygen would increase the oxygen content only by about 2 vol% (see Figure 7–2).

The level of saturation of hemoglobin with oxygen also affects the carbon dioxide dissociation curve. When the hemoglobin is 97% saturated with oxygen,

TABLE 8–1. Carbon Dioxide Transport Mechanisms

CARBON DIOXIDE TRANSPORT MECHANISMS	APPROX. % OF TOTAL CO$_2$ TRANSPORTED TO THE LUNGS	APPROX. QUANTITY OF TOTAL CO$_2$ TRANSPORTED TO THE LUNGS
IN PLASMA		
Carbamino Compound	1%	2 ml/min
Bicarbonate	5%	10 ml/min
Dissolved CO$_2$	5%	10 ml/min
IN RED BLOOD CELLS		
Dissolved	5%	10 ml/min
Carbamino-Hb	21%	42 ml/min
Bicarbonate	63%	126 ml/min
Total	100%	Total 200 ml/min

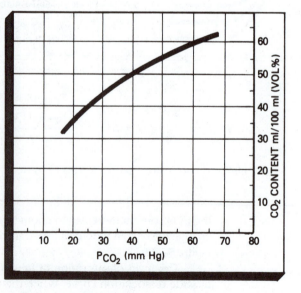

FIGURE 8–3. Carbon dioxide dissociation curve.

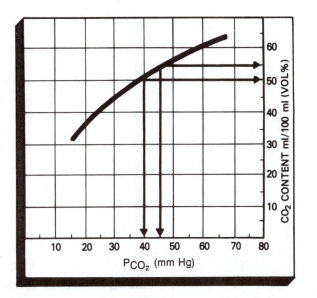

FIGURE 8–4. Carbon dioxide dissociation curve. An increase in the P_{CO_2} from 40 mm Hg to 46 mm Hg raises the CO_2 content by about 5 vol%. P_{CO_2} changes have a greater effect on CO_2 content levels than P_{O_2} changes have on O_2 levels.

for example, there is less CO_2 content for any given P_{CO_2} than if the hemoglobin is, say, 75% saturated with oxygen (Figure 8–5).The fact that deoxygenated blood enhances the loading of carbon dioxide is called the **Haldane effect**. It should also be noted that the Haldane effect works the other way—that is, the oxygenation of blood enhances the unloading of CO_2.

Figure 8–6 compares both the oxygen and the carbon dioxide dissociation curves in terms of partial pressure, content, and shape.

ACID-BASE BALANCE

To fully understand acid-base balance, a working definition of the following terms and phrases is essential.

Electrolytes—charged species (ions) that can conduct a current in solution.
Buffer—a substance that is capable of neutralizing both acids and bases without causing an appreciable change in the original pH.
Strong acid—an acid that dissociates completely into H^+ and an anion (an acid is a hydrogen ion donor).
Weak acid—an acid that dissociates only partially into ions.

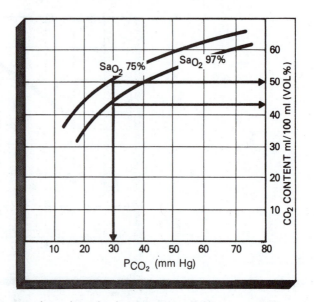

FIGURE 8–5. Carbon dioxide dissociation curve at two different oxygen/hemoglobin saturation levels (Sa_{O_2} of 97 percent and 75 percent). When the saturation of O_2 increases in the blood, the CO_2 content decreases at any given P_{CO_2}. This is known as the *Haldane effect.*

Strong base—a base that dissociates completely.

Weak base—a base that reacts with water to form OH^- in an equilibrium; partial dissociation.

Dissociation constant—refers to weak acid or base systems that have an equilibrium between the molecular form and its ions. For example,

$$HA \rightleftharpoons [H^+] + [A^-]$$
$$\text{(molecule)} \qquad \text{(ions)}$$

$$K_a = \frac{[H^+][A^-]}{[HA]}$$

where K_a is the concentration of all species at equilibrium, [   ] means concentration in terms of molarity (M), H^+ is hydrogen ion, A^- is the anion, and HA is the molecular weak acid.

HA is said to be in the *un-ionized* (undissociated) state. $[H^+]$ and $[A^-]$ are said to be in the *ionized* (dissociated) state.

The pH Scale

Because the transport of carbon dioxide can affect the hydrogen ion concentration $[H^+]$, and because hydrogen ion activity can significantly affect the

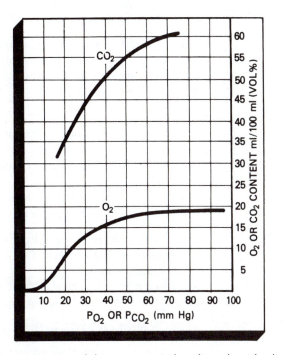

FIGURE 8–6. Comparison of the oxygen and carbon dioxide dissociation curves in terms of partial pressure, content, and shape.

metabolic function of the cells, it is important to understand the quantitative measurement of the hydrogen ion concentration. Clinically, the pH scale is used. A pH of 7 is neutral, a pH of less than 7 is acidic, and a pH greater than 7 is basic.

In chemistry, the pH is defined as the *negative logarithm, to the base 10, of the hydrogen ion concentration:*

$$pH = -\log_{10}[H^+]$$

Thus, a pH of 7 (e.g., pure water) is equal to 10^{-7} mole/L (0.0000001 mole/L) of hydrogen ions. The normal pH range in the human body is 7.35 to 7.45. An **acid** is a substance that donates $[H^+]$ and therefore increases the hydrogen ion concentration of a solution and causes the numerical value of the pH to decrease. A **base** is a substance that accepts $[H^+]$ and therefore decreases the hydrogen ion concentration and causes the pH value to increase.

The narrow pH range is maintained by (1) the buffer systems of the blood and tissues, (2) the respiratory system's ability to regulate the elimination of CO_2 (see Chapter Ten), and (3) the renal system's ability to regulate the excretion of hydrogen and the reabsorption of bicarbonate ions (see Chapter Twelve).

The Buffer Systems

The ability of an acid-base mixture to resist large changes in pH is called its buffer action. There are numerous acid-base combinations, or buffer combinations, in the body that can do this. The following are buffers of special interest to the respiratory care practitioner:

- Plasma
  - Carbonic acid/sodium bicarbonate (H_2CO_3/$NaHCO_3$)
  - Sodium acid phosphate/sodium alkaline phosphate (NaH_2PO_4/$NaHPO_4$)
  - Acid proteinate/sodium proteinate (H_{prot}/Na_{prot})
- Erythrocytes
  - Acid hemoglobin/potassium hemoglobin (HHb/KHb)
  - Potassium acid phosphate/potassium alkaline phosphate (KH_2PO_4/K_2HPO_4)

In regard to the above buffer examples, the carbonic acid/sodium bicarbonate combination (H_2CO_3/$NaHCO_3$) is the most important and, therefore, is used in the following discussion.

When a strong acid like hydrochloric acid (HCl) is added to the H_2CO_3/$NaHCO_3$, the following chain of events occurs:

$$HCl + NaHCO_3{}^- \rightleftharpoons H_2CO_3 + NaCl$$

As shown, this reaction reduces the strong acid into a weak acid (H_2CO_3) and a neutral salt (NaCl). Because of this chemical process, the pH movement toward the acidic range is minimal.

In contrast, when a strong base like sodium hydroxide (NaOH) is added to a H_2CO_3/$NaHCO_3$ system, the following reaction occurs:

$$NaOH + H_2CO_3 \rightleftharpoons NaHCO_3 + H_2O$$

As can be seen, this reaction causes the formation of sodium bicarbonate and the loss of H_2CO_3. Because the carbonic acid (H_2CO_3) is a weak acid, the increase in pH is small.

The Henderson-Hasselbalch Equation

The **Henderson-Hasselbalch equation** uses the components of the H_2CO_3/$HCO_3{}^-$ system in the following way:

$$pH = pK + \log \frac{[HCO_3{}^-]}{[H_2CO_3]}$$

pK is derived from the dissociation constant of the acid portion of the buffer combination. Normally, the pK is 6.1.

Under normal conditions, when the $HCO_3{}^-$ is 24 mEq/L and the H_2CO_3 is 1.2 mEq/L, use of the Henderson-Hasselbalch equation allows us to calculate a pH of 7.4 as follows:

$$pH = pK + \log \frac{[HCO_3^-]}{[H_2CO_3]}$$

$$= 6.1 + \log \frac{24 \text{ mEq/L}}{1.2 \text{ mEq/L}}$$

$$= 6.1 + \log \frac{20}{1}$$

$$= 6.1 + 1.3$$

$$= 7.4$$

As the above equation illustrates, the major component of the Henderson-Hasselbalch formula is the ratio of HCO_3^- to H_2CO_3, which is normally 20 to 1.

Thus, when the HCO_3^- to H_2CO_3 ratio changes, the pH will also change: for example, when the ratio increases to, say, 25 to 1, the pH increases as follows:

$$pH = 6.1 + \log \frac{25}{1}$$

$$= 6.1 + 1.4$$

$$= 7.5$$

In contrast, when the HCO_3^- to H_2CO_3 ratio decreases to, say, 15 to 1, the pH decreases as follows:

$$pH = 6.1 + \log \frac{15}{1}$$

$$= 6.1 + 1.18$$

$$= 7.29$$

THE ROLE OF THE P_{CO_2}/HCO$_3^-$/pH RELATIONSHIP IN ACID-BASE BALANCE

Respiratory Acid-base Imbalances

The bulk of CO_2 is transported from the tissues to the lungs as HCO_3^-. As the CO_2 level increases, the plasma P_{CO_2}, HCO_3^-, and H_2CO_3 increase. The converse is also true: as the level of CO_2 decreases, the plasma P_{CO_2}, HCO_3^-, and H_2CO_3 decrease.

Because the blood pH is dependent on the ratio between the plasma HCO_3^- (base) and the plasma H_2CO_3 (acid), acute ventilatory changes will immediately alter the pH. The normal HCO_3^- to H_2CO_3 ratio is 20 : 1. It should be noted that even though both plasma HCO_3^- and plasma H_2CO_3 move in the same direction during acute ventilatory changes, acute changes in the H_2CO_3 level play a much more powerful role in altering the pH status than acute changes in the HCO_3^- level. This is due to the 20 : 1 ratio between HCO_3^- to H_2CO_3. *In other words, for every H_2CO_3 molecule increase or decrease, twenty HCO_3^- molecules must also increase or decrease, respectively, in order to maintain a 20 : 1 ratio between HCO_3^- and H_2CO_3 (the normal pH status).*

Acute Ventilatory Failure.   During **acute ventilatory failure** (e.g., acute hypoventilation caused by an overdose of narcotics or barbiturates), the $P_{A_{CO_2}}$ progressively increases. This action necessarily increases the blood P_{CO_2}, H_2CO_3, and HCO_3^- levels (Figure 8–7). Because acute changes in H_2CO_3 levels are more significant than acute changes in HCO_3^- levels, a decreased HCO_3^- to H_2CO_3 ratio develops (a ratio less than 20 : 1). This action causes the patient's blood pH to decrease, or become less alkaline. The *normal buffer line* on the $P_{CO_2}/HCO_3^-/pH$ nomogram in Figure 8–8 illustrates the expected HCO_3^- and pH changes that develop as a result of CO_2 changes only.

Chronic Ventilatory Failure and Kidney Compensation.   If the patient hypoventilates for a long period of time (e.g., more than 24 to 48 hours), the kidneys will work to correct the decreased pH by retaining HCO_3^- in the blood. Renal compensation in the presence of chronic hypoventilation can be verified when the calculated HCO_3^- and pH readings are higher than expected for a particular P_{CO_2}

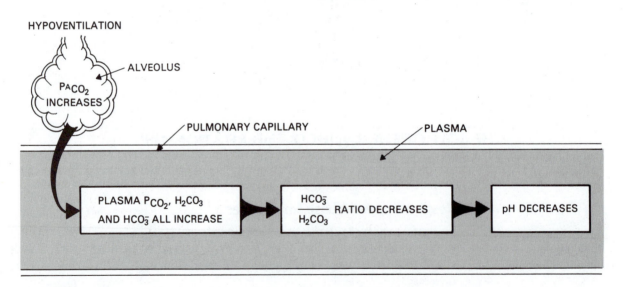

FIGURE 8–7.   Alveolar hypoventilation causes the $P_{A_{CO_2}}$ and the plasma P_{CO_2}, H_2CO_3, and HCO_3^- to increase. This action decreases the HCO_3^-/H_2CO_3 ratio, which in turn decreases the blood pH.

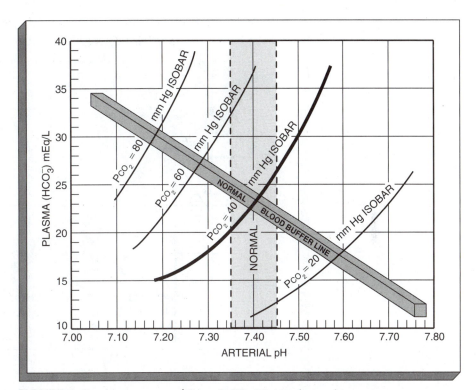

FIGURE 8–8.   Nomogram of P_{CO_2}/HCO$_3^-$/pH relationship.

level. For example, in terms of the absolute P_{CO_2}/HCO$_3^-$/pH relationship, when the P_{CO_2} is about 80 mm Hg, the pH level should be less than 7.2, and the HCO$_3^-$ level should be about 30 mEq/L, according to the normal blood buffer line (Figure 8–9). If the HCO$_3^-$ and pH levels are greater than these values (i.e., the pH and HCO$_3^-$ readings cross the P_{CO_2} *isobar** above the normal blood buffer line in the upper left-hand corner of the nomogram), renal retention of HCO$_3^-$ (**partial renal compensation**) has likely occurred. When the HCO$_3^-$ level increases enough to return the acidic pH to normal, **complete renal compensation** is said to have occurred (see Figure 8–9).

Acute Alveolar Hyperventilation.   During **acute alveolar hyperventilation** (e.g., hyperventilation due to pain and/or anxiety), the $P_{A_{CO_2}}$ will decrease and allow more CO_2 molecules to leave the pulmonary blood. This action necessarily

---

*The isobars on the P_{CO_2}/HCO$_3^-$/pH nomogram illustrate the pH changes that develop in the blood as a result of (1) metabolic changes (i.e., HCO$_3^-$ changes), or (2) a combination of metabolic and respiratory (CO_2) changes.

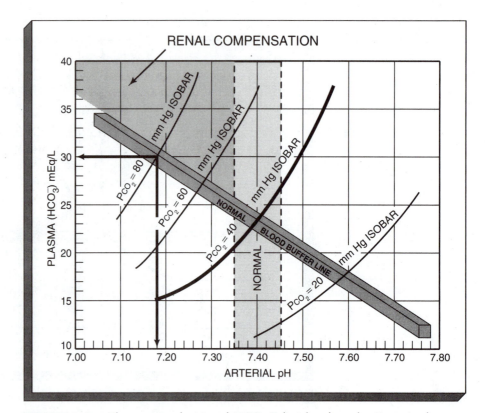

FIGURE 8–9. The expected pH and HCO_3^- levels when the P_{CO_2} is about 80 mm Hg. When the HCO_3^- and pH lines cross an isobar in the shaded area, renal compensation is present.

decreases the blood P_{CO_2}, H_2CO_3, and HCO_3^- levels (Figure 8–10). Because acute changes in H_2CO_3 levels are more significant than acute changes in HCO_3^- levels, an increased HCO_3^- to H_2CO_3 ratio develops (a ratio greater than 20 : 1). This action causes the patient's blood pH to increase, or become more alkaline. The normal buffer line on the P_{CO_2}/HCO_3^-/pH nomogram illustrates this relationship (see Figure 8–8).

Chronic Alveolar Hyperventilation and Renal Compensation. If the patient hyperventilates for a long period of time (e.g., a patient who has been mechanically hyperventilated for more than 24 to 48 hours), the kidneys will attempt to correct the increased pH by excreting excess HCO_3^- in the urine. Renal compensation in the presence of chronic hyperventilation can be verified when the calculated HCO_3^- and pH readings are lower than expected for a particular P_{CO_2} level. For example, in terms of the absolute P_{CO_2}/HCO_3^-/pH relationship, when the P_{CO_2} is

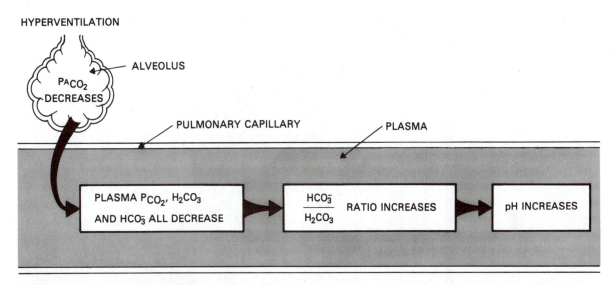

FIGURE 8–10. Alveolar hyperventilation causes the P_{ACO_2} and the plasma P_{CO_2}, H_2CO_3, and HCO_3^- to decrease. This action increases the HCO_3^-/H_2CO_3 ratio, which in turn increases the blood pH.

about 25 mm Hg, the pH level should be greater than 7.5, and the HCO_3^- level should be about 19 mEq/L. If the HCO_3^- and pH levels are lower than these values (i.e., the pH and HCO_3^- readings cross a P_{CO_2} isobar below the normal blood buffer line in the lower right-hand corner), renal excretion of HCO_3^- (**partial renal compensation**) has likely occurred. When the HCO_3^- level decreases enough to return the alkalotic pH to normal, **complete renal compensation** is said to have occurred (Figure 8–11).

As a general rule, the kidneys do not overcompensate for an abnormal pH. That is, if the patient's blood pH becomes acidic for a long period of time due to hypoventilation, the kidneys will not retain enough HCO_3^- for the pH to climb higher than 7.4. The opposite is also true: should the patient's blood pH become alkalotic for a long period of time due to hyperventilation, the kidneys will not excrete enough HCO_3^- for the pH to fall below 7.4.

There is one important exception to this rule. In persons chronically hypoventilating for a long period of time (e.g., in chronic obstructive pulmonary disease), it is not uncommon to find a pH greater than 7.4. This is believed to be due to water and chloride ion shifts between the intercellular and extracellular spaces that occur when the renal system works to compensate for a decreased blood pH.

To summarize: the lungs play an important role in maintaining the P_{CO_2}, HCO_3^-, and pH levels on a moment-to-moment basis. The kidneys, on the other hand, play an important role in balancing the HCO_3^- and pH levels during long periods of hyperventilation or hypoventilation.

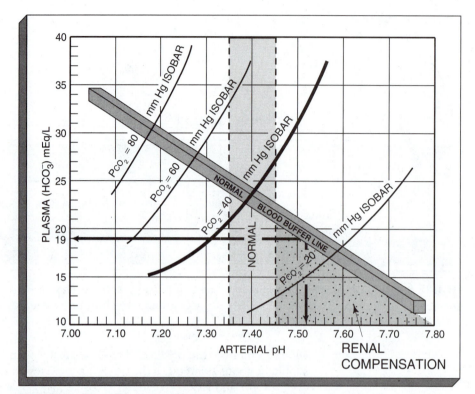

FIGURE 8–11. The expected pH and HCO_3^- levels when the P_{CO_2} is about 25 mm Hg. When the HCO_3^- and pH lines cross an isobar in the shaded area, renal compensation is present.

Metabolic Acid-base Imbalances

Metabolic Acidosis. By using the isobars of the $P_{CO_2}/HCO_3^-/pH$ nomogram, the presence of other acids, not related to an increased P_{CO_2} level or to renal compensation, can be identified. This condition is referred to as **metabolic acidosis**.

When metabolic acidosis is present, the calculated HCO_3^- reading and pH will both be lower than expected for a particular P_{CO_2} level in terms of the absolute $P_{CO_2}/HCO_3^-/pH$ relationship. For example, a HCO_3^- reading of 17 mEq/L and a pH of 7.25 would both be less than expected in a patient who has a P_{CO_2} of 40 mm Hg, according to the normal blood buffer line (Figure 8–12).

Common Causes of Metabolic Acidosis.

- **Lactic Acidosis.** When the oxygen level is inadequate to meet tissue needs, alternate biochemical reactions are activated that do not utilize oxygen. This is

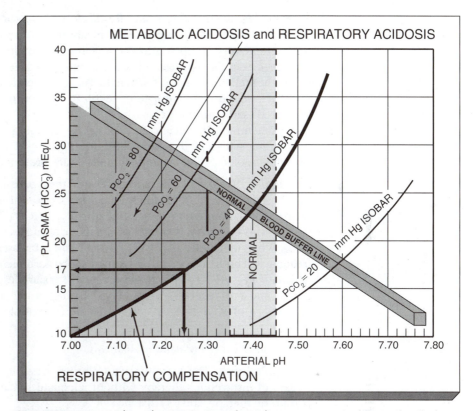

FIGURE 8–12. When the HCO_3^- and pH lines cross an isobar in the darker shaded area, both metabolic and respiratory acidosis are present. When the HCO_3^- and pH lines cross an isobar in the lighter shaded area, the metabolic acidosis is partially corrected by means of respiratory compensation (*hyperventilation*).

known as **anaerobic metabolism** (non-oxygen-utilizing). Lactic acid is the end-product of this process. When these ions move into the blood, and a patient has both a reduced oxygen level and a decreased pH level, lactic acidosis is present.

- **Keto-acidosis.** When blood insulin is low in the diabetic patient, serum glucose cannot easily enter the tissue cells for metabolism. This condition activates alternate metabolic processes that produce **ketones** as metabolites. Ketone accumulation in the blood causes keto-acidosis. The absence of glucose because of starvation can also cause keto-acidosis. Keto-acidosis may also be seen in patients with excessive alcohol intake.
- **Renal Failure.** During renal failure, an accumulation of hydrogen ions can cause metabolic acidosis.

Chronic Metabolic Acidosis and Respiratory Compensation.   Normally, the immediate compensatory response for metabolic acidosis is an increased ventilatory rate (respiratory compensation) that causes the patient's Pa_{CO_2} to decline. This process causes the hydrogen ion concentration to decrease and therefore works to offset the metabolic acidosis. When the Pa_{CO_2} decreases enough to move the acidic pH back to normal, **complete respiratory compensation** is said to have occurred (see Figure 8–12).

When the pH is acidic and the HCO_3^- reading is below the normal blood buffer line while, at the same time, the P_{CO_2} level is above 40 mm Hg, both metabolic acidosis and respiratory acidosis are present (see Figure 8–12).

Metabolic Alkalosis.   The presence of other bases, not related to either a decreased P_{CO_2} level or to kidney compensation, can also be identified by using the isobars of a nomogram illustrating the $P_{CO_2}/HCO_3^-/pH$ relationship (Figure 8–13). This condition is known as metabolic alkalosis.

When metabolic alkalosis is present, the calculated HCO_3^- reading and pH reading will both be higher than expected for a particular P_{CO_2} level in terms of the absolute $P_{CO_2}/HCO_3^-/pH$ relationship. For example, a HCO_3^- reading of 31 mEq/L and a pH level of 7.5 would both be higher than expected in a patient who has a P_{CO_2} of 40 mm Hg, according to the normal blood buffer line (see Figure 8–13).

Common Causes of Metabolic Alkalosis.

- **Hypokalemia.** The depletion of total body potassium can occur from (1) several days of intravenous therapy without adequate replacement of potassium, (2) diuretic therapy, and (3) diarrhea.

   Whenever the potassium level is low, the normal kidney attempts to save potassium by excreting hydrogen ions. This mechanism causes the blood base to increase. In addition, as the potassium level in the blood decreases, intracellular potassium moves into the extracellular space in an effort to offset the reduced potassium level in the blood serum. As the potassium cation (K^+) leaves the cell, however, a hydrogen cation (H^+) enters the cell. This mechanism causes the blood serum to become more alkalotic.

   Patients with hypokalemia frequently demonstrate the clinical triad of (1) metabolic alkalosis, (2) muscular weakness, and (3) cardiac dysrhythmias.

- **Hypochloremia.** When the chloride ion (Cl^-) concentration decreases, bicarbonate ions increase in an attempt to maintain a normal cation balance in the blood serum. As the bicarbonate ion increases, the patient's blood serum becomes alkalotic. The kidneys, moreoever, usually excrete potassium ions when chloride ions are unavailable which, as described above, will also contribute to the patient's metabolic alkalosis.

- **Gastric Suction or Vomiting.** Excessive gastric suction or vomiting causes a loss of hydrochloric acid (HCl) and the result is an increase in blood base; i.e., metabolic alkalosis.

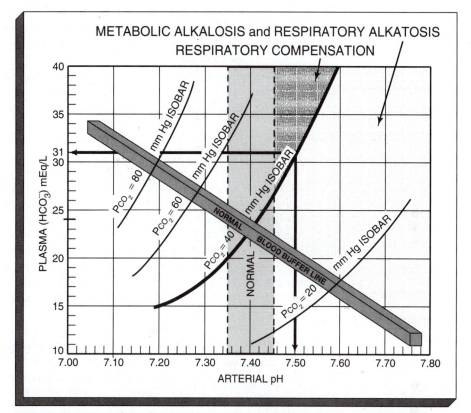

FIGURE 8–13. When the HCO_3^- and pH lines cross an isobar in the darker shaded area, both metabolic and respiratory alkalosis are present. When the HCO_3^- and pH lines cross an isobar in the lighter shaded area, the metabolic acidosis is partially corrected by means of respiratory compensation (*hypoventilation*).

- **Excessive Administration of Steroids.** Large doses of sodium-retaining steroids can cause the kidneys to accelerate the excretion of hydrogen ions and potassium. Excessive excretion of either one or both of these ions will cause metabolic alkalosis.
- **Excessive Administration of Sodium Bicarbonate.** If an excessive amount of sodium bicarbonate is administered, metabolic alkalosis will occur. This used to happen frequently during cardiopulmonary resuscitation.

Chronic Metabolic Alkalosis and Respiratory Compensation. Normally, the immediate compensatory response to metabolic alkalosis is a decreased ventilatory rate (*respiratory compensation*) which causes the patient's Pa_{CO_2} to increase.

The excess hydrogen ions produced by the elevated blood Pa_{CO_2} work to offset the patient's metabolic alkalosis. When the Pa_{CO_2} increases enough to move the alkalotic pH back to normal, *complete respiratory compensation* is said to have occurred (see Figure 8–13).

When the pH is alkalotic and the HCO_3^- reading is above the normal blood buffer line, while at the same time the P_{CO_2} level is below 40 mm Hg, both metabolic alkalosis and respiratory alkalosis are present (see Figure 8–13).

Base Excess/Deficit

Clinically, the $P_{CO_2}/HCO_3^-/pH$ nomogram also serves as an excellent tool to calculate the patient's total **base excess/deficit**. By knowing the base excess/deficit, non-respiratory acid-base imbalances can be quantified and managed. The base excess/deficit is reported in milliequivalents per liter (mEq/L) of base above or below the normal buffer base line of the $P_{CO_2}/HCO_3^-/pH$ nomogram.

For example, if the patient has a pH of 7.25 and a HCO_3^- of 17 mEq/L, the $P_{CO_2}/HCO_3^-/pH$ nomogram will confirm that the patient has (1) metabolic acidosis and (2) a base excess of a −7 (more properly called a *base deficit* of 7) (see Figure 8–12). Metabolic acidosis may be treated by the careful intravenous infusion of sodium bicarbonate ($NaHCO_3$).

In contrast, if the patient has a pH of 7.5 and a HCO_3^- of 31 mEq/L, the $P_{CO_2}/HCO_3^-/pH$ nomogram will verify that the patient has (1) metabolic alkalosis and (2) a base excess of 7 mEq/L (see Figure 8–13). Metabolic alkalosis is commonly treated by (1) correcting the underlying electrolyte problem (e.g., hypokalemia or hypochloremia), or (2) administering ammonium chloride (NH_4Cl).

Example of Clinical Use of $P_{CO_2}/HCO_3^-/pH$ Nomogram

It has been shown that the $P_{CO_2}/HCO_3^-/pH$ nomogram is an excellent clinical tool to confirm the presence of (1) respiratory acid-base imbalances, (2) metabolic acid-base imbalances, or (3) a combination of a respiratory and metabolic acid-base imbalance. To demonstrate the clinical usefulness of the $P_{CO_2}/HCO_3^-/pH$ nomogram consider the following case:

CASE STUDY: CARBON MONOXIDE POISONING

A 36-year-old man, who had been working in his car while the motor was running, suddenly experienced confusion, disorientation, and nausea. After calling for help, he started to vomit. About 60 seconds later he collapsed and lost consciousness. The emergency medical technicians who transported the patient to the hospital stated that the patient continued to vomit intermittently while en route to the hospital. In the emergency room, the following data were found:

Respiratory rate: 36 breaths/minute
Heart rate: 122 beats/minute
Blood pressure: 165/105
Breath sounds: clear
Skin color: cherry red
Blood Gases (on room air):
  pH   7.52
  Pa_{CO_2} 25 mm Hg
  HCO_3^- 19 mEq/L
  Pa_{O_2} 119 mm Hg
Carboxyhemoglobin level
(COHb)   55%

Even though the patient's Pa_{O_2} is very high (due to the hyperventilation), the carboxyhemoglobin of 55% has seriously reduced the ability of the patient's hemoglobin to carry oxygen. The increased respiratory rate, heart rate, and blood pressure are compensatory mechanisms activated to counteract the decreased arterial oxygenation (i.e., these mechanisms increase the total oxygen delivery). The "cherry red" skin color is a classic sign of COHb poisoning.

Because it was reported that the patient had vomited excessively prior to the arterial blood gas sample, it is not easily determined if the high pH is a result of (1) the acute hyperventilation only (caused by the reduced arterial oxygenation) or (2) a combination of both the acute hyperventilation and the loss of stomach acids (caused by the vomiting). By using the $P_{CO_2}/HCO_3^-/pH$ nomogram, this question can be answered. In this case, when the pH, HCO_3^-, and Pa_{CO_2} values listed above are applied to the $P_{CO_2}/HCO_3^-/pH$ nomogram, it can be seen that the elevated pH is due solely to the decreased P_{CO_2} level, since all three variables cross through the normal buffer line (see Figure 8–11).*

SELF-ASSESSMENT QUESTIONS

    1. During acute alveolar hypoventilation, the blood
        I. H_2CO_3 increases
        II. pH increases
        III. HCO_3^- increases

---

*See Appendix VI for a credit-card size $P_{CO_2}/HCO_3^-/pH$ nomogram that can be copied and laminated for use as a handy clinical reference tool.

    IV. P_{CO_2} increases
      a. II only
      b. IV only
      c. II and III only
      d. I and IV only
      e. I, III, and IV only

2. The bulk of the CO_2 produced in the cells is transported to the lungs as
      a. H_2CO_3
      b. HCO_3^-
      c. CO_2 and H_2O
      d. Carbonic anhydrase
      e. HHb

3. During acute alveolar hyperventilation, the blood
    I. P_{CO_2} increases
    II. H_2CO_3 decreases
    III. HCO_3^- increases
    IV. pH decreases
      a. II only
      b. IV only
      c. I and III only
      d. II and IV only
      e. II, III, and IV only

4. In chronic hypoventilation, renal compensation has likely occurred when the
    I. HCO_3^- is higher than expected for a particular P_{CO_2}
    II. pH is lower than expected for a particular P_{CO_2}
    III. HCO_3^- is lower than expected for a particular P_{CO_2}
    IV. pH is higher than expected for a particular P_{CO_2}
      a. I only
      b. II only
      c. I and IV only
      d. III and IV only
      e. I and II only

5. When metabolic acidosis is present, the patient's blood
    I. HCO_3^- is higher than expected for a particular P_{CO_2}
    II. pH is lower than expected for a particular P_{CO_2}
    III. HCO_3^- is lower than expected for a particular P_{CO_2}
    IV. pH is higher than expected for a particular P_{CO_2}
      a. I only
      b. II only
      c. I and IV only
      d. III and IV only
      e. II and III only

6. Keto-acidosis can develop from
    I. an inadequate oxygen level

    II. renal failure

    III. an inadequate insulin level

    IV. anerobic metabolism

    V. an inadequate glucose level

      a. I only

      b. II and III only

      c. IV and V only

      d. III and V only

      e. II, III, and V only

7. Metabolic alkalosis can develop from

    I. hyperchloremia

    II. hypokalemia

    III. hypochloremia

    IV. hyperkalemia

      a. I only

      b. IV only

      c. I and III only

      d. I and IV only

      e. II and III only

8. Which of the following HCO_3^- to H_2CO_3 ratios represent an acidic pH?

    I. $18 : 1$

    II. $28 : 1$

    III. $12 : 1$

    IV. $22 : 1$

      a. I only

      b. II only

      c. III only

      d. II and III only

      e. I and III only

9. If a patient has a P_{CO_2} level of 70 mm Hg, what is the H_2CO_3 concentration?

      a. 0.7 mEq/L

      b. 1.3 mEq/L

      c. 1.5 mEq/L

      d. 1.7 mEq/L

      e. 2.1 mEq/L

10. The value of the pK in the Henderson-Hasselbalch equation is

      a. 1.0

      b. 6.1

      c. 7.4

      d. 20.1

      e. 24

Answers appear in Appendix VII.

CHAPTER 9

VENTILATION-PERFUSION RELATIONSHIPS

VENTILATION-PERFUSION RATIO

Ideally, each alveolus in the lungs should receive the same amount of ventilation and pulmonary capillary blood flow. In reality, however, this is not the case. Overall, alveolar ventilation is normally about 4 L/min and pulmonary capillary blood flow is about 5 L/min, making the average overall ratio of ventilation to blood

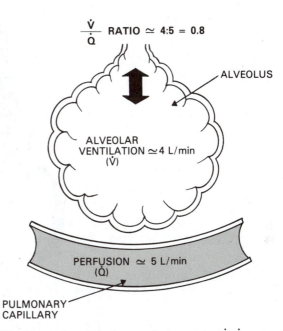

$$\frac{\dot{V}}{\dot{Q}} \ \text{RATIO} \ \simeq \ 4:5 \ = \ 0.8$$

ALVEOLUS

ALVEOLAR
VENTILATION $\simeq$ 4 L/min
($\dot{V}$)

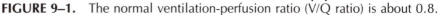

PERFUSION $\simeq$ 5 L/min
($\dot{Q}$)

PULMONARY
CAPILLARY

FIGURE 9–1. The normal ventilation-perfusion ratio ($\dot{V}/\dot{Q}$ ratio) is about 0.8.

flow 4 : 5, or 0.8. This relationship is called the **ventilation-perfusion ratio** ($\dot{V}/\dot{Q}$ ratio) (Figure 9–1).

Although the overall $\dot{V}/\dot{Q}$ ratio is about 0.8, the ratio varies remarkably throughout the lung. For example, in the normal individual in the upright position, the alveoli in the upper portions of the lungs (apices) receive a moderate amount of ventilation and little blood flow. As a result, the $\dot{V}/\dot{Q}$ ratio in the upper lung region is higher than 0.8.

In the lower regions of the lung, however, alveolar ventilation is moderately increased and blood flow is greatly increased, since blood flow is gravity dependent. As a result, the $\dot{V}/\dot{Q}$ ratio is lower than 0.8. In summary, the $\dot{V}/\dot{Q}$ ratio progressively decreases from top to bottom in the upright lung, and the average $\dot{V}/\dot{Q}$ ratio is about 0.8 (Figure 9–2).

How the Ventilation-perfusion Ratio Affects the Alveolar Gases

The $\dot{V}/\dot{Q}$ ratio profoundly affects the oxygen and carbon dioxide pressures in the alveoli ($P_{A_{O_2}}$ and $P_{A_{CO_2}}$). Although the normal $P_{A_{O_2}}$ and $P_{A_{CO_2}}$ are typically about 100 mm Hg and 40 mm Hg, respectively, this is not the case throughout most of the alveolar units. These figures merely represent an average.

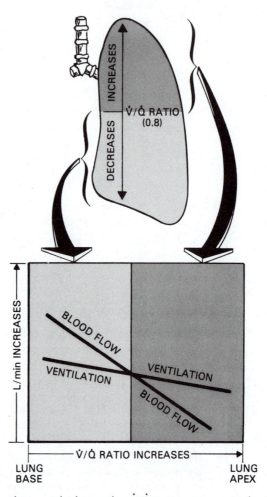

FIGURE 9–2. In the upright lung, the $\dot{V}/\dot{Q}$ ratio progressively decreases from the apex to the base.

The $P_{A_{O_2}}$ is determined by the balance between (1) the amount of oxygen entering into the alveoli and (2) its removal by capillary blood flow. The $P_{A_{CO_2}}$, on the other hand, is determined by the balance between (1) the amount of carbon dioxide that diffuses into the alveoli from the capillary blood and (2) its removal out of the alveoli by means of ventilation. Thus, changing $\dot{V}/\dot{Q}$ ratios alter the $P_{A_{O_2}}$ and $P_{A_{CO_2}}$ levels for the reasons discussed below.

Increased $\dot{V}/\dot{Q}$ Ratio. When the $\dot{V}/\dot{Q}$ ratio increases, the $P_{A_{O_2}}$ rises and the $P_{A_{CO_2}}$ falls. The $P_{A_{CO_2}}$ decreases because it washes out of the alveoli faster than it is replaced by the venous blood. The $P_{A_{O_2}}$ increases because it does not diffuse into

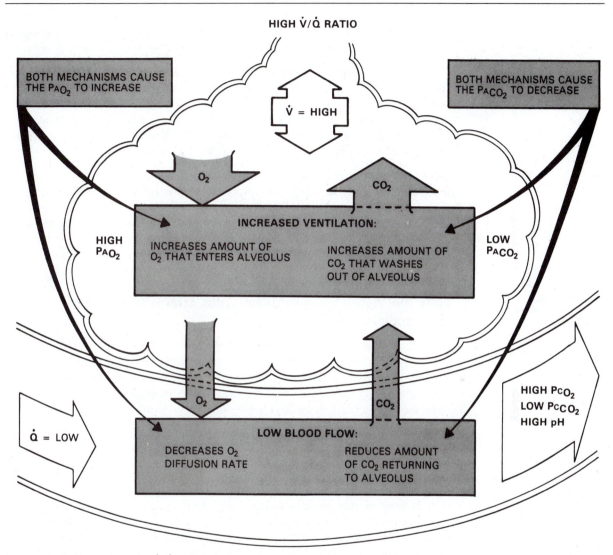

FIGURE 9–3. When the $\dot{V}/\dot{Q}$ ratio is high, the alveolar oxygen pressure ($P_{A_{O_2}}$) increases and the alveolar carbon dioxide pressure ($P_{A_{CO_2}}$) decreases.

the blood* as fast as it enters (or is ventilated into) the alveolus (Figure 9–3). The $P_{A_{O_2}}$ also increases because the $P_{A_{CO_2}}$ decreases and therefore allows the $P_{A_{O_2}}$ to move closer to the partial pressure of atmospheric oxygen, which is about 159 mm

*See how oxygen can be classified as either perfusion or diffusion limited, in Chapter Three.

Hg at sea level (see Table 3–2).[†] This $\dot{V}/\dot{Q}$ relationship is present in the upper segments of the upright lung (see Figure 9–2).

Decreased $\dot{V}/\dot{Q}$ Ratio.   When the $\dot{V}/\dot{Q}$ ratio decreases, the $P_{A_{O_2}}$ falls and the $P_{A_{CO_2}}$ rises. The $P_{A_{O_2}}$ decreases because oxygen moves out of the alveolus and into the pulmonary capillary blood faster than it is replenished by ventilation. The $P_{A_{CO_2}}$ increases because it moves out of the capillary blood and into the alveolus faster than it is washed out of the alveolus (Figure 9–4). This $\dot{V}/\dot{Q}$ relationship is present in the lower segments of the upright lung (see Figure 9–2).

O_2–CO_2 Diagram.   The effect of changing $\dot{V}/\dot{Q}$ ratios on the $P_{A_{O_2}}$ and $P_{A_{CO_2}}$ levels is summarized in the O_2–CO_2 diagram (Figure 9–5). The line in this diagram represents all the possible alveolar gas compositions as the $\dot{V}/\dot{Q}$ ratio decreases or increases. For example, the O_2–CO_2 diagram (nomogram) shows that in the upper lung regions, the $\dot{V}/\dot{Q}$ ratio is high, the $P_{A_{O_2}}$ is up, and the $P_{A_{CO_2}}$ is down. In contrast, the diagram shows that in the lower lung regions, the $\dot{V}/\dot{Q}$ ratio is low, the $P_{A_{O_2}}$ is down, and the $P_{A_{CO_2}}$ is up.

How the Ventilation-perfusion Ratio Affects the End-capillary Gases

The oxygen and carbon dioxide pressures in the end-capillary blood ($P_{c_{O_2}}$ and $P_{c_{CO_2}}$) mirror the $P_{A_{O_2}}$ and $P_{A_{CO_2}}$ changes that occur in the lungs. Thus, as the $\dot{V}/\dot{Q}$ ratio progressively decreases from the top to the bottom of the upright lung, causing the $P_{A_{O_2}}$ to decrease and the $P_{A_{CO_2}}$ to increase, the $P_{c_{O_2}}$ and $P_{c_{CO_2}}$ also decrease and increase, respectively (see Figures 9–3 and 9–4).

Downstream, in the pulmonary veins, the different $P_{c_{O_2}}$ and $P_{c_{CO_2}}$ levels mix together and, under normal circumstances, produce a P_{O_2} of 100 mm Hg and a P_{CO_2} of 40 mm Hg (Figure 9–6, page 281). Clinically, the result of the $P_{c_{O_2}}$ and $P_{c_{CO_2}}$ mixture that occurs in the pulmonary veins is reflected downstream in the $P_{a_{O_2}}$ and $P_{a_{CO_2}}$ of an arterial blood gas sample (see Table 7–1).

It should also be noted that as the $P_{A_{CO_2}}$ decreases from the bottom to the top of the lungs, the progressive reduction of the CO_2 level in the end-capillary blood causes the pH to become more alkaline. The overall pH mixture in the pulmonary veins and, subsequently, in the arterial blood is normally about 7.35 to 7.45 (see Figure 7–1).

Figure 9–7 (page 282) summarizes the important effects of changing $\dot{V}/\dot{Q}$ ratios.

Respiratory Quotient

Gas exchange between the systemic capillaries and the cells is called **internal respiration**. Under normal circumstances, about 250 ml of oxygen are

---

†See The Ideal Alveolar Gas Equation, Chapter Three.

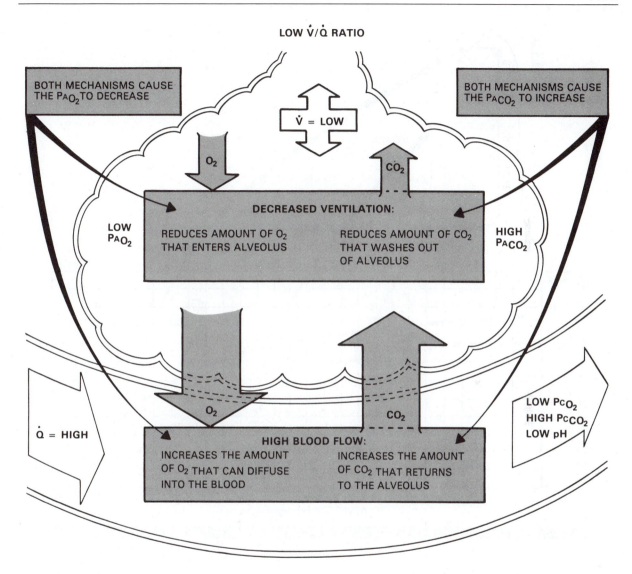

FIGURE 9–4.

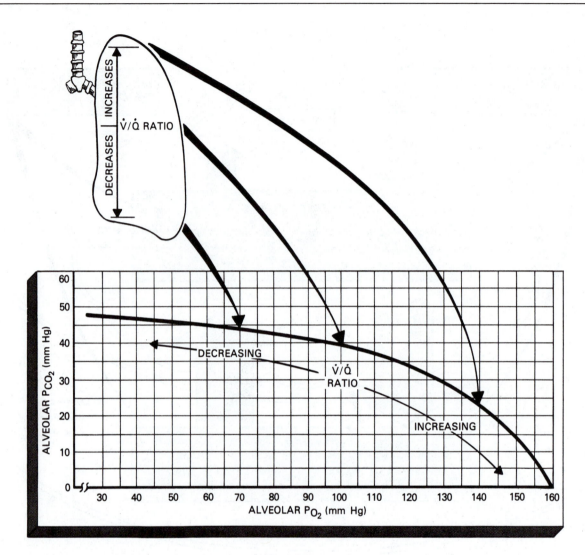

FIGURE 9–5. The O_2–CO_2 diagram.

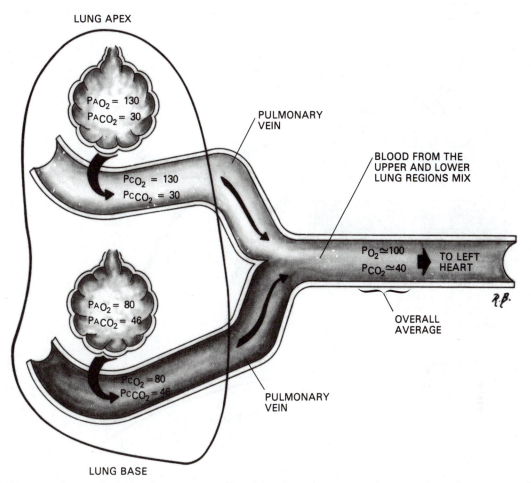

FIGURE 9–6.   The mixing of pulmonary capillary blood gases (Pc_{O_2} and Pc_{CO_2}) from the upper and lower lung regions.

consumed by the tissues during one minute. In exchange, the cells produce about 200 ml of carbon dioxide. Clinically, the ratio between the volume of oxygen consumed ($\dot{V}_{O_2}$) and the volume of carbon dioxide produced ($\dot{V}_{CO_2}$) is called the **respiratory quotient** (RQ) and is expressed as follows:

$$RQ = \frac{\dot{V}_{CO_2}}{\dot{V}_{O_2}}$$

$$= \frac{200 \text{ ml } CO_2/\text{min}}{250 \text{ ml } O_2/\text{min}}$$

$$= 0.8$$

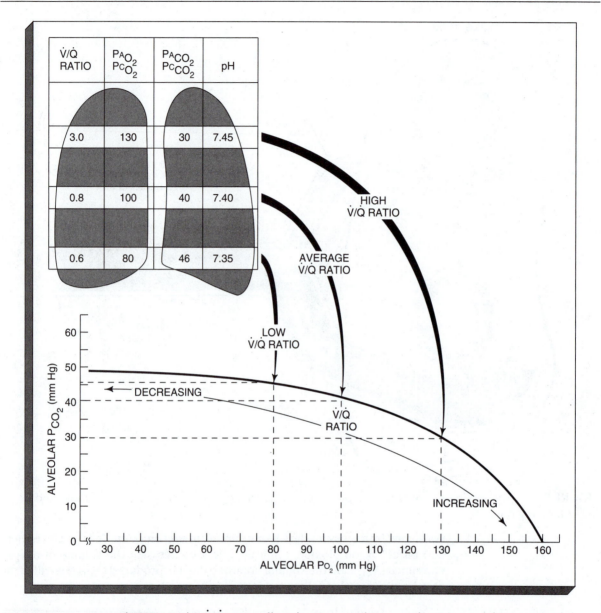

FIGURE 9–7. How changes in the $\dot{V}/\dot{Q}$ ratio affect the $P_{A_{O_2}}$ and $P_{c_{CO_2}}$, the $P_{A_{CO_2}}$ and $P_{c_{CO_2}}$, and the pH of the pulmonary blood.

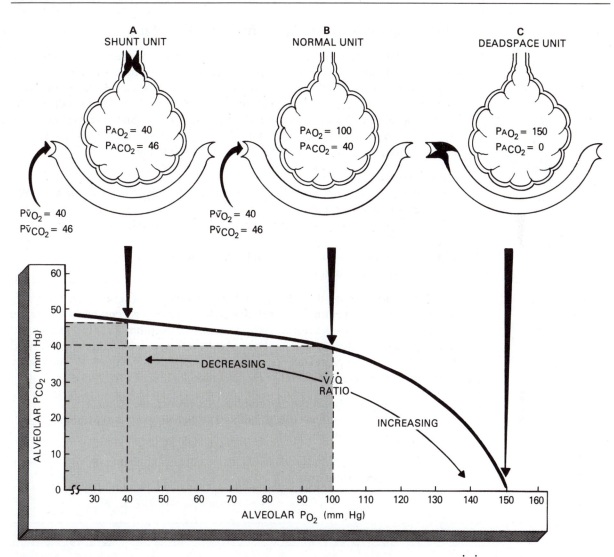

FIGURE 9–8. Alveolar O_2 and CO_2 pressure changes that occur as a result of $\dot{V}/\dot{Q}$ ratio changes caused by respiratory disorders. *A*) shunt unit; *B*) normal unit; *C*) deadspace unit.

Respiratory Exchange Ratio

Gas exchange between the pulmonary capillaries and the alveoli is called **external respiration**, since this gas exchange is between the body and the external environment. The quantity of oxygen and carbon dioxide exchanged during a period of one minute is called the **respiratory exchange ratio** (RR). Under normal conditions, the RR equals the RQ.

How Respiratory Disorders Affect the $\dot{V}/\dot{Q}$ Ratio

In respiratory disorders, the $\dot{V}/\dot{Q}$ ratio is always altered. For example, in disorders that diminish pulmonary perfusion, the affected lung area receives little or no blood flow in relation to ventilation. This condition causes the $\dot{V}/\dot{Q}$ ratio to increase. As a result, a larger portion of the alveolar ventilation will not be physiologically effective and is said to be **wasted** or **deadspace** ventilation. When the $\dot{V}/\dot{Q}$ ratio increases, the $P_{A_{O_2}}$ increases and the $P_{A_{CO_2}}$ decreases. Pulmonary disorders that increase the $\dot{V}/\dot{Q}$ ratio include the following:

- Pulmonary emboli
- Partial or complete obstruction in the pulmonary artery or some of the arterioles (e.g., atherosclerosis, collagen disease)
- Extrinsic pressure on the pulmonary vessels (e.g., pneumothorax, hydrothorax, tumors)
- Destruction of the pulmonary vessels (e.g., emphysema)
- Decreased cardiac output

In disorders that diminish pulmonary ventilation, the affected lung area receives little or no ventilation in relation to blood flow. This condition causes the $\dot{V}/\dot{Q}$ ratio to decrease. As a result, a larger portion of the pulmonary blood flow will not be physiologically effective in terms of gas exchange, and is said to be **shunted blood**. When the $\dot{V}/\dot{Q}$ ratio decreases, the $P_{A_{O_2}}$ decreases and the $P_{A_{CO_2}}$ increases. Pulmonary disorders that decrease the $\dot{V}/\dot{Q}$ ratio include the following:

- Obstructive lung disorders (e.g., emphysema, bronchitis, asthma)
- Restrictive lung disorders (e.g., pneumonia, silicosis, pulmonary fibrosis)
- Hypoventilation from any cause

Figure 9–8 summarizes the O_2–CO_2 effects of changing $\dot{V}/\dot{Q}$ ratios in response to respiratory disorders.

SELF-ASSESSMENT QUESTIONS

1. Overall, the normal $\dot{V}/\dot{Q}$ ratio is about
   - a. 0.2
   - b. 0.4
   - c. 0.6
   - d. 0.8
   - e. 1.0
2. In the healthy individual in the upright position, the
   - I. $\dot{V}/\dot{Q}$ ratio is highest in the lower lung regions
   - II. $P_{A_{O_2}}$ is lowest in the upper lung regions

III. $\dot{V}/\dot{Q}$ ratio is lowest in the upper lung regions

IV. $P_{A_{CO_2}}$ is highest in the lower lung regions

    a. I only

    b. II only

    c. IV only

    d. I and IV only

    e. II and IV only

3. When the $\dot{V}/\dot{Q}$ ratio decreases, the

    I. $P_{A_{O_2}}$ falls

    II. $P_{c_{CO_2}}$ increases

    III. $P_{A_{CO_2}}$ rises

    IV. $P_{c_{O_2}}$ decreases

        a. I only

        b. III only

        c. I and II only

        d. II, III, and IV only

        e. I, II, III, and IV

4. When alveolar ventilation is 7 L/min and the pulmonary blood flow is 9.5 L/min, the $\dot{V}/\dot{Q}$ ratio is about

    a. 0.4

    b. 0.5

    c. 0.6

    d. 0.7

    e. 0.8

5. If a patient's tissue cells consume 275 ml of O_2 per minute and produce 195 ml of CO_2 per minute, what is the RQ?

    a. 0.65

    b. 0.7

    c. 0.8

    d. 0.96

    e. 1.25

Answers appear in Appendix VII.

CHAPTER 10

CONTROL OF VENTILATION

OBJECTIVES

By the end of this chapter, the student should be able to:

1. Describe the function of the following *respiratory neurons* of the *medulla oblongata:*
   —The dorsal respiratory group
   —The ventral respiratory group
2. Describe the influence of the following *pontine respiratory centers* on the respiratory neurons of the medulla oblongata:
   —Apneustic center
   —Pneumotaxic center
3. List conditions that can depress the respiratory neurons.
4. Describe how the following regulate the respiratory neurons:
   —Central chemoreceptors
   —Peripheral chemoreceptors
   —Reflexes that influence ventilation
     • Hering-Breuer inflation reflex
     • Deflation reflex
     • Irritant reflex
     • Juxtapulmonary-capillary receptor reflex
     • Reflexes from the aortic and carotid sinus baroreceptors
     • Other stimuli that affect ventilation
5. Complete the self-assessment questions at the end of this chapter.

The intrinsic rhythmicity of respiration is primarily controlled by specific neural areas located in the reticular substance of the medulla and pons of the brain. These neural areas possess monitoring, stimulating, and inhibiting properties that continually adjust the ventilatory pattern to meet specific metabolic needs. Also received and coordinated in these respiratory neural areas are the voluntary signals transmitted by the cerebral cortex during a variety of ventilatory maneuvers such as talking, singing, sniffing, coughing, or blowing into a woodwind instrument.

To fully understand this subject, a basic knowledge of (1) the function of the major respiratory components of the medulla, (2) the influence of the pontine respiratory centers on the respiratory components of the medulla, (3) the major monitoring systems that influence the respiratory components of the medulla, and (4) the reflexes that influence ventilation is necessary.

THE RESPIRATORY COMPONENTS OF THE MEDULLA

Although knowledge concerning this subject is incomplete, it is now believed that two groups of **respiratory neurons** in the medulla oblongata are responsible for coordinating the intrinsic rhythmicity of respiration: these are (1) the **dorsal respiratory group** (DRG), and (2) the **ventral respiratory group** (VRG) (Figure 10–1).

Dorsal Respiratory Group

The dorsal respiratorygroup (DRG) consists chiefly of **inspiratory neurons**. The DRG neurons are believed to be responsible for the basic rhythm of

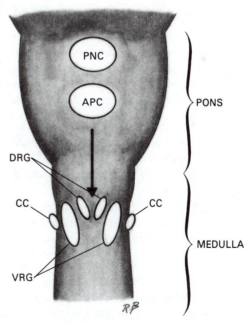

FIGURE 10–1. Schematic illustration of the respiratory components of the lower brainstem (pons and medulla). PNC = pneumotaxic center; APC = apneustic center; DRG = dorsal respiratory group; VRG = ventral respiratory group; CC = central chemoreceptors.

ventilation (see Figure 10–1). They (1) receive numerous signals from the body regarding the respiratory needs; (2) evaluate and prioritize the various signals; and, depending on the respiratory needs, (3) emit neural impulses every few seconds to the muscles of inspiration, primarily the diaphragm. The signals released by the DRG continue for about 1 to 2 seconds and then cease abruptly, causing the muscles of inspiration to relax. During exhalation, which lasts for about 2 to 3 seconds, the natural elastic recoil forces of the lungs cause the lungs to deflate.

Ventral Respiratory Group

The ventral respiratory group (VRG) contains both **inspiratory** and **expiratory neurons**. During normal quiet breathing, the VRG is almost entirely dormant, since the lungs passively return to their original size by virtue of their own elastic recoil forces. During heavy exercise or stress, however, the expiratory neurons of the VRG actively send impulses to the muscles of exhalation (e.g., abdominal muscles) and the accessory muscles of inspiration innervated by the vagus nerve (e.g., sternocleidomastoid) (see Figure 10–1).

The Influence of the Pontine Respiratory Centers on the Respiratory Components of the Medulla

The pontine respiratory centers consist of the **apneustic center** and the **pneumotaxic center**. Although these centers are known to exist and can be made to operate under experimental conditions, their functional significance in man is still not fully understood. It appears that these centers function to some degree to modify and fine-tune the rhythmicity of respirations.

Apneustic Center.   The apneustic center is located in the middle and lower pons (see Figure 10–1). If unrestrained, the apneustic center continually sends neural impulses to the DRG and VRG in the medulla. This action causes a prolonged, gasping type of inspiratory maneuver called **apneustic breathing**. Under normal conditions, however, the apneustic center receives numerous signals that suppress its function, thus permitting expiration to occur. Such signals include the strong inhibitory impulses transmitted by the pneumotaxic center and the Hering-Breuer inflation reflex.

Pneumotaxic Center.   The pneumotaxic center is located in the reticular substance of the upper one-third of the pons (see Figure 10–1). By varying the neural impulses that suppress the apneustic center, the pneumotaxic area enhances the rhythmicity of the breathing pattern. Neural impulses from the pneumotaxic center simultaneously cause (1) the depth of breathing to decrease and (2) the rate of breathing to increase, by almost an equal amount. Because these two respiratory maneuvers (rapid and shallow breaths) offset each other, the total change in minute ventilation is unremarkable.

Some investigators believe the pneumotaxic center is closely related to the so-called **panting center** in animals such as dogs. For example, when the dog becomes overheated, the panting center causes the dog to breathe with rapid, shallow breaths that evaporate large amounts of water from the dog's upper airways, thus cooling the animal. In man, the pneumotaxic center appears to have an effect similar to the Hering-Breuer inflation reflex.*

Failure of the Respiratory Components of the Medulla

There are several clinical conditions that can depress the function of the respiratory components of the medulla. Such conditions include (1) reduced blood flow through the medulla as a result of excess pressure caused by a cerebral edema or some other intracerebral abnormality, (2) acute poliomyelitis, and (3) ingestion of drugs that depress the central nervous system.

MONITORING SYSTEMS THAT INFLUENCE THE RESPIRATORY COMPONENTS OF THE MEDULLA

From moment to moment, the respiratory components of the medulla (DRG and VRG) activate specific ventilatory patterns based upon information received from several different monitoring systems throughout the body. The major known monitoring systems are the (1) **central chemoreceptors** and (2) **peripheral chemoreceptors**. Certain neural impulses transmitted to the respiratory neurons during exercise and certain reflexes also influence ventilation.

Central Chemoreceptors

The most powerful stimulus known to influence the respiratory components (DRG and VRG) of the medulla is an excess concentration of hydrogen ions $[H^+]$ in the cerebrospinal fluid (CSF). The central chemoreceptors, which are located bilaterally and ventrally in the substance of the medulla, are responsible for monitoring the H^+ ion concentration of the CSF. In fact, a portion of the central chemoreceptors is actually in direct contact with the CSF. It is believed that the central chemoreceptors transmit signals to the respiratory components of the medulla by the following mechanism:

1. As the CO_2 level increases in the arterial blood (e.g., during hypoventilation), the CO_2 molecules diffuse across a semipermeable membrane, called the

---

*The Hering-Breuer inflation reflex is described in further detail later in this chapter, page 297.

blood–brain barrier, which separates the blood from the CSF. The blood–brain barrier is very permeable to CO_2 molecules but relatively impermeable to H^+ and HCO_3^- ions.

2. As CO_2 moves into the CSF, it forms carbonic acid by means of the following reaction:

$$CO_2 + H_2O \rightleftharpoons H_2CO_3 \rightleftharpoons H^+ + HCO_3^-$$

3. Because the CSF lacks hemoglobin and carbonic anhydrase and has a relatively low bicarbonate and protein level, the overall buffering system in the CSF is very slow. Because of the inefficient CSF buffering system, the H^+ generated from the above reaction rapidly increases and therefore significantly reduces the pH level in the CSF.

4. The liberated H^+ ions cause the central chemoreceptors to transmit signals to the respiratory component in the medulla, which, in turn, increases the alveolar ventilation.

5. The increased ventilation reduces the Pa_{CO_2} and, subsequently, the P_{CO_2} in the CSF. As the P_{CO_2} in the CSF decreases, the H^+ ion concentration of the CSF also falls. This action decreases the stimulation of the central chemoreceptors. Thus, the neural signals to the respiratory components in the medulla also diminish; this, in turn, causes alveolar ventilation to decrease.

6. In view of the above sequences, it should be understood that the central chemoreceptors regulate ventilation through the indirect effects of CO_2 on the pH level of the CSF (Figure 10–2).

Peripheral Chemoreceptors.   The peripheral chemoreceptors are special oxygen-sensitive cells that react to reductions of oxygen levels in the arterial blood. They are located high in the neck at the bifurcation of the internal and external carotid arteries and on the aortic arch (Figure 10–3). They are near to, but distinct from, the *baroreceptors* (pressoreceptors) (see Figure 5–10). The peripheral chemoreceptors are also called the *carotid and aortic bodies*.

The carotid and aortic bodies are composed of epithelial-like cells and neuron terminals in intimate contact with the arterial blood. When activated by a low Pa_{O_2}, *afferent* (sensory) signals are transmitted to the respiratory components in the medulla by way of the glossopharyngeal nerve (9th cranial nerve) from the carotid bodies and by way of the vagus nerve (10th cranial nerve) from the aortic bodies. This action, in turn, causes *efferent* (motor) signals to be transmitted to the respiratory muscles, causing ventilation to increase (Figure 10–4). Compared to the aortic bodies, the carotid bodies play a much greater role in initiating an increased ventilatory rate in response to reduced arterial oxygen levels.

As shown in Figure 10–5, page 294, the peripheral chemoreceptors are not significantly activated until the oxygen content of the inspired air is low enough to reduce the Pa_{O_2} to 60 mm Hg (Sa_{O_2} about 90 percent). Beyond this point, any

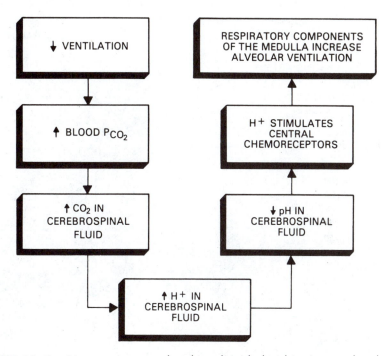

FIGURE 10–2. How an increased carbon dioxide level increases alveolar ventilation.

further reduction in the Pa_{O_2} causes a marked increase in ventilation. *Suppression* of the peripheral chemoreceptors is seen, however, when the Pa_{O_2} falls below 30 mm Hg.

In the patient with a low Pa_{O_2} and a chronically high Pa_{CO_2} level (e.g., the end-stages of emphysema), the peripheral chemoreceptors may be totally responsible for the control of ventilation. This is because a chronically high CO_2 concentration in the CSF inactivates the H^+ sensitivity of the central chemoreceptor—that is, HCO_3^- moves into the CSF via the active transport mechanism and combines with H^+, thus returning the pH to normal. A compensatory response to a chronically high CO_2 concentration, however, is the enhancement of the sensitivity of the peripheral chemoreceptors at higher CO_2 levels (Figure 10–6).

Finally, it is important to understand that the peripheral chemoreceptors are specifically sensitive to the P_{O_2} of the blood and relatively insensitive to the oxygen content of the blood. The precise mechanism for this exclusive P_{O_2} sensitivity is not fully understood. It is known, however, that the blood flow through the peripheral chemoreceptors is very high in relation to metabolism. Thus, the overall extraction of oxygen is relatively low, and therefore the difference between the oxygen content in the arterial blood and the venous blood $[C(a - \bar{v})_{O_2}]$ is small.

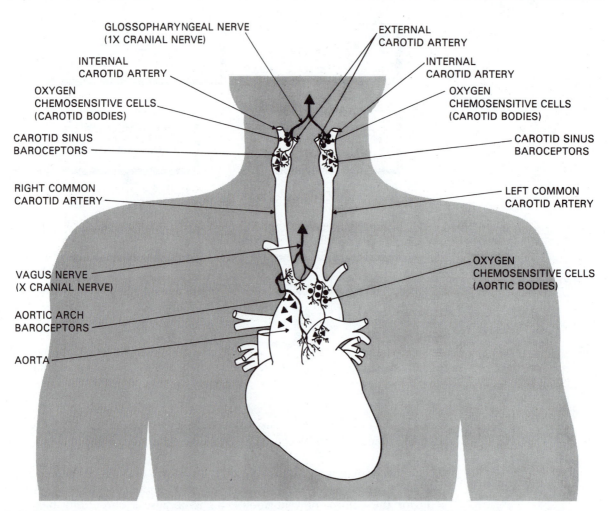

FIGURE 10–3. Location of the carotid and aortic bodies (the peripheral chemoreceptors).

Clinically, this exclusive Pa_{O_2} sensitivity can be misleading. There are certain conditions in which the Pa_{O_2} is normal (and therefore the peripheral chemoreceptors are not stimulated), yet the oxygen content of the blood is dangerously low. Such conditions include chronic anemia, carbon monoxide poisoning, and methemoglobinemia.

Other Factors That Stimulate the Peripheral Chemoreceptors. Although the peripheral chemoreceptors are primarily stimulated by a reduced Pa_{O_2} level, they are also activated by a decreased pH (increased H^+ level). This is an important feature of the peripheral chemoreceptors, since there are many situations in which

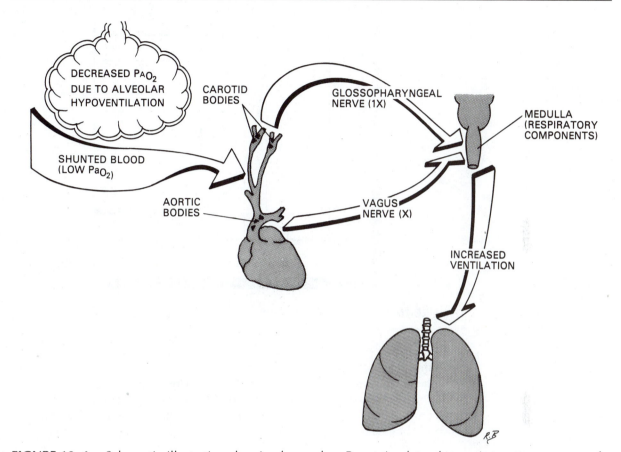

FIGURE 10–4. Schematic illustration showing how a low Pa_{O_2} stimulates the respiratory components of the medulla to increase alveolar ventilation.

a change in arterial H^+ ion levels can occur by means other than a primary change in the P_{CO_2}. In fact, because the H^+ ions do not readily move across the blood–brain barrier, the peripheral chemoreceptors play a major role in initiating ventilation whenever the H^+ ion concentration increases for reasons other than an increased Pa_{CO_2}. For example, the accumulation of lactic acid in the blood stimulates hyperventilation almost entirely through the peripheral chemoreceptors (Figure 10–7, page 296).

The peripheral chemoreceptors are also stimulated by (1) hypoperfusion (e.g., stagnant hypoxia), (2) increased temperature, (3) nicotine, and (4) the direct effect of Pa_{CO_2}. The response of the peripheral chemoreceptors to Pa_{CO_2} stimulation, however, is minor and not nearly so great as the response generated by the central chemoreceptors. The peripheral chemoreceptors do respond faster

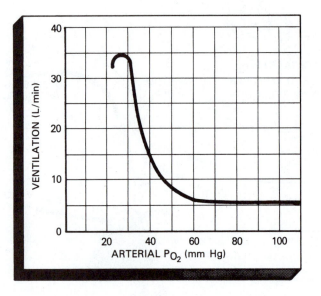

FIGURE 10–5. The effect of low Pa_{O_2} levels on ventilation.

than the central chemoreceptors to an increased Pa_{CO_2}. This occurs because the peripheral chemoreceptors are stimulated directly by the CO_2 molecule, whereas the central chemoreceptors are stimulated by the H^+ generated by the CO_2 hydration reaction in the CSF—a reaction that occurs slowly in the absence of carbonic anhydrase (see Figure 10–2).

Other Responses Activated by the Peripheral Chemoreceptors.   In addition to the increased ventilation activated by the peripheral chemoreceptors, other responses can occur as a result of peripheral chemoreceptor stimulation, including the following:

• Peripheral vasoconstriction
• Increased pulmonary vascular resistance
• Systemic arterial hypertension
• Tachycardia
• Increase in left ventricular performance

How Environmental Changes Can Influence the Peripheral and Central Chemoreceptors.   To facilitate the understanding of how the peripheral and central chemoreceptors control the ventilatory pattern, consider the following chain of events that develops when an individual who normally resides at sea level ascends to a high altitude (say, to the mountains to ski) for a period of two weeks.

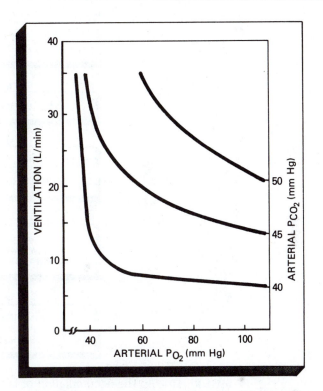

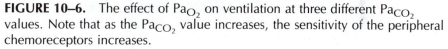

FIGURE 10–6. The effect of Pa_{O_2} on ventilation at three different Pa_{CO_2} values. Note that as the Pa_{CO_2} value increases, the sensitivity of the peripheral chemoreceptors increases.

Stimulation of the Peripheral Chemoreceptors.

1. As the individual ascends the mountain, the barometric pressure, and therefore the P_{O_2}, of the atmosphere progressively decrease. (Remember, however, that the oxygen percentage is still 21 percent.)
2. As the atmospheric P_{O_2} decreases, the individual's oxygen pressure in the arterial blood (Pa_{O_2}) also decreases.
3. As the individual continues to ascend the mountain, the Pa_{O_2} eventually falls low enough (about 60 mm Hg) to stimulate the peripheral chemoreceptors, which, in turn, transmit signals to the medulla to increase ventilation.
4. The increased ventilation initiated by the peripheral chemoreceptors causes a secondary decrease in the Pa_{CO_2}. The individual hyperventilates in response to the reduced Pa_{O_2} level.
5. Because the peripheral chemoreceptors do not acclimate to a decreased oxygen concentration, hyperventilation will continue for the entire time the individual remains at the high altitude.

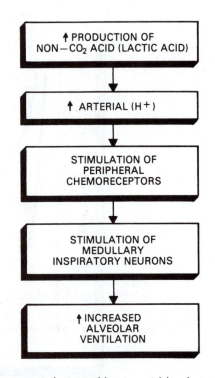

FIGURE 10–7.   The accumulation of lactic acid leads to an increased alveolar ventilation primarily through the stimulation of the peripheral chemoreceptors.

Readjustment of the Central Chemoreceptors at High Altitudes.   **In response to the hyperventilation that occurs while the individual is at the high altitude, the central chemoreceptors readjust to the lower CO_2 level because of the following chain of events:**

1. As the individual hyperventilates to offset the low atmospheric P_{O_2}, the individual's Pa_{CO_2} level decreases.
2. In response to the decreased Pa_{CO_2}, the CO_2 molecules in the CSF move into the blood until equilibrium occurs.
3. This reaction causes the pH of the CSF to increase.
4. Over the next 48 hours, however, HCO_3^- will also leave the CSF (via the active transport mechanism) to correct the pH back to normal. In short, the individual's CSF readjusts to the low CO_2 level.

Stimulation of the Central Chemoreceptors After Leaving a High Altitude.   Interestingly, even after the individual returns to a lower altitude, hyperventilation continues for a few days. The reason for this is as follows:

1. As the individual moves down the mountain, the barometric pressure steadily increases, and therefore the atmospheric P_{O_2} increases.
2. As the atmospheric P_{O_2} increases, the individual's Pa_{O_2} also increases and eventually ceases to stimulate the individual's peripheral chemoreceptors.
3. As the stimulation of the peripheral chemoreceptors decreases, the individual's ventilatory rate decreases.
4. As the ventilatory rate declines, however, the individual's Pa_{CO_2} progressively increases.
5. As the Pa_{CO_2} increases, CO_2 molecules move across the blood–brain barrier into the CSF.
6. As CO_2 moves into the CSF, H^+ ions are formed, causing the pH of the CSF to decrease.
7. The H^+ ions liberated in the above reaction stimulate the central chemoreceptors to increase the individual's ventilatory rate.
8. Eventually, HCO_3^- ions move across the blood–brain barrier into the CSF to correct the pH back to normal. When this occurs, the individual's ventilatory pattern will be as it was before the trip to the mountains.

REFLEXES THAT INFLUENCE VENTILATION

A number of reflexes are known to influence the rate of ventilation.

Hering-Breuer Inflation Reflex

The Hering-Breuer inflation reflex is generated by stretch receptors located in the walls of the bronchi and bronchioles that become excited when the lungs overinflate. Signals from these receptors travel through the vagus nerve to the respiratory components in the medulla, causing inspiration to cease. In essence, the lungs themselves provide a feedback mechanism to terminate inspiration. Instead of a reflex to control ventilation, the Hering-Breuer reflex appears to be a protective mechanism that prevents pulmonary damage caused by excessive lung inflation. The significance of the Hering-Breuer reflex in the adult at normal tidal volumes is controversial; it appears to have more significance in the control of ventilation in the newborn.

Deflation Reflex

When the lungs are compressed or deflated, an increased rate of breathing results. The precise mechanism responsible for this reflex is not known. Some workers believe that the increased rate of breathing may be due to the reduced stimulation of receptors serving the Hering-Breuer inflation reflex rather than to the stimulation of specific deflation receptors. Others, however, think that the deflation reflex is not due to the absence of receptor stimulation of the Hering-Breuer reflex, since the reflex is still seen when the temperature of the bronchi and bronchioles is less than 8°C. The Hering-Breuer reflex is not seen when the bronchi and bronchioles are below this temperature.

Irritant Reflex

When the lungs are exposed to noxious gases, the irritant receptors may also be stimulated. The irritant receptors are subepithelial mechanoreceptors located in the trachea, bronchi, and bronchioles. When the receptors are activated, a reflex response causes the ventilatory rate to increase. Stimulation of the irritant receptors may also produce a reflex cough and bronchoconstriction.

Juxtapulmonary-capillary Receptors

Juxtapulmonary-capillary receptors, or *J receptors*, are located in the interstitial tissues between the pulmonary capillaries and the alveoli. It is believed that the J receptors are activated by the following:

- Pulmonary capillary congestion
- Capillary hypertension
- Edema of the alveolar walls
- Humoral agents (serotonin)
- Lung deflation
- Emboli

When the J receptors are stimulated, a reflex response triggers rapid, shallow breathing.

Reflexes from the Aortic and Carotid Sinus Baroreceptors

The normal function of the aortic and carotid sinus baroreceptors, located near the aortic and carotid peripheral chemoreceptors, is to initiate reflexes that causes (1) a decreased heart and ventilatory rate in response to an elevated systemic blood pressure and (2) an increased heart and ventilatory rate in response to a reduced systemic blood pressure (see Figure 5–10).

Other Stimuli That Affect Ventilation

Many stimuli can influence ventilation, including the following:

1. A sudden cold stimulus, such as plunging into very cold water, may cause respiration to temporarily cease.
2. A sudden pain may cause a temporary cessation of breathing. Prolonged pain, however, activates the general adaptation syndrome and increases the breathing rate.

3. Irritation of the pharynx or larynx by touch or chemicals can trigger an immediate cessation of breathing, followed by an episode of coughing.

4. The stretching of the anal sphincter triggers an increased respiratory rate. Clinically, this technique is sometimes used to activate respirations during emergencies—for example, during periods of apnea in newborn infants.

5. Light pressure applied to the thorax may increase ventilation. The significance of this chest wall reflex in humans is unknown.

SELF-ASSESSMENT QUESTIONS

1. The respiratory components of the medulla consist of which of the following?
   - I. Dorsal respiratory group
   - II. Apneustic center
   - III. Ventral respiratory group
   - IV. Pneumotaxic center
     - a. I only
     - b. II only
     - c. I and III only
     - d. II and IV only
     - e. I, II, III, and IV

2. Which of the following has the most powerful effect on the respiratory components of the medulla?
   - a. Decreased O_2
   - b. Increased H^+
   - c. Decreased CO_2
   - d. Increased pH
   - e. Decreased HCO_3^-

3. Which of the following may cause a temporary cessation in breathing?
   - I. Sudden pain
   - II. Pharynx or larynx irritation
   - III. Sudden cold
   - IV. Inhalation of noxious gases
     - a. I only
     - b. II only
     - c. IV only
     - d. III and IV only
     - e. I, II, and III only

4. Which of the following will readily diffuse across the blood–brain barrier?
   - I. CO_2
   - II. H^+
   - III. HCO_3^-

IV. H_2CO_3
   a. I only
   b. II only
   c. III only
   d. II and IV only
   e. II, III, and IV only

5. When the systemic blood pressure increases, the aortic and carotid sinus baroreceptors initiate reflexes that cause a/an:
   I. increased heart rate
   II. decreased ventilatory rate
   III. increased ventilatory rate
   IV. decreased heart rate
   a. I only
   b. II only
   c. III only
   d. II and IV only
   e. I and III only

6. The peripheral chemoreceptors are significantly activated when the P_{O_2} decreases to about
   a. 80 mm Hg
   b. 75 mm Hg
   c. 70 mm Hg
   d. 65 mm Hg
   e. 60 mm Hg

7. Stimulation of the peripheral chemoreceptors can cause which of the following?
   I. Tachycardia
   II. Decreased left ventricular performance
   III. Increased pulmonary vascular resistance
   IV. Systemic arterial hypertension
   a. I only
   b. II only
   c. IV only
   d. I, III, and IV only
   e. I, II, III, and IV

8. Suppression of the peripheral chemoreceptors begins when the P_{O_2} falls below
   a. 50 mm Hg
   b. 40 mm Hg
   c. 30 mm Hg
   d. 20 mm Hg
   e. 10 mm Hg

9. In addition to a low P_{O_2}, the peripheral chemoreceptors are also sensitive to a/an:

      I. decreased H^+

      II. increased P_{CO_2}

      III. decreased pH

      IV. increased temperature

        a. I only

        b. II only

        c. III only

        d. I, II, and III only

        e. II, III, and IV only

10. Which of the following protects the lungs from excessive inflation?

        a. Juxtapulmonary-capillary receptors

        b. Hering-Breuer inflation reflex

        c. Deflation reflex

        d. Irritant reflex

        e. Reflexes from the aortic and carotid sinus baroreceptors

Answers appear in Appendix VII.

CHAPTER 11

CARDIOPULMONARY PHYSIOLOGY OF THE FETUS AND THE NEWBORN

OBJECTIVES

By the end of this chapter, the student should be able to:

1. Describe the developmental events that occur during the following periods of fetal life:
   —Embryonic period
   —Pseudoglandular period
   —Canalicular period
   —Terminal sac period
2. Describe how the following components relate to the placenta:
   —Umbilical arteries
   —Cotyledons
   —Fetal vessels
   —Chorionic villi
   —Intervillous space
   —Spiral arterioles
   —Umbilical vein
3. List the three major reasons why oxygen transfers from maternal to fetal blood.
4. List the factors believed to cause the wide variance between the maternal and fetal P_{O_2} and P_{CO_2}.
5. Describe how the following components relate to the fetal circulation:
   —Umbilical vein
   —Liver
   —Ductus venosus
   —Inferior vena cava
   —Right atrium
   —Superior vena cava
   —Foramen ovale

—Pulmonary veins

　　　—Left ventricle

　　　—Right ventricle

　　　—Ductus arteriosus

　　　—Common iliac arteries

　　　—External and internal iliacs

　6. Describe what happens to the following special structures of fetal circulation after birth:

　　　—Placenta

　　　—Umbilical arteries

　　　—Umbilical vein

　　　—Ductus venosus

　　　—Foramen ovale

　　　—Ductus arteriosus

　7. Describe how the fetal lung fluid is removed from the lungs at birth.

　8. List the number of alveoli at birth and at 12 years of age.

　9. Describe the pressure-volume changes of the lungs of the newborn during the first two weeks of life.

　10. Identify the average newborn values for the following:

　　　—Compliance

　　　—Airway resistance

　11. Describe how the following circulatory changes develop at birth:

　　　—Decrease in pulmonary vascular resistance

　　　—Closure of the foramen ovale

　　　—Constriction of the ductus arteriosus

　12. Describe the role of the following in the control of ventilation of the newborn:

　　　—Peripheral chemoreceptors

　　　—Central chemoreceptors

　　　—Infant reflexes

　　　　• Trigeminal reflex

　　　　• Irritant reflex

　　　　• Head paradoxical reflex

　13. List the following normal clinical parameters of the newborn:

　　　—Lung volumes and capacities

　　　—Respiratory rate

　　　—Heart rate

　　　—Blood pressure

　14. Complete the self-assessment questions at the end of this chapter.

FETAL LUNG DEVELOPMENT

During fetal life, the development of the lungs is arbitrarily divided into four periods: **embryonic, pseudoglandular, canalicular,** and **terminal sac.**

Embryonic Period. This period encompasses the developmental events that occur during the first 5 weeks after fertilization. The lungs first appear as a small bud arising from the esophagus on the 24th day of embryonic life (Figure 11–1). On about the 28th day of gestation, it branches into the right and left lung buds. Between the 30th and 32nd day, primitive lobar bronchi begin to appear—two on the left lung bud and three on the right lung bud. By the end of the 5th week, cartilage can be seen in the trachea, and the mainstem bronchi are surrounded by primitive cellular mesoderm, which gradually differentiates into bronchial smooth muscle, connective tissue, and cartilaginous plates, as the lungs develop.

Pseudoglandular Period. This period includes the developmental processes that occur between the 5th and the 16th week of gestation. By the 6th week, all the segments are present and the subsegmental bronchi are also well represented. The subsegmental bronchi continue to undergo further branching throughout this developmental stage, and by the 16th week all the subsegmental bronchi are present.

By the 10th week, ciliated columnar epithelial cells, a deeper basal layer of irregular cells, and a primitive basement membrane appear in the conducting airways. Goblet cells also begin to appear at this time in the trachea and large bronchi. Between the 10th and 14th weeks, there is a sudden burst of bronchial branching. It is estimated that as much as 75 percent of the conducting airways develop at this time.

At 11 weeks of gestation, cartilage begins to appear in the lobar bronchi. Cartilaginous airways continue to form until about 24 weeks gestation. By the 12th week, the bronchial mucous glands start to appear. Immature smooth muscle cells are also noted at this time in the pulmonary arteries. As the tracheobronchial tree develops, new bronchial glands form until 25 to 26 weeks gestation. At birth, the concentration of bronchial glands is about 17 glands per square millimeter (mm^2). In the adult, the concentration drops to about 1 gland/mm^2, as a result of bronchial elongation and widening. By the 16th week, there are about 20 generations of bronchial airways.

Canalicular Period. This period includes the developmental events between the 17th and 24th week of gestation. During this time, the terminal bronchioles continue to proliferate and primitive respiratory bronchioles begin to appear. The lung mass becomes highly vascularized and the lung lobes are clearly recognizable. At about the 20th week of gestation, the lymphatic vessels begin to appear.

Terminal Sac Period. This period begins at the 24th week of gestation and continues until term (between the 38th and 41st week of gestation). The

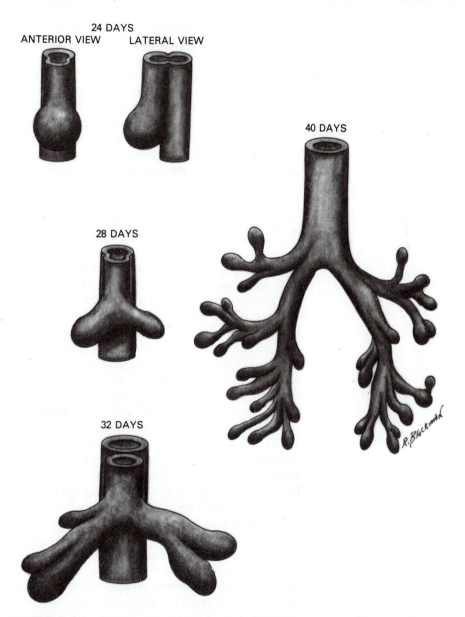

FIGURE 11–1. Schematic representation of the developmental events that occur in the human lung during the embryonic and pseudoglandular periods (see text for explanation).

structures that appeared in the canalicular period continue to proliferate and the entire acinus (respiratory bronchioles, alveolar ducts, alveolar sacs, and alveoli) develops. The type I and type II alveolar cells can be identified at this time, and pulmonary surfactant begins to appear. Although pulmonary capillaries begin to appear at the 24th week, the air–blood interface between the alveoli and the pulmonary capillaries is poorly defined. By the 28th week, the air–blood interface and the quantity of pulmonary surfactant are usually sufficient to support life. By the 34th week, the respiratory acini are well developed. The smooth muscle fibers in the conducting airways begin to appear during the last few weeks of gestation. These muscles continue to mature after birth.

PLACENTA

Following conception, the fertilized egg moves down the **uterine tube** (Fallopian tube) and implants into the wall of the uterus. The placenta develops at the point of implantation. Throughout fetal life, the placenta transfers maternal oxygen and nutrients to the fetus and transfers waste products out of the fetal circulation. When fully developed, the placenta appears as a reddish-brown disk about 20 cm long and 2.5 cm thick. Anatomically, the placenta consists of about 15 to 20 segments called **cotyledons** (Figure 11–2). Each cotyledon is composed of **fetal vessels, chorionic villi,** and **intervillous spaces** (Figure 11–3). Functionally, the cotyledons provide an interface between the maternal and fetal circulation.

Deoxygenated blood is carried from the fetus to the placenta by way of two **umbilical arteries**, which are wrapped around the **umbilical vein** (see Figure 11–3). Normally, the P_{O_2} in the umbilical arteries is about 20 mm Hg and the P_{CO_2} is about 55 mm Hg. Once in the placenta, the umbilical arteries branch and supply each cotyledon. As the umbilical arteries enter the cotyledon, they again branch into the fetal vessels, which then loop around the internal portion of the finger-like projections of the chorionic villi. Externally, the chorionic villi are surrounded by the intervillous space (see Figure 11–3).

Maternal blood from the uterine arteries enters the intervillous space through the **spiral arterioles**. The spiral arterioles continuously spurt jets of oxygenated blood and nutrients around the chorionic villi. Although the maternal blood P_{O_2} is usually normal during the last trimester of pregnancy (80 to 100 mm Hg), the P_{CO_2} is frequently lower than expected (about 33 mm Hg). This decreased maternal P_{CO_2} is caused by the alveolar hyperventilation that develops as the growing infant restricts the mother's diaphragmatic excursion.

Once in the intervillous space, oxygen and nutrients in the maternal blood move through the tissues of the chorionic villi and enter the fetal blood. Oxygen transfers from the maternal to fetal blood because of the (1) maternal–fetal P_{O_2}

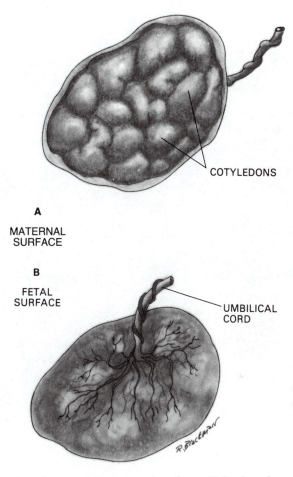

COTYLEDONS

A

MATERNAL
SURFACE

B

FETAL
SURFACE

UMBILICAL
CORD

FIGURE 11–2.   The placenta. *A)* maternal surface; *B)* fetal surface.

gradient, (2) higher hemoglobin concentration in the fetal blood as compared to maternal blood, and (3) greater affinity of fetal hemoglobin (Hb F) for oxygen as compared to adult hemoglobin (Hb A). While the maternal oxygen and nutrients are moving into the fetal blood, carbon dioxide (P_{CO_2} of about 55 mm Hg) and other waste products are moving out of the fetal blood and enter the maternal blood. The blood-to-blood barrier (chorionic villi) is about 3.5 microns (μ) thick.

Oxygenated fetal blood (actually a P_{O_2} of about 30 mm Hg and a P_{CO_2} of about 40 mm Hg) flows out of the chorionic villi (via the fetal vessels) and returns to the

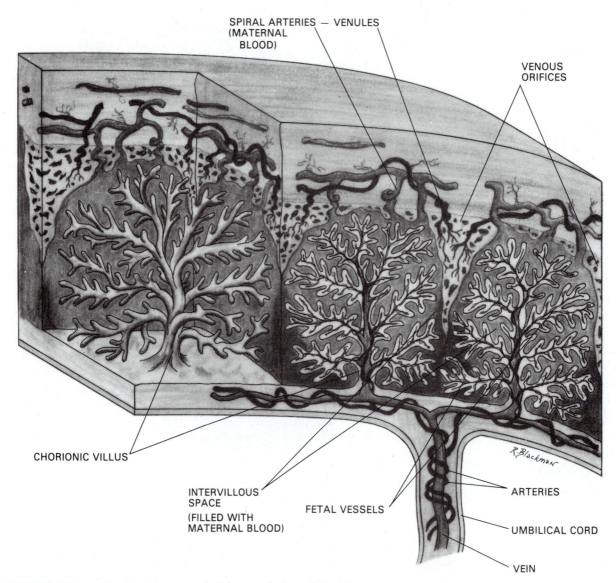

FIGURE 11–3. Anatomic structure of the cotyledon of the placenta.

fetus by way of the umbilical vein (see Figure 11–3). The wide variance between the maternal and fetal P_{O_2} and P_{CO_2} is thought to be due to the following factors:

- The placenta itself is an actively metabolizing organ
- The permeability of the placenta varies from region to region with respect to respiratory gases

- There are fetal and maternal vascular shunts

The fetal waste products in the maternal blood move out of the intervillous space by virtue of the arteriovenous pressure gradient. The pressure in the spiral arteries is about 75 mm Hg and the pressure of the **venous orifices**, which are found adjacent to the spiral arteries, is about 8 mm Hg.

FETAL CIRCULATION

The **umbilical vein** carries oxygenated blood and nutrients from the placenta to the fetus (Figure 11–4). The umbilical vein enters the navel of the fetus and ascends anteriorly to the liver. About one-half of the blood enters the liver, and the rest flows through the **ductus venosus** and enters the **inferior vena cava**. This results in oxygenated fetal blood mixing with deoxygenated blood from the lower parts of the fetal body. The newly mixed fetal blood then travels up the inferior vena cava and enters the **right atrium**, where it again mingles with deoxygenated blood from the **superior vena cava**.

Once in the right atrium, most of the blood flows directly into the left atrium through the **foramen ovale**. While in the left atrium, the fetal blood again mingles with a small amount of deoxygenated blood from the pulmonary veins. The blood then enters the left ventricle and is pumped primarily to the heart and brain.

The rest of the blood in the right atrium moves into the right ventricle and is pumped into the pulmonary artery. Once in the pulmonary artery, most of the blood bypasses the lungs and flows directly into the aorta through the **ductus arteriosus**. A small amount of blood (about 15 percent) flows through the lungs and returns to the left atrium via the pulmonary veins. The Pa_{O_2} in the descending aorta is about 20 mm Hg. Downstream, the **common iliac arteries** branch into the **external** and **internal iliacs**. The blood in the internal iliac branch passes into the umbilical arteries and again flows back to the placenta to pick up oxygen and to drop off waste products.

After birth—and once the lungs and the renal, digestive, and liver functions are established—the special structures of the fetal circulation are no longer required. These special structures go through the following changes:

- The placenta is passed by the mother
- The umbilical arteries atrophy and become the lateral umbilical ligaments
- The umbilical vein becomes the round ligament (*ligamentum teres*) of the liver
- The ductus venosus becomes the *ligamentum venosum*, which is a fibrous cord in the liver
- The flap on the foramen ovale usually closes and becomes a depression in the interatrial septum called the *fossa ovalis*
- The ductus arteriosus atrophies and becomes the *ligamentum arteriosum*

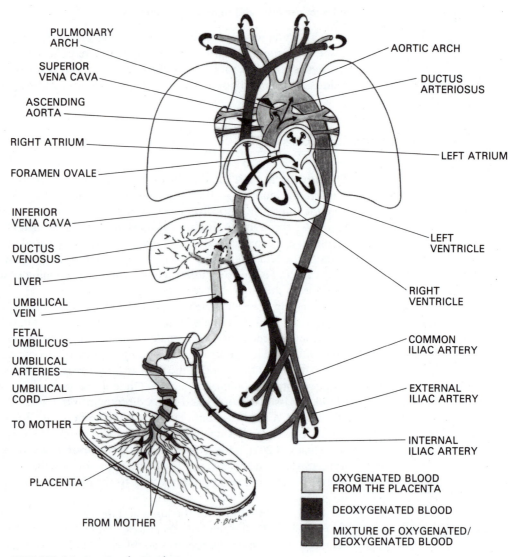

FIGURE 11–4. Fetal circulation.

Fetal Lung Fluids

It is estimated that, at birth, the lungs are partially inflated with liquid approximately equal to the newborn's functional residual capacity. It was once thought that this liquid originated from the aspiration of amniotic fluid, since the fetus normally demonstrates periods of rapid and irregular breathing during the last trimester of gestation. It is now known, however, that this is not the case. The fluid apparently originates from the alveolar cells during fetal development. At birth the fluid is removed from the lungs during the first 24 hours of life primarily by the following mechanisms:

- About one-third of the fluid is squeezed out of the lungs as the infant passes through the birth canal
- About one-third of the fluid is absorbed by the pulmonary capillaries
- About one-third of the fluid is removed by the lymphatic system

Number of Alveoli at Birth

About 24 million primitive alveoli are present at birth. This number, however, represents only about 10 percent of the adult gas exchange units. The number of alveoli continue to increase until about 12 years of age. Thus, it is important to note that respiratory problems during childhood can have a dramatic effect on the anatomy and physiology of the mature pulmonary system.

BIRTH

Moments after birth, an intriguing and dramatic sequence of anatomic and physiologic events occurs. The function of the placenta is suddenly terminated, the lungs rapidly establish themselves as the organ of gas exchange, and all the features of adult circulation are set in place.

First Breath

At birth, the infant is bombarded by a variety of external sensory stimuli (e.g., thermal, tactile, and visual). At the same time, the placenta ceases to function, causing the fetal blood P_{O_2} to decrease, the P_{CO_2} to increase, and the pH to decrease. Although the exact mechanism is unknown, the sensitivity of both the central and the peripheral chemoreceptors of the newborn increases dramatically at birth. In response to all these stimuli, the infant *inhales*.

To initiate the first breath, however, the infant must generate a remarkable negative intrapleural pressure to overcome the viscous fluid in the lungs. It is estimated that the intrapleural pressure has to decrease to about -40 cm H_2O before any air enters the lungs. Intrapleural pressures as low as -100 cm H_2O have been reported. About 40 ml of air enter the lungs during the first breath. On exhalation, the infant expels about one-half of the volume obtained on the first breath, thus establishing the first portion of the residual volume. Figure 11–5 illustrates the typical pressure-volume changes of the lungs that occur in the

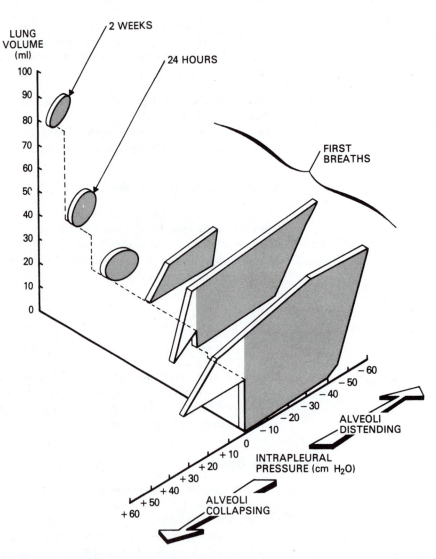

FIGURE 11–5. The pressure-volume changes of the newborn lungs during the first two weeks of life.

newborn during the first 2 weeks of life. The average *lung compliance* of the newborn is about .005 L/cm H_2O (5 ml/cm H_2O); the *airway resistance* is about 30 cm H_2O/L/sec.

Circulatory Changes at Birth

As the infant inhales for the first time, the pulmonary vascular resistance falls dramatically. Two major mechanisms account for the decreased pulmonary vascular resistance: (1) the sudden increase in the alveolar P_{O_2}, which offsets the hypoxic vasoconstriction, and (2) the mechanical increase in lung volume, which widens the caliber of the extra-alveolar vessels.

As the pulmonary vascular resistance decreases, a greater amount of blood flows through the lungs, and therefore more blood returns to the left atrium. This causes the pressure in the left atrium to increase and the flap of the foramen ovale to close functionally. The closure of the foramen ovale is further aided by the fall in pressure that occurs in the right atrium as the umbilical flow ceases. A few minutes later, the smooth muscles of the ductus arteriosus constrict in response to the increased P_{O_2}.

Clinically, however, the newborn's P_{O_2} must increase to more than 45 to 50 mm Hg in order for the ductus arteriosus to close. If this P_{O_2} level is not reached, the ductus arteriosus will remain open, and the pulmonary vascular resistance will remain elevated, producing the syndrome known as **persistent pulmonary hypertension of the neonate (PPHN)** (previously known as persistent fetal circulation). Furthermore, should the fetal P_{O_2} increase sufficiently to close the ductus arteriosus but then fall within the first 24 to 48 hours after birth, the ductus arteriosus will reopen.

It is believed that other substances released at birth (such as bradykinin, serotonin, and prostaglandin inhibitors) contribute to the constriction of the ductus arteriosus.

CONTROL OF VENTILATION IN THE NEWBORN

Within moments after birth, the newborn infant initiates the first breath. Although they are inhibited during fetal life, the peripheral and central chemoreceptors play a major role in activating the first breath. It is not precisely understood why these chemoreceptors are dormant during fetal life but are suddenly activated at birth.

Peripheral Chemoreceptors

The exact role of the peripheral chemoreceptors in the newborn is not clearly defined. It is known, however, that in both the pre-term and term infant, hypoxia elicits a transient rise in ventilation, followed by a marked fall. The magnitude of the increase is similar whether the infant is in the rapid eye-movement (REM) state, quiet sleep state, or awake state. However, the late fall is less marked or is absent when the infant is in the quiet sleep state. One to two weeks after birth, the infant demonstrates the adult response of sustained hyperventilation. The response to hypoxia is greater and more sustained in the term infant that in the pre-term infant. While it is known that the peripheral chemoreceptors of the adult are responsive to CO_2, little information is available about the peripheral chemoreceptors' sensitivity to changes in CO_2 and pH during the newborn period.

Central Chemoreceptors

The central chemoreceptors of the newborn respond to the elevated CO_2 levels in a manner similar to that of the adult. The response to an increased CO_2 level is primarily an increased tidal volume, with little change in inspiratory time or ventilatory rate. The response of the central chemoreceptors may be more marked with increasing gestational age, although not all researchers agree.

Infant Reflexes

Trigeminal Reflex. Stimulation of the newborn's trigeminal nerve (i.e., the face and nasal and nasopharyngeal mucosa) causes a decrease in the infant's respiration and heart rate. In fact, it has been reported that even gentle stimulation of the malar region in both the pre-term and term infant may cause significant respiratory slowing. Thus, the various procedures (such as nasopharyngeal suctioning) may be hazardous to the newborn. Clinically, facial cooling has been used as a means of terminating paroxysms of supraventricular tachycardia in the newborn.

Irritant Reflex. Epithelial irritant receptors, located throughout the airways, respond to direct tactile stimulation, lung deflation, and irritant gases. This response is mediated by myelinated vagal fibers. Based upon gestational age, these receptors elicit different responses. In pre-term infants of less than 35 weeks gestation, tracheal stimulation (e.g., endotracheal suctioning or intubation) is commonly followed by respiratory slowing or apnea. In the term infant, however,

TABLE 11–1. Approximate Lung Volumes and Capacities of the Newborn

Tidal volume (V_T)	15 ml	Vital capacity (VC)	115 ml
Residual volume (RV)	40 ml	Functional residual capacity (FRC)	80 ml
Expiratory reserve volume (ERV)	40 ml	Inspiratory capacity (IC)	75 ml
Inspiratory reserve volume (IRV)	60 ml	Total lung capacity (TLC)	155 ml

stimulation causes marked hyperventilation. The inhibitory response seen in the pre-term infant may be due to vagal nerve immaturity (i.e., the vagal nerves are not adequately myelinated). Unmyelinated neurons are unable to transmit high-frequency discharges.

TABLE 11–2. Normal Vital Sign Ranges of the Newborn	
Respiratory rate (RR)	35–50/min
Heart rate (HR)	130–150/min
Blood pressure (BP)	60/40–70/45

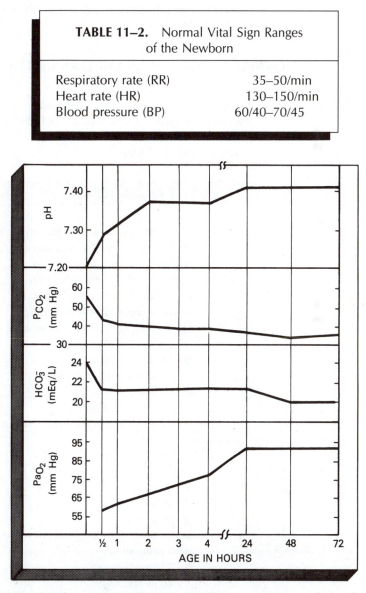

FIGURE 11–6. The average pH, Pa_{CO_2}, HCO_3^-, and Pa_{O_2} values of the normal infant during the first 72 hours of life.

Head Paradoxical Reflex. The head paradoxical reflex is a deep inspiration that is elicited by lung inflation. In other words, the infant inhales and then tops the inspiration with a deep breath before exhalation occurs. This reflex is seen in the term infant and is thought to be mediated by the irritant receptors. The head parodoxical reflex may play a role in sighing, which is frequently seen in the newborn. This reflex is thought to be valuable in maintaining lung compliance by offsetting alveolar collapse.

NORMAL CLINICAL PARAMETERS IN THE NEWBORN

Table 11–1 lists the average pulmonary function findings of the newborn. The normal vital signs of the newborn are listed in Table 11–2. Figure 11–6 illustrates graphically the average pH, Pa_{CO_2}, HCO_3^-, and Pa_{O_2} values of the normal infant over a period of 72 hours after birth.

SELF-ASSESSMENT QUESTIONS

1. During the embryonic period, the lungs first appear at about the
   a. 10th day after fertilization
   b. 24th day after fertilization
   c. 6th week after fertilization
   d. 12th week after fertilization
   e. 16th week after fertilization
2. The lungs are usually sufficiently mature to support life by the
   a. 24th week of gestation
   b. 28th week of gestation
   c. 32nd week of gestation
   d. 36th week of gestation
   e. 40th week of gestation
3. At birth, the number of alveoli represent about how much of the total adult gas exchange units?
   a. 10%
   b. 20%
   c. 30%
   d. 40%
   e. 50%
4. The number of alveoli continues to increase until about
   a. 6 years of age
   b. 8 years of age
   c. 10 years of age
   d. 12 years of age
   e. 16 years of age

5. The average P_{O_2} in the umbilical arteries during fetal life is about
   a. 20 mm Hg
   b. 40 mm Hg
   c. 60 mm Hg
   d. 80 mm Hg
   e. 100 mm Hg

6. The average P_{O_2} in the umbilical vein during fetal life is about
   a. 10 mm Hg
   b. 20 mm Hg
   c. 30 mm Hg
   d. 40 mm Hg
   e. 50 mm Hg

7. The average P_{CO_2} in the umbilical arteries during fetal life is about
   a. 25 mm Hg
   b. 35 mm Hg
   c. 45 mm Hg
   d. 55 mm Hg
   e. 65 mm Hg

8. In the placenta, maternal blood is continuously pumped through the
   a. umbilical arteries
   b. chorionic villi
   c. fetal vessels
   d. umbilical vein
   e. intervillous space

9. In the fetal circulation, once blood enters the right atrium, most of the blood enters the left atrium by passing through the
   a. ductus arteriosus
   b. pulmonary veins
   c. ductus venosus
   d. pulmonary arteries
   e. foramen ovale

10. Shortly after birth the ductus arteriosus constricts in response to
    I. increased P_{O_2}
    II. decreased P_{CO_2}
    III. increased pH
    IV. prostaglandins
       a. I only
       b. II only
       c. III and IV only
       d. I and IV only
       e. II and IV only

Answers appear in Appendix VII.

CHAPTER 12

RENAL FAILURE AND ITS EFFECTS ON THE CARDIOPULMONARY SYSTEM

OBJECTIVES

By the end of this chapter, the student should be able to:

1. Describe how the following relate to the kidneys:
   —Hilum
   —Ureters
   —Cortex
   —Medulla
   —Renal pelvis
   —Major calyces
   —Minor calyces
   —Renal papillae
   —Renal pyramid
   —Nephron
2. Describe how the following relate to the nephron:
   —Glomerulus
   —Bowman's capsule
   —Renal corpuscle
   —Proximal convoluted tubule
   —Descending limb of the loop of Henle
   —Ascending limb of the loop of Henle
   —Distal convoluted tubule
   —Collecting duct
3. Describe how the following blood vessels relate to the nephron:
   —Renal arteries
   —Interlobar arteries
   —Arcuate arteries
   —Interlobular arteries
   —Afferent arterioles
   —Efferent arterioles

—Peritubular capillaries
—Interlobular veins
—Arcuate vein
—Interlobar vein
—Renal vein

4. Describe the role of the following in the formation of urine:
—Glomerular filtration
—Tubular reabsorption
—Tubular secretion

5. Describe the role of the following in the control of urine concentration and volume:
—Countercurrent mechanism
—Selective permeability

6. Describe the role of the kidneys in the regulation of the following:
—Sodium
—Potassium
—Calcium, magnesium, and phosphate
—Acid-base balance

7. Describe the role of the following in controlling the blood volume:
—Capillary fluid shift system
—The renal system

8. Identify common causes of renal disorders, including the following:
—Congenital disorders
—Infections
—Obstructive disorders
—Inflammation and immune responses
—Neoplasms

9. Identify causes of the following types of renal disorders:
—Prerenal conditions
—Intrarenal conditions
—Postrenal conditions

10. Describe how mechanical ventilation alters urinary output.

11. Describe cardiopulmonary problems that can develop with renal failure, including the following:
—Hypertension and edema
—Metabolic acidosis
—Electrolyte abnormalities
  • Chloride
  • Potassium
—Anemia
—Bleeding
—Cardiovascular problems

12. Complete the self-assessment questions at the end of this chapter.

The composition of blood is largely determined by what the kidneys retain and excrete. The kidneys filter dissolved particles from the blood and selectively reabsorb the substances that are needed to maintain the normal composition of body fluids. When the renal system fails, a variety of indirect cardiopulmonary problems develop, including hypertension, congestive heart failure, pulmonary edema, anemia, and changes in acid-base balance. Because of this fact, a basic understanding of the etiology, classification, and clinical manifestations associated with renal failure is essential in respiratory care.

THE KIDNEYS

The kidneys are two bean-shaped organs that are located against the posterior wall of the abdominal cavity, one on each side of the vertebral column (Figure 12–1). In the adult, each kidney is about 12 cm long, 6 cm wide, and 3 cm thick. Medially, in the central concave portion of each kidney there is a longitudinal fissure called the **hilum**. The renal artery, renal vein, and nerves enter and leave kidneys through the hilum. The **ureters**, which transport urine from the kidneys to the bladder, also exit the kidneys through the hilum.

As shown in Figure 12–2, the **cortex**, which is the outer one-third of the kidney, is a dark brownish-red layer. The middle two-thirds of the kidney, the **medulla**, can be seen as a light-colored layer. Within the kidney, the ureter expands to form a funnel-shaped structure called the **renal pelvis**. The renal pelvis subdivides into two or three tubes called **major calyces** (singular, **calyx**). These, in turn, divide into several smaller tubes called **minor calyces**. A series of small structures called **renal papillae** (or *papillary ducts*) extend from the calyx toward the cortex of the kidney to form a triangular-shaped structure called the **renal pyramid**. The peripheral portions of the papillary ducts serve as collecting ducts for the waste products selectively filtered and excreted by the **nephrons**.

The Nephron

The nephrons are the functional units of the kidneys (Figure 12–3, page 323). Each kidney contains about one million nephrons. Each nephron consists of a **glomerulus, proximal tubule, loop of Henle,** and **distal tubule**. The distal tubules empty into the collecting ducts. Although the collecting ducts are, technically, not part of the renal pyramid, they are considered a functional part of the nephron because of their role in urine concentration, ion salvaging, and acid-base balance.

The glomerulus consists of a network of interconnected capillaries encased in a thin-walled saclike structure called **Bowman's capsule**. The glomerulus and Bowman's capsule constitute what is known as a **renal corpuscle**. Urine formation begins with the filtration of fluid and low-molecular-weight particles through the

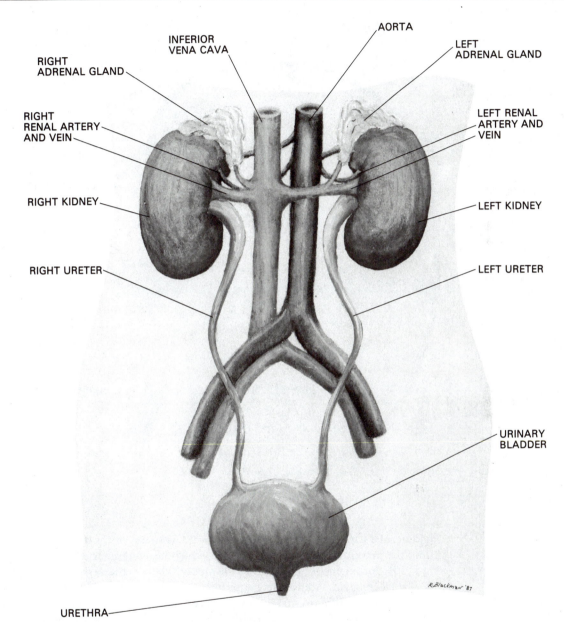

FIGURE 12–1.   The organs of the urinary system. Urine is formed by the kidneys and flows through the ureters to the bladder, where it is eliminated via the urethra.

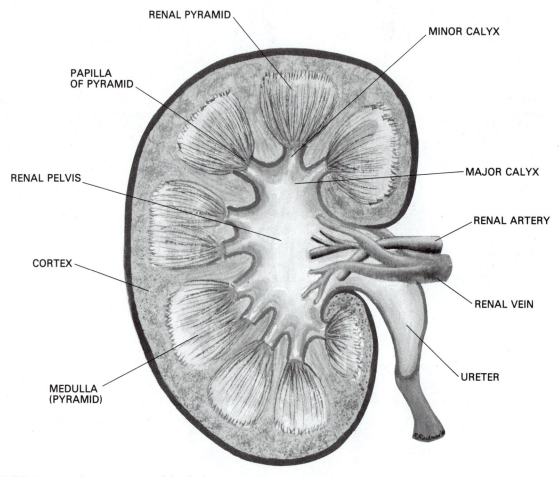

FIGURE 12–2.   Cross section of the kidney.

glomerular capillaries into Bowman's capsule. The substances that are filtered pass into the **proximal convoluted tubule**, which lies in the cortex.

The proximal tubule dips into the medulla to form the *descending* limb of the loop of Henle. The tubule then bends into a U-shaped structure to form the loop of Henle. As the tubule straightens, it ascends back toward the cortex as the *ascending* limb of the loop of Henle. The tubule again becomes convoluted as it enters the cortex. This portion of the nephron is called the **distal convoluted tubule** (see Figure 12–3). The distal convoluted tubule empties into the **collecting duct**. The collecting duct then passes through the renal pyramid to empty into the minor and major calyces, which in turn drain into the renal pelvis (see Figure 12–2). From the renal pelvis, the mixture of waste products (collectively referred

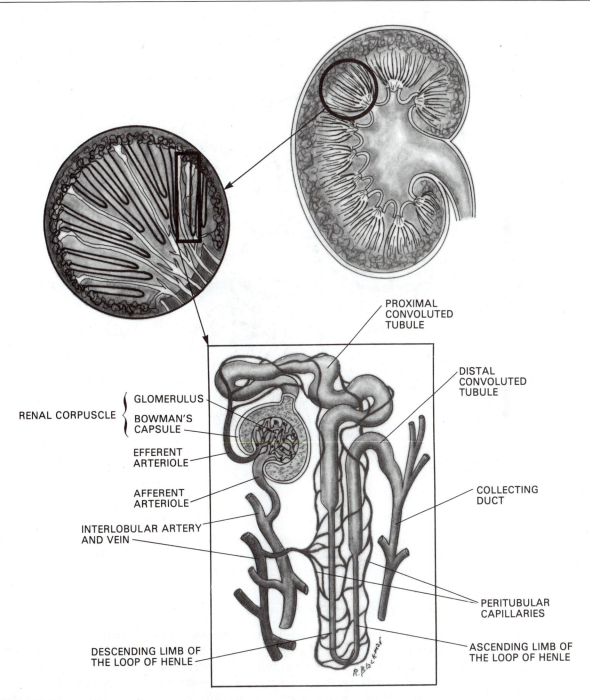

PROXIMAL CONVOLUTED TUBULE

DISTAL CONVOLUTED TUBULE

RENAL CORPUSCLE { GLOMERULUS

BOWMAN'S CAPSULE

EFFERENT ARTERIOLE

AFFERENT ARTERIOLE

INTERLOBULAR ARTERY AND VEIN

COLLECTING DUCT

PERITUBULAR CAPILLARIES

DESCENDING LIMB OF THE LOOP OF HENLE

ASCENDING LIMB OF THE LOOP OF HENLE

FIGURE 12–3. The nephron.

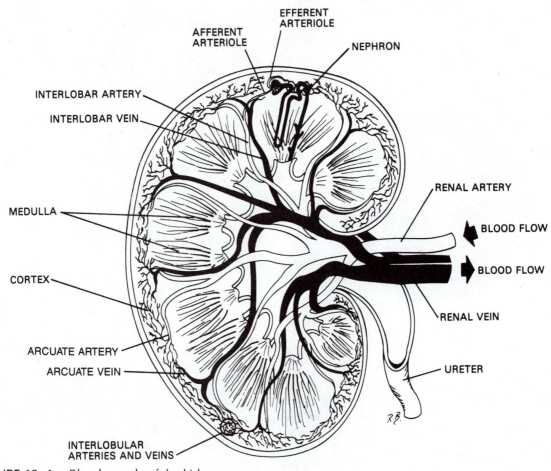

FIGURE 12–4.   Blood vessels of the kidney.

to as urine) drains into the ureter where it is carried by peristalsis to the urinary bladder. The urine is stored in the urinary bladder until it is discharged from the body through the urethra (see Figure 12–1).

Blood Vessels of the Kidneys

As shown in Figure 12–4, the right and left **renal arteries** carry blood to the kidneys. Shortly after passing through the hilum of the kidney, the renal artery divides into several branches called the **interlobar arteries**. At the base of the renal pyramids, the interlobar arteries become the **arcuate arteries**. Divisions of the arcuate arteries form a series of **interlobular arteries**, which enter the cortex and branch into the **afferent arterioles**.

The afferent arterioles deliver blood to the capillary cluster that forms the glomerulus. After passing through the glomerulus, the blood leaves by way of the efferent arterioles. The efferent arterioles then branch into a complex network of capillaries called the **peritubular capillaries**, which surround the various portions of the renal tubules of the nephron (see Figure 12–3).

The peritubular capillaries eventually reunite to form the **interlobular veins**, followed by the **arcuate vein**, the **interlobar vein**, and the **renal vein**. The renal vein eventually joins the inferior vena cava as it courses through the abdominal cavity.

URINE FORMATION

The formation of urine involves glomerular filtration, tubular reabsorption, and tubular secretion.

Glomerular Filtration

Urine formation begins at the renal corpuscle. Water and dissolved substances such as electrolytes, are forced out of the glomerular capillaries by means of the blood pressure (*hydrostatic pressure*). The filtration of substances through the capillary membrane of the glomerulus is similar to the filtration of other capillaries throughout the body. The permeability of the glomerular capillary, however, is much greater than that of the capillaries in other tissues. As the filtrate leaves the glomerular capillaries, it is received in Bowman's capsule.

The rate of filtration is directly proportional to the hydrostatic pressure of the blood. The hydrostatic pressure in the glomerular capillary is about 55 mm Hg. This pressure, however, is partially offset by the hydrostatic pressure in Bowman's capsule of about 15 mm Hg. The osmotic pressure of the plasma is another important factor that offsets glomerular filtration. In other words, in the capillaries the hydrostatic pressure acting to move water and dissolved particles outward is opposed by the inward osmotic pressure generated by the presence of protein in the plasma. Under normal conditions, the magnitude of the osmotic pressure is about 30 mm Hg. As shown in Table 12–1, the net filtration pressure, which is the algebraic sum of the three relevant forces, is about 10 mm Hg. The glomeruli filter about 125 ml of fluid per minute (about 180 L/day). Of the 125 ml, however, only about 1 ml is excreted as urine. The average urine output is about 60 ml per hour, or 1440 ml per day.

Tubular Reabsorption

As the glomerular filtrate passes through the (1) proximal convoluted tubule, (2) loop of Henle, and (3) distal convoluted tubule, water, sodium, glucose, and other substances leave the tubule and enter the blood in the peritubular capillaries. Some substances, such as glucose and amino acids, are completely reabsorbed.

TABLE 12–1. Forces of Glomerular Filtration

FACTORS	FORCE
Enhances Filtration	
Glomerular capillary blood pressure	+55 mm Hg
Opposes Filtration	
Fluid pressure in Bowman's capsule	−15 mm Hg
Osmotic force (caused by the protein concentration difference)	−30 mm Hg
Net Filtration Pressure	+10 mm Hg

About 99 percent of the filtered water and sodium are reabsorbed. About 50 percent of urea is reabsorbed and the electrolyte reabsorption is generally a function of need.

Although tubular reabsorption occurs throughout the entire renal tubule system, the bulk of it occurs in the proximal convoluted portion. Certain sections of the tubule, however, reabsorb specific substances, using particular modes of transport. For example, the proximal tubule reabsorbs glucose by means of *active transport*, while water reabsorption occurs throughout the renal tubule by *osmosis*.

Tubular Secretion

Tubular secretion is the mechanism by which various substances are transported from the plasma to the peritubular capillaries to the fluid of the renal tubule (the *opposite* direction of tubular reabsorption). In essence, this mechanism constitutes a second pathway through which fluid can gain entrance into the renal tubule (the first being *glomerular filtration*). The most important substances transported into the tubules by means of secretion are hydrogen (H^+) and potassium (K^+) ions. In fact, most of the hydrogen and potassium ions found in the urine enter the tubules by secretion. Thus, the mechanisms that control the rates of hydrogen and potassium tubular secretion regulate the level of these substances in the blood.

URINE CONCENTRATION AND VOLUME

The composition and volume of extracellular fluids are controlled by the kidney's ability to produce either a dilute or concentrated urine. The kidneys are able to do this by virtue of two mechanisms: the **countercurrent mechanism** and the **selective permeability of the collecting ducts.**

Countercurrent Mechanism

The countercurrent mechanism controls water reabsorption in the distal tubules and collecting ducts. It accomplishes this function through the unique anatomic position of various nephrons. About one out of every five nephrons descends deep into the renal medulla. These nephrons are called **juxtamedullary nephrons**. The normal osmolality of the glomerular filtrate is approximately 300 mOsm/L.* The osmolality of the interstitial fluid increases from about 300 mOsm/L in the cortex to about 1200 mOsm/L as the juxtamedullary nephron descends into the renal medulla. This sets up a strong active transport of sodium out of the descending limb of Henle. The increased amount of sodium in the interstitial fluid, in turn, prevents water from returning to the peritubular capillaries surrounding the tubules.

Selective Permeability

The permeability of the collecting ducts is regulated by the antidiuretic hormone (ADH). ADH is produced in the hypothalamus and is released by the pituitary gland. The hypothalamic cells manufacture ADH in response to input from numerous vascular baroreceptors, particularly a group found in the left atrium (Figure 12–5). For example, when the atrial blood volume and, therefore, pressure increase, the baroreceptors are activated to transmit neural impulses to the hypothalamus, causing the production of ADH to be inhibited. This causes tubules to be impermeable to water and the urine to be greater in volume and more dilute.

In contrast, decreased atrial pressure (*dehydration*) decreases the neural impulses originating from the baroreceptors and causes the production of ADH to increase. The result is the rapid movement of water out of these portions of the tubules of the nephron and into the interstitium of the medullary area by osmosis. This causes the urine volume to decrease and its concentration to increase.

The specific gravity (*osmolality*) of urine varies with its concentration of solutes. The urine produced by the healthy kidney has a specific gravity of about 1.018 to 1.040 under normal conditions. During periods of diminished renal function, the urine specific gravity may fall to levels of 1.008 to 1.012.

REGULATION OF ELECTROLYTE CONCENTRATION

The kidneys play a major role in maintaining a normal cellular environment by regulating the concentration of various ions. Some of the more important ions

---

*Milliosmols (mOsm/L) = 1000 milliosmols equal 1 osmol which is the unit in which osmotic pressure is expressed. We speak of osmols or milliosmols per liter.

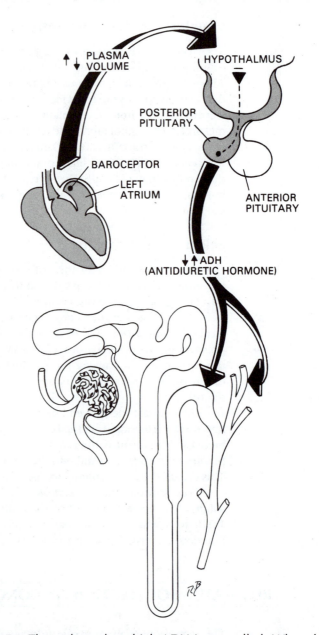

FIGURE 12–5. The pathway by which ADH is controlled. When the baroreceptors in the left atrium sense an increased pressure (increased plasma volume), they send neural impulses to the hypothalamus that cause the production of ADH to decrease. In contrast, a decreased pressure (decreased plasma volume) causes the production of ADH to increase.

regulated by the kidneys are sodium, potassium, calcium, magnesium, and phosphate.

Sodium Ions

Sodium ions (Na^+) account for over 90 percent of the positively charged ions in the extracellular fluid. Because the sodium ions cause almost all of the osmotic pressure of the fluids, it follows that the sodium ion concentration directly affects the osmolality of the fluids. Thus, when the sodium concentration increases, there is a corresponding increase in the extracellular fluid osmolality. In contrast, the extracellular fluid osmolality decreases when there is a decreased sodium concentration.

The kidneys control the concentration of sodium primarily by regulating the amount of water in the body. When the sodium level becomes too high, the amount of water in the body increases by (1) secretion of antidiuretic hormone (ADH), which causes the kidney to retain water, and (2) stimulation of thirst, which causes the individual to drink liquids.

Potassium Ions

A balanced potassium (K^+) level is essential for normal nerve and muscle function. Clinically, when the potassium level becomes too low, muscle weakness, diarrhea, metabolic alkalosis, and tachycardia develop. An excessively high potassium concentration causes muscle weakness, metabolic acidosis, and life-threatening arrhythmias. In response to a high K^+ level, the kidneys work to return the concentration to normal by means of two negative feedback control mechanisms. The *first* is the direct effect the excess potassium has on the epithelial cells of the renal tubules to cause an increased transport of potassium out of the peritubular capillaries and into the tubules of the nephrons, where it is subsequently passed in the urine. The *second* is the stimulating effect the elevated potassium level has on the adrenal cortex, causing it to release increased quantities of *aldosterone*. Aldosterone stimulates the tubular epithelial cells to transport potassium ions into the nephron tubules and, hence, into the urine. The extracellular potassium concentration is normally 3.5 to 5 mEq/L.

Calcium, Magnesium, and Phosphate Ions

The precise mechanisms by which calcium, magnesium, and phosphate concentrations are regulated by the kidneys are not well understood. It is known, however, that elevated levels of any one of these ions in the extracellular fluid cause the tubules to decrease reabsorption and to pass the substances into the urine. In contrast, when any one of these substances is low in concentration, the tubules rapidly reabsorb the substance until its concentration in the extracellular fluids returns to normal.

Role of the Kidneys in Acid-base Balance

In addition to the natural acid-base buffers (see Chapter Eight) of the body fluids (e.g., HCO_3^-, phosphate, and protein buffers), and the respiratory system's ability to regulate the elimination of CO_2, the renal system also plays an important role in maintaining a normal acid-base balance by virtue of its ability to regulate the excretion of hydrogen ions and the reabsorption of bicarbonate ions.

All the renal tubules are capable of secreting hydrogen ions. The rate of secretion is directly proportional to the hydrogen ion concentration in the blood. Thus, when the extracellular fluids become too acidic, the kidneys excrete hydrogen ions into the urine. In contrast, when the extracellular fluids become too alkaline, the kidneys excrete basic substances (primarily sodium bicarbonate) into the urine.

This principle is illustrated in Figure 12–6, which shows that at point A, the extracellular fluid is 7.55. Because this is on the alkaline side, the pH of the urine is also alkaline (pH 7.5), since the kidneys excrete alkaline substances from the body fluids. In contrast, the extracellular pH at point B is 7.25 and the pH of the urine is very acidic (pH 5.25), because of excretion of large quantities of acidic substances (primarily hydrogen ions) from the body fluids. In both of these examples, the excretion of acidic or alkaline substances moves the pH toward normal.

Blood Volume

In the adult, the normal blood volume is about 5 liters, and it rarely increases or decreases more than a few hundred milliliters from that value. The capillary fluid shift system and the renal system are the two major mechanisms responsible for this constancy of the blood volume.

Capillary Fluid Shift System.   Under normal circumstances, the pressure in the capillaries of the systemic system is about 17 mm Hg. When the pressure rises above this value, fluid begins to leak into the tissue spaces, causing the blood volume to decrease toward normal. In contrast, when the blood volume falls, the capillary pressure decreases and fluid is then absorbed from the interstitial spaces, causing the blood volume to move back toward normal. This mechanism, however, has its limitations, since the tissue spaces cannot expand indefinitely when the blood volume becomes too high, nor can the tissue spaces supply an inexhaustible amount of fluid when the blood volume is low.

The Renal System.   When the blood volume increases, the glomerular pressure in the kidney rises, causing the amount of the glomerular filtrate and the volume of the urine to increase. In addition, the pressure in the peritubular capillaries decreases fluid reabsorption from the tubules, which further increases the volume of urine.

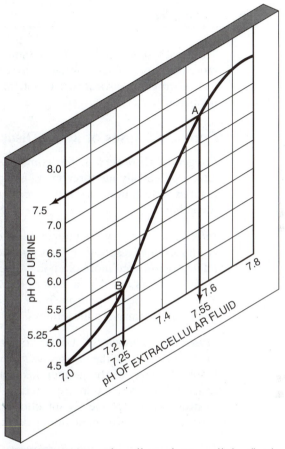

FIGURE 12–6. The effect of extracellular fluid pH on the urine pH.

An increased blood volume increases the glomerular pressure (normally 60 mm Hg) by means of two mechanisms. *First*, the increased blood volume increases the blood flow through the afferent arterioles that lead into the kidneys and thus increases the intrarenal pressure. *Second*, the increased blood volume stretches the atria of the heart, which contain stretch receptors called **volume receptors**. When the volume receptors in the atria are stretched, a neural reflex is initiated that causes the renal afferent arterioles to dilate. This causes the blood flow into the kidneys to increase and thus increases the amount of urine formed. Furthermore, when the volume receptors are stretched, the secretion of ADH by the posterior pituitary gland is inhibited, which in turn increases the urine output.

RENAL FAILURE

The renal system is subject to the same types of disorders as other body parts. The more common causes of renal failure are (1) congenital disorders, (2) infections, (3) obstructive disorders, (4) inflammation and immune responses, and (5) neoplasms.

Common Causes of Renal Disorders

Congenital Disorders.   Approximately 10 percent of the infants born each year have a potentially life-threatening malformation of the renal system. Such abnormalities include unilateral renal agenesis, renal dysplasia, and polycystic disease of the kidney.

Infections.   Urinary tract infections are the second most common type of bacterial infections (respiratory tract infections are the most common). Urinary tract infections are seen more often in women than men. Approximately 20 percent of all females will develop at least one urinary tract infection during their lifetime. These infections range from bacteriuria to severe kidney infections that cause irreversible damage to the kidneys.

Obstructive Disorders.   Urinary obstruction can affect all age groups and can occur at any part of the urinary tract. About 90 percent of obstructions are located below the level of the glomerulus. Some factors that predispose individuals to urinary flow obstruction are listed in Table 12–2. Persons who have a urinary obstruction are prone to infections, a heightened susceptibility to calculus formation, and permanent kidney damage.

Inflammation and Immune Responses.   Kidney inflammation is caused by altered immune responses, drugs and related chemicals, and radiation. Inflammation can

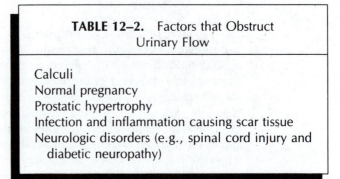

TABLE 12–2.   Factors that Obstruct
Urinary Flow

Calculi
Normal pregnancy
Prostatic hypertrophy
Infection and inflammation causing scar tissue
Neurologic disorders (e.g., spinal cord injury and
   diabetic neuropathy)

cause significant alterations in the glomerulus, tubules, and interstitium. The various forms of glomerulonephritis are believed to be caused by natural immune responses.

Neoplasms.   Cancer of the kidneys accounts for 1 to 2 percent of all cancers. Although cancer of the kidneys is relatively rare in the adult, one form of cancer—Wilms' tumor—accounts for about 70 percent of all cancers of early childhood.

Classification of Renal Disorders

Renal disorders are commonly classified according to the anatomic portion of the renal system responsible for the renal decline. The major classifications are (1) prerenal, (2) renal, and (3) postrenal.

Prerenal Conditions.   Prerenal conditions consist of abnormalities that impair blood flow to the kidneys. Prerenal problems are the most common and, generally, are reversible if identified and treated early. Table 12–3 lists some common prerenal causes of renal failure.

Normally, about 20 to 25 percent of the cardiac output is filtered by the kidneys. When the volume of blood falls (e.g., in cardiac failure or hemorrhage), the blood flow to the kidneys may decrease sharply. Thus, one of the early clinical manifestations of prerenal failure is a sharp reduction in urine output.

Renal Conditions.   Renal abnormalities involve conditions that obstruct flow through the kidneys. Table 12–4 lists the five categories of renal abnormalities.

Postrenal Conditions.   An obstruction of the urinary tract at any point between the calyces and the urinary meatus is known as a postrenal obstruction. Table 12–5 lists some abnormalities included in the postrenal category.

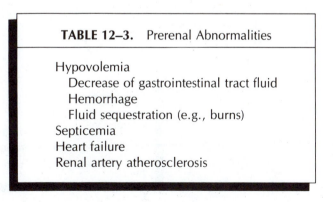

TABLE 12–3.   Prerenal Abnormalities

Hypovolemia
   Decrease of gastrointestinal tract fluid
   Hemorrhage
   Fluid sequestration (e.g., burns)
Septicemia
Heart failure
Renal artery atherosclerosis

TABLE 12–4.   Renal Abnormalities

Renal ischemia
Injury to the glomerular membrane caused by nephrotoxic agents
   Aminoglycoside agents (e.g., gentamicin, kanamycin)
   Heavy metals (e.g., lead, mercury)
   Organic solvents (e.g., ethylene glycol)
   Radiopaque contrast media
   Sulfonamides
Acute tubular necrosis
Intratubuluar obstruction
   Uric acid cystals
   Hemolytic reactions (e.g., blood transfusion reactions)
Acute inflammatory conditions
   Acute pyelonephritis
   Necrotizing papillitis

Mechanical Ventilation as Cause of Renal Failure

It is well documented that mechanical ventilation can alter urinary output. *Positive pressure ventilation* decreases urinary output, whereas *negative pressure ventilation* increases urinary output. It is believed that this is due in part to the blood pressure changes that occur in response to mechanical ventilation. For example, in positive pressure ventilation, the venous return is often impeded, causing the blood volume and, therefore, the pressure in the atria to diminish. The reduced pressure stimulates the volume receptors in the atria to send more impulses to the pituitary gland. This causes more ADH to be released. As the concentration of ADH increases, the amount of urine formed by the kidneys decreases.

TABLE 12–5.   Postrenal Abnormalities

Ureteral obstruction (e.g., calculi, tumors)
Bladder outlet obstruction (e.g., prostatic
   hypertrophy)

CARDIOPULMONARY PROBLEMS CAUSED BY RENAL FAILURE

In chronic renal failure, a variety of cardiopulmonary problems can develop. In acute renal failure, the body's ability to eliminate nitrogenous wastes, water, and electrolytes is impaired. As the renal system declines further, the BUN, creatinine, potassium, and phosphate levels rapidly increase, and metabolic acidosis develops. Water retention gives rise to peripheral edema and pulmonary congestion. During the end stages, virtually every portion of the body is affected. In terms of specific cardiopulmonary problems, the following problems can be expected in patients with renal failure:

Hypertension and Edema

When the renal function is impaired, the kidneys lose their ability to excrete sodium. Consequently, the ingestion of excess sodium commonly leads to hypertension and edema.

Metabolic Acidosis

With the decline in renal function, the kidney's ability to secrete hydrogen ions (H^+) and to conserve bicarbonate (HCO_3^-) progressively decreases. Furthermore, during the more advanced stages of renal failure, hyperkalemia is a frequent finding. Thus, because of the increased H^+ and K^+ ion levels and the loss of HCO_3^-, *metabolic acidosis* is an almost inevitable clinical manifestation in severe renal failure.

Renal Acid-base Disturbances Caused by Electrolyte Abnormalities

Chloride (Cl^-) abnormalities can lead to acid-base disturbances through the renal system. For example, when the plasma Cl^- level falls below normal, the amount of Cl^- available for glomerular filtration decreases. Under normal circumstances, when the positive sodium ion (Na^+) is reabsorbed by the tubules, the negative Cl^- ion must also be reabsorbed to maintain electrical neutrality. In the absence of adequate amounts of Cl^-, however, the electrical balance is maintained by the secretion of hydrogen ions (H^+). The loss of H^+ results in *hypochloremic alkalosis*. In contrast, when the plasma Cl^- level is higher than normal, the secretion of H^+ ions is reduced. This in turn causes a reduction in bicarbonate reabsorption and *hyperchloremic acidosis*.

Potassium (K^+) abnormalities can also lead to acid-base disturbances through the renal system. For example, under normal conditions the K^+ ion behaves similar to the H^+ ion in that it is secreted in the renal tubules in exchange for Na^+. In the absence of Na^+, neither K^+ nor H^+ can be secreted. When the K^+

level is higher than normal, however, the competition with H^+ for Na^+ exchange increases. When this happens, the amount of H^+ ions secreted is reduced, which in turn decreases the amount of bicarbonate reabsorption. The end-product of this process is *hyperkalemic acidosis*. When the K^+ level is lower than normal, the competition with H^+ for Na^+ exchange decreases. Consequently, the amount of H^+ secreted is increased, which in turn increases the amount of HCO_3^- reabsorption. The end-product of this process is *hypokalemic alkalosis*.

Anemia

The kidneys are a primary source of the hormone *erythropoietin*, which stimulates the bone marrow to produce red blood cells. When the renal system fails, the production of erythropoietin is often inadequate to stimulate the bone marrow to produce a sufficient amount of red blood cells. In addition, the toxic wastes that accumulate as a result of renal failure also suppress the ability of bone marrow to produce red blood cells. Both of these mechanisms contribute to the anemia seen in chronic renal failure.

Bleeding

Approximately 20 percent of persons with chronic renal failure have a tendency to bleed as a result of platelet abnormalities. Clinically, this is manifested by epistaxis, gastrointestinal bleeding, and bruising of the skin and subcutaneous tissues.

Cardiovascular Problems

Hypertension is often an early sign of renal failure. In severe cases, the increased extracellular fluid volume, caused by sodium and water retention, gives rise to edema, congestive heart failure, and pulmonary edema. Pericarditis is also seen in about 50 percent of persons with chronic renal failure. This condition develops as a result of the pericardium being exposed to the metabolic end-products associated with renal decline.

SELF-ASSESSMENT QUESTIONS

1. The outer one-third of the kidney is called the
   a. renal pelvis
   b. medulla
   c. minor calyces
   d. renal pyramid
   e. cortex

2. Glomerular filtration is directly proportional to
    a. blood cell size
    b. hydrostatic pressure
    c. osmotic pressure
    d. protein size
    e. the patient's fluid intake

3. Tubular reabsorption occurs primarily in the
    a. renal corpuscle
    b. proximal convoluted tubule
    c. loop of Henle
    d. distal convoluted tubule
    e. collecting duct

4. The major substance(s) transported by means of tubular secretion is/are:
    I. H^+
    II. Cl^-
    III. K^+
    IV. HCO_3^-
    V. Na^+
        a. I only
        b. IV only
        c. V only
        d. I and III only
        e. IV and V only

5. The urine produced by the healthy kidney has a specific gravity of about
    a. 1.000 to 1.001
    b. 1.006 to 1.020
    c. 1.018 to 1.040
    d. 1.060 to 1.080
    e. 1.080 to 1.100

6. Which of the following can be classified as a prerenal condition?
    I. Heart failure
    II. Intratubular obstruction
    III. Bladder outlet obstruction
    IV. Hypovolemia
        a. I only
        b. II only
        c. IV only
        d. II and III only
        e. I and IV only

7. Which of the following is the functional unit(s) of the kidneys?
    a. Cortex
    b. Collecting ducts
    c. Major calyces

    d. Peritubular capillaries
    e. Nephrons
8. Which of the following empties urine into the bladder?
    a. Collecting ducts
    b. Ureters
    c. Distal convoluted tubules
    d. Urethra
    e. Major calyces
9. Normally, the net glomerular filtration pressure is about
    a. 5 mm Hg
    b. 10 mm Hg
    c. 15 mm Hg
    d. 20 mm Hg
    e. 25 mm Hg
10. Which of the following is/are part of the nephron?
    I. Proximal convoluted tubules
    II. Loop of Henle
    III. Glomerulus
    IV. Distal convoluted tubules
       a. II only
       b. III only
       c. II, III, and IV only
       d. I, II, and III only
       e. I, II, III, and IV

Answers appear in Appendix VII.

CHAPTER 13

AGING AND ITS EFFECTS ON THE CARDIOPULMONARY SYSTEM

OBJECTIVES

By the end of this chapter, the student should be able to:

1. Describe the effects of aging on the following components of the *respiratory system:*
   —Static mechanical properties
   - Elastic recoil of the lungs
   - Lung compliance
   - Thoracic compliance
   —Lung volumes and capacities
   —Dynamic maneuvers of ventilation
   —Pulmonary diffusing capacity
   —Alveolar deadspace ventilation
   —Pulmonary gas exchange
   —Arterial blood gases
   —Arterial-venous oxygen content difference
   —Hemoglobin concentration
   —Control of ventilation
   —Exercise tolerance
   —Pulmonary diseases in the aged
2. Describe the effects of aging on the following components of the *cardiovascular system:*
   —Structure of the heart
   —Work of the heart
   —Heart rate
   —Stroke volume
   —Cardiac output
   —Peripheral vascular resistance
   —Blood pressure
3. Complete the self-assessment questions at the end of this chapter.

The aging process is normal, progressive, and physiologically irreversible. Aging occurs in spite of optimal nutrition, genetic background, environmental surroundings, and activity patterns. The biological aging process, however, may demonstrate altered rates of progression in response to an individual's genetic background and day-to-day living habits.

Assuming that the death rate remains the same in the United States, the number of people 74 to 85 years of age will double (to 10.6 million) by the year 2000. The number of people older than 85 will increase by more than 80 percent (to 3.8 million). Between the years 2010 and 2030, those born 1946 to 1964 during the post–World War II baby boom (the biggest baby boom in history) will be turning 65. During this period, it is estimated that the number of people over 65 years of age will increase from the present 25 million to some 50 million. By the year 2020, the 75-and-over population, who have specific activity limitations due to chronic ailments, will increase 2.5 times (to 10.7 million). Figure 13–1 illustrates the actual and projected population of persons 55 years and older for four different age groups between the years of 1900 and 2040.

It is also projected that the number of short-stay hospital days of persons 65 years and older will increase from the 105,358 in 1980 to over 286,000 by the year 2050 (Figure 13–2). Because the mortality and morbidity rates rise sharply after age 65, the large size of this population will undoubtedly pose a tremendous challenge to the health care industry. A basic understanding of how the aging process influences the cardiopulmonary system is critical for the respiratory care practitioner.

THE INFLUENCE OF AGING ON THE RESPIRATORY SYSTEM

The growth and development of the lungs is essentially complete by about 20 years of age. Most of the pulmonary function indices reach their maximum levels between 20 and 25 years of age and then progressively decline. The precise influence of aging on the respiratory system is difficult to determine, since changes associated with time are often indistinguishable from those of disease. For example, factors such as chronic exposure to environmental pollutants, repeated pulmonary infections, smoking, and some working conditions can cause alterations in the respiratory system that are not easily differentiated from changes due to aging alone. In spite of these difficulties, the conclusions reached here appear to be well founded.

Static Mechanical Properties

The **functional residual capacity** is the volume remaining in the lungs when the elastic recoil of the lungs exactly balances the natural tendency of the

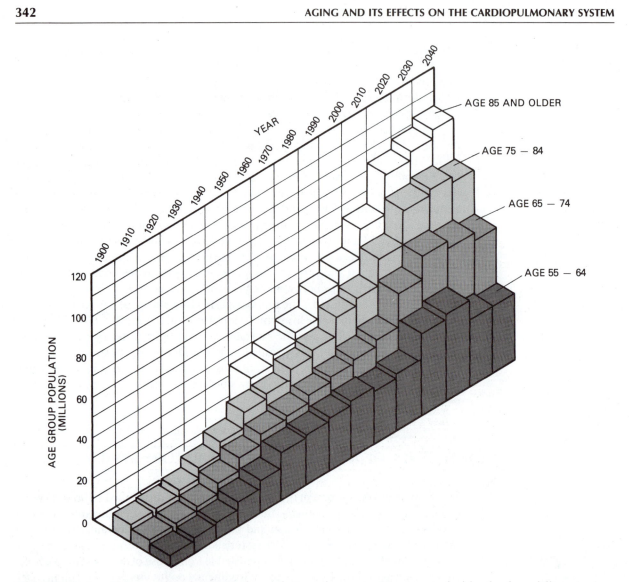

FIGURE 13–1.   The actual and projected population of persons 55 years and older for four different age groups between the years 1900 and 2040.

chest wall to expand. With aging, the elastic recoil of the lungs decreases, causing lung compliance to increase. This is illustrated graphically as a shift to the left (steeper slope) of the volume-pressure curve (Figure 13–3). The decrease in lung elasticity develops because the alveoli progressively deteriorate and enlarge after age 30. Structurally, the alveolar changes resemble the air sac changes associated with emphysema.

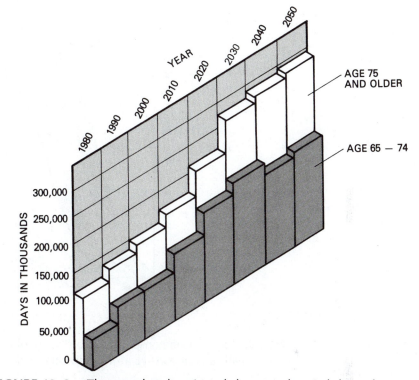

FIGURE 13–2. The actual and projected short-stay hospital days of persons 65 years and older between the years 1980 and 2050.

Even though the potential for greater lung expansion exists as an individual becomes older, it cannot be realized because of the structural limitations that develop in the chest wall. With aging the costal cartilages of the thoracic wall progressively calcify, causing the ribs to slant downward, and this structural change causes the thorax to become less compliant. Because of these anatomic changes, the transpulmonary pressure difference, which is responsible for holding the airways open, is diminished with age.

Finally, the reduction in chest wall compliance is slightly greater than the increase in lung compliance, resulting in an overall moderate decline in total compliance of the respiratory system. It is estimated that the work expenditure of a 60-year-old individual to overcome static mechanical forces during normal breathing is 20 percent greater than that of a 20-year-old person. The decreased compliance of the respiratory system associated with age is offset by increased respiratory frequency rather than by increased tidal volume during exertion.

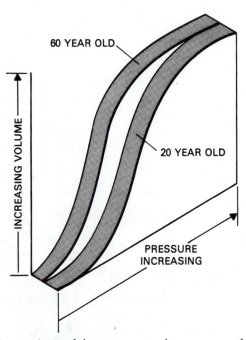

FIGURE 13–3. Comparison of the pressure-volume curve of a 60-year-old person with that of a 20-year-old individual. With aging, the curve shifts to the left.

Lung Volumes and Capacities

Figure 13–4 shows the changes that occur in the lung volumes and capacities with aging. Although studies are in conflict, it is generally agreed that the total lung capacity (TLC) essentially remains the same throughout life. Should the TLC decrease, however, it is probably due to the decreased height that typically occurs with age.

It is well documented that the residual volume (RV) increases with age. This is primarily due to age-related alveolar enlargement and to small airway closure. As the RV increases, the RV/TLC ratio also increases. The RV/TLC ratio increases from approximately 20 percent at age 20 to about 35 percent at age 60. This increase occurs predominantly after the age of 40. As the RV increases, moreover, the expiratory reserve volume (ERV) decreases. Most studies show that the functional residual capacity (FRC) increases with age, but not as much as the RV and the RV/TLC. Since the FRC typically increases with age, the inspiratory capacity (IC) decreases.

Because the vital capacity (VC) is equal to the TLC minus the RV, the VC inevitably decreases as the RV increases. It is estimated that in the male, the VC

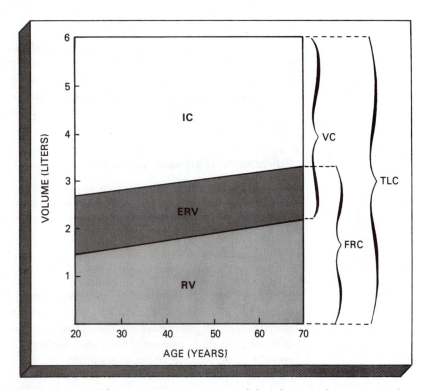

FIGURE 13–4. Schematic representation of the changes that occur in lung volumes and capacities with aging.

decreases about 25 ml/year. In the female, the VC decreases about 20 ml/year. In general, the VC decreases about 40 to 50 percent by age 70.

Dynamic Maneuvers of Ventilation

Because of the loss of lung elasticity associated with aging, there inevitably is a marked effect on the dynamics of ventilation. In fact, one of the most prominent physiologic changes associated with age is the reduced efficiency in forced air expulsion. This normal deterioration is reflected by a progressive decrease in the following dynamic lung functions:

- Forced vital capacity (FVC)
- Peak expiratory flow rate (PEFR)
- Forced expiratory flow$_{25-75\%}$ (FEF$_{25-75\%}$)
- Forced expiratory volume in 1 second (FEV$_1$)
- Forced expiratory volume in 1 second/Forced vital capacity ratio (FEV$_1$/FVC ratio)

• Maximum voluntary ventilation (MVV)

It is estimated that these dynamic lung functions decrease approximately 20 to 30 percent throughout the average adult's life. Precisely what causes the flow rates to decline is still controversial. Since, however, gas flow is dependent upon (1) the applied pressure and (2) the airway resistance, changes in either or both of these factors could be responsible for the reduction of gas flow rates seen in the elderly.

Pulmonary Diffusing Capacity

The pulmonary diffusing capacity ($D_{L_{CO}}$) progressively decreases with age. It is estimated that the $D_{L_{CO}}$ falls about 20 percent over the course of adult life. This is probably the result of decreased alveolar surface area and decreased pulmonary capillary blood flow, both of which are known to occur with aging.

Alveolar Deadspace Ventilation

Alveolar deadspace ventilation increases with advancing age. This is probably due to the decreased cardiac index associated with aging and to the structural alterations of the pulmonary capillaries that occur as a result of the normal alveolar deterioration. It is estimated that the alveolar deadspace ventilation increases about 1 ml per year throughout adult life.

PULMONARY GAS EXCHANGE

The alveolar-arterial oxygen tension difference $P_{(A-a)O_2}$ progressively increases with age. Although controversial, factors that may increase the $P_{(A-a)O_2}$ include the physiologic shunt, the mismatching of ventilation and perfusion, and a decreased diffusing capacity.

ARTERIAL BLOOD GASES

The Pa_{O_2} progressively decreases with age. Because lung degeneration and relative hypoxemia are a normal part of aging, an acceptable Pa_{O_2} range for individuals between 60 and 90 years of age can be calculated by subtracting 1 mm Hg from the minimal 80 mm Hg level for every year over 60 (see Table 7–1). Thus, a Pa_{O_2} of 65 mm Hg should be acceptable for a 75-year-old individual.

The Pa_{CO_2} remains constant throughout life. A possible explanation for this is the greater diffusion ability of carbon dioxide through the alveolar-capillary barrier. Because the Pa_{CO_2} remains the same in the healthy adult with age, the pH and HCO_3^- levels also remain constant.

Arterial-venous Oxygen Content Difference

The maximum arterial-venous oxygen content difference $C(a - \bar{v})_{O_2}$ tends to decrease with age. Contributory factors include (1) decline in physical fitness, (2) less efficient peripheral blood distribution, and (3) reduction in tissue enzyme activity.

Hemoglobin Concentration

Anemia is a common finding among the elderly. Several factors predispose the aged to anemia. Red bone marrow has a tendency to be replaced by fatty marrow, especially in the long bones. Gastrointestinal atrophy, which is commonly associated with advancing age, may slow the absorption of iron or vitamin B_{12}. Gastrointestinal bleeding is also more prevalent in the elderly. Perhaps the most important reasons for anemia in the aged are sociologic rather than medical—for example, insufficient income to purchase food or decreased interest in cooking and eating adequate meals.

Control of Ventilation

The ventilatory response to both hypoxia and hypercapnia diminishes with age. This is probably due to a reduced sensitivity of the peripheral and central chemoreceptors. The incidence of snoring and obstructive sleep apnea also increases with aging.

Exercise Tolerance

In healthy individuals of any age, the respiratory function does not limit exercise tolerance. The oxygen transport system is more critically dependent on the cardiovascular system than on respiratory function. The maximal oxygen uptake ($\dot{V}_{O_2max}$), which is the parameter most commonly used to evaluate an individual's aerobic exercise tolerance, peaks at age 20 and progressively and linearly decreases with age. Although there is considerable variation among individuals, it is estimated that from 20 to 60 years of age, a person's maximal oxygen uptake decreases by approximately 35 percent. Evidence indicates, however, that regular physical conditioning throughout life increases oxygen uptake and therefore enhances the capacity for exertion during work and recreation.

Pulmonary Diseases in the Aged

Although the occurrence of pulmonary diseases increases with age, it is difficult to determine the precise relationship aging has to pulmonary disease. This is because aging is also associated with the presence of chronic diseases (e.g., lung cancer, bronchitis, and emphysema). It is known, however, that the incidence of serious infectious pulmonary diseases is significantly greater in the elderly. While the incidence has decreased dramatically in recent years, the mortality from pneumonia is still a major cause of death in the elderly. Evidence suggests that this is partly due to the impaired defense mechanisms in the aged.

THE INFLUENCE OF AGING ON THE CARDIOVASCULAR SYSTEM

A variety of adverse changes develops in the cardiovascular system with age. In fact, the major causes of death in the aging population are diseases of the cardiovascular system. The major changes in the cardiovascular system that develop as a function of age are as follows.

Structure of the Heart

Between 30 and 80 years of age, the thickness of the left ventricular wall increases by about 25 percent. Cardiac hypertrophy, however, is not considered a primary change associated with aging. In the ventricles, the muscle fiber size progressively increases. Fibrosis develops in the lining of the chambers and fatty infiltration occurs in the wall of the chambers. The amount of connective tissue increases, causing the heart to become less elastic. Thus, the compliance of the heart is reduced and the heart functions less efficiently as a pump. The heart valves thicken from calcification and fibrosis. This structural change causes the valves to be more rigid and less effective. As the valves become more rigid and distorted, the blood flow may be impeded and systolic murmurs may develop.

Work of the Heart

The work of the heart, which is defined as stroke volume times mean systolic blood pressure, decreases approximately 1 percent per year (Figure 13–5).

Heart Rate

Although the effect of age on the resting heart rate is controversial, it is known that the increase in heart rate in response to stress is less in the elderly. The maximum heart rate can be estimated by the following formula:

maximum heart rate = 220 − age

Thus, the maximum heart rate for a 60-year-old is about 160 (220 − 60 = 160). (Recent research has shown that some older subjects can achieve

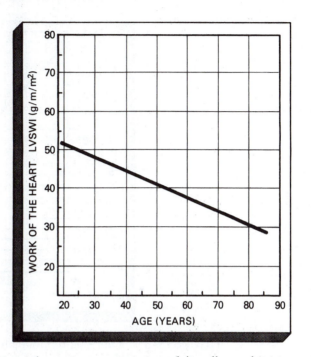
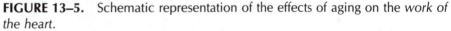

FIGURE 13–5. Schematic representation of the effects of aging on the *work of the heart.*

higher heart rates than those predicted by this method.) The reasons for the decreased maximum heart rate are unclear (Figure 13–6). It may be due to the diminished myocardial oxygen supply associated with advanced age. Another possibility is the decreased compliance of the heart in the aged. The increase in heart rate in response to stress may be impaired because of increased connective tissue in the sino-atrial and atrioventricular nodes and in the bundle branches. The number of catecholamine receptors on the muscle fibers may also be reduced.

With aging, moreover, it not only takes more time for the heart to accelerate, but it also takes more time to return to normal after a stressful event. Because of this, the expected increase in pulse rate in response to certain clinical situations (e.g., anxiety, pain, hemorrhage, and infectious processes) is often not as evident in the elderly.

Stroke Volume

The stroke volume diminishes with age. The precise reason for the reduction in the stroke volume is unknown. It is suggested, however, that the decline in

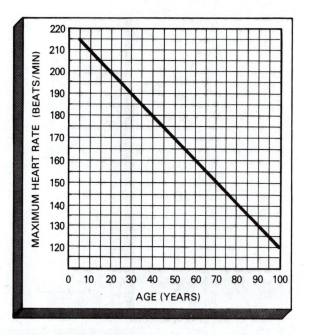

FIGURE 13–6.   Schematic representation of the effects of aging on the *maximum heart rate.*

stroke volume may be a reflection of poor myocardial perfusion, decreased cardiac compliance, and poor contractility. As the stroke volume declines, the *stroke volume index* (stroke volume divided by body surface area) also decreases.

Cardiac Output

As the stroke volume diminishes, the cardiac output inevitably declines. After the age of 20, the cardiac output decreases in a linear fashion about 1 percent per year (Figure 13–7). Between the ages of 30 and 80, the cardiac output decreases about 40 percent in both men and women. As the cardiac output declines, the *cardiac index* (cardiac output divided by body surface area) also decreases.

Peripheral Vascular Resistance

It is well documented that the elasticity of the major blood vessels decreases with advancing age. Both the arteries and veins undergo age-related changes. The intima thickens and the media becomes more fibrotic (see Figure 1–24). Collagen and extracellular materials accumulate in both the intima and media. As the

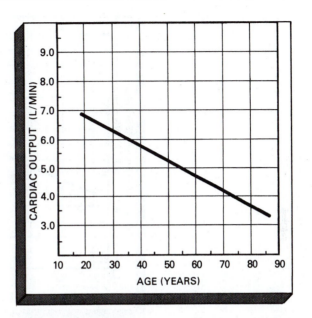

FIGURE 13–7. Schematic representation of the effects of aging on the *cardiac output*.

peripheral vascular system stiffens, its ability to accept the cardiac stroke volume declines. This age-related development increases the *resting pulse pressure* and the *systolic blood pressure*. It is estimated that the *total* peripheral resistance increases about 1 percent per year (Figure 13–8).

As the peripheral resistance increases, the perfusion of the body organs decreases. This progressive decline in organ perfusion partly explains the many organ debilities seen in the elderly. As the vascular system stiffens with age, its tolerance to change diminishes. For example, a sudden move from the horizontal to the vertical position may cause a marked drop in systemic blood pressure, causing dizziness, confusion, weakness, and fainting. Arterial stiffening also makes the baroreceptors, located in the carotid sinuses and aortic arch, sluggish and less able to moderate blood pressure changes.

Blood Pressure

As described previously, factors associated with aging that increase blood pressure are increasing stiffness of large arteries and increasing total peripheral resistance. Other factors, such as obesity, salt intake, and stress, can also elevate the blood pressure.

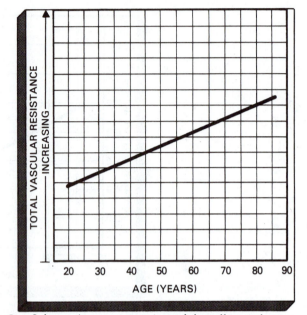

FIGURE 13–8.   Schematic representation of the effects of aging on the *total vascular resistance*.

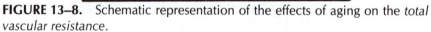

SELF-ASSESSMENT QUESTIONS

1. As an individual grows older, the
   a. residual volume decreases
   b. expiratory reserve volume increases
   c. functional residual capacity decreases
   d. inspiratory reserve volume increases
   e. vital capacity decreases
2. Most of the lung function indices reach their maximum levels between
   a. 1–5 years of age
   b. 5–10 years of age
   c. 10–15 years of age
   d. 15–20 years of age
   e. 20–25 years of age
3. With advancing age, the
   I. lung compliance decreases
   II. chest wall compliance increases

    III. lung compliance increases

    IV. chest wall compliance decreases

       a. I only

       b. II only

       c. III only

       d. I and II only

       e. III and IV only

4. As an individual grows older, the

      I. forced vital capacity increases

     II. peak expiratory flow rate decreases

    III. forced expiratory volume in 1 second increases

    IV. maximum voluntary ventilation increases

       a. I only

       b. II only

       c. II and IV only

       d. III and IV only

       e. II, III, and IV only

5. With advancing age, the

      I. Pa_{CO_2} increases

     II. Pa_{O_2} decreases

    III. $P_{(A-a)O_2}$ decreases

    IV. $C(a - \bar{v})_{O_2}$ decreases

       a. I only

       b. II only

       c. III only

       d. II and IV only

       e. III and IV only

6. The maximum heart rate of a 45-year-old person is

       a. 155 beats/min

       b. 165 beats/min

       c. 175 beats/min

       d. 185 beats/min

       e. 195 beats/min

7. Over the course of life, the diffusion capacity decreases by about

       a. 5%

       b. 10%

       c. 15%

       d. 20%

       e. 25%

8. Between 30 and 80 years of age, the cardiac output decreases by about

       a. 10%

       b. 20%

    c. 30%

    d. 40%

    e. 50%

9. With advancing age, the

    I. blood pressure increases

    II. stroke volume decreases

    III. cardiac output increases

    IV. heart work decreases

      a. I only

      b. II only

      c. III and IV only

      d. II and III only

      e. I, II, and IV only

10. Between 20 and 60 years of age, the RV/TLC ratio

      a. increases from 20% to 25%

      b. increases from 20% to 30%

      c. increases from 20% to 35%

      d. increases from 20% to 40%

      e. remains the same

Answers appear in Appendix VII.

CHAPTER 14

EXERCISE AND ITS EFFECTS ON THE CARDIOPULMONARY SYSTEM

OBJECTIVES

By the end of this chapter, the student should be able to:

1. Describe the effects of exercise on the following components of the cardiopulmonary system:
   —Ventilation
   —Oxygen consumption
   —Arterial blood gases
   —Oxygen diffusion capacity
   —Alveolar-arterial oxygen tension difference
   —Circulation
   • Sympathetic discharge
   • Increased cardiac output
   • Increased arterial blood pressure
   • Pulmonary vascular pressures
   • Opening of muscle capillaries
2. Describe the interrelationships between muscle work, oxygen consumption, and cardiac output.
3. Describe the influence of training on the heart and on cardiac output.
4. Differentiate between stroke volume and heart rate in increasing the cardiac output.
5. Describe how body temperature and cutaneous blood flow relate to a number of symptoms collectively referred to as heat stroke.
6. List the benefits of cardiovascular rehabilitation.
7. Complete the self-assessment questions at the end of this chapter.

During heavy exercise, components of the cardiopulmonary system may be stressed close to their limit. Alveolar ventilation may increase as much as 20-fold, oxygen diffusion capacity as much as 3-fold, cardic output as much as 6-fold, muscle blood flow as much as 25-fold, oxygen consumption as much as 20-fold, and heat production as much as 20-fold.

Muscle training can increase muscle size and strength 30 to 60 percent. The efficiency of intracellular metabolism may increase by 30 to 50 percent. The size of the heart chambers and the heart mass of well-trained athletes, such as marathon runners, may be increased by 40 percent. When the level of exercise is greater, however, than the ability of the cardiopulmonary system to provide a sufficient supply of oxygen to the muscles, anaerobic metabolism ensues. The point at which anaerobic metabolism develops is called the **anaerobic threshold**.

VENTILATION

Control of Ventilation

The precise mechanism responsible for increased alveolar ventilation during exercise is not well understood. Exercise causes the body to consume a large amount of oxygen and, simultaneously, to produce a large amount of carbon dioxide. However, alveolar ventilation increases so much that the concentration of these gases in the body does not change significantly. In addition, no oxygen or carbon dioxide chemoreceptors have been identified on the venous side of circulation, or in the lungs, that could account for the increased alveolar ventilation during exercise. Thus it is unlikely that the increased ventilation seen in exercise is caused by either of these gases.

It has been suggested that the increased ventilation is caused by neural impulses sent to the medulla by way of the following pathways (Figure 14–1):

1. The cerebral cortex sending neural signals to the exercising muscles may also send collateral signals to the medulla to increase the rate and depth of breathing.
2. Proprioceptors in the moving muscles, tendons, and joints transmit sensory signals via the spinal cord to the respiratory centers of the medulla.
3. The increase in body temperature during exercise may also contribute to increased ventilation.

Alveolar Ventilation

During normal quiet breathing, an adult exchanges about 6 liters of air per minute. During strenuous exercise, this can increase to 120 liters per minute, a 20-fold increase. Depending on the intensity and duration of the exercise, alveolar ventilation must increase to (1) supply sufficient oxygen to the blood, and (2)

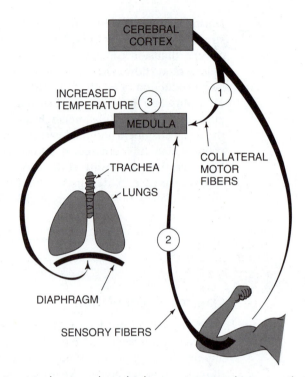

FIGURE 14–1. Mechanisms by which exercise stimulates ventilation. (*1*) Colateral fibers from the motor neurons go to the medulla; (*2*) sensory signals from the exercising limbs are sent to the medulla; (*3*) the increase in body temperature during exercise may also increase ventilation.

eliminate the excess carbon dioxide produced by the skeletal muscles. The increased alveolar ventilation is produced mainly by an increased depth of ventilation (increased tidal volume) rather than by an increased rate of ventilation. During very heavy exercise, however, both an increased depth and frequency of ventilation is seen. The tidal volume is usually about 50 percent of the vital capacity, and the respiratory rate is usually between 40 and 50 breaths per minute.

There are three distinct consecutive breathing patterns seen during mild and moderate exercise. The **first stage** is characterized by an increase in alveolar ventilation, within seconds after the onset of exercise. The **second stage** is typified by a slow, gradual further increase in alveolar ventilation developing over approximately the first 3 minutes of exercise. Alveolar ventilation during this period increases almost linearly with the amount of work performed. During the **third stage**, alveolar ventilation stabilizes. When an individual stops exercising, alveolar ventilation decreases abruptly (Figure 14–2).

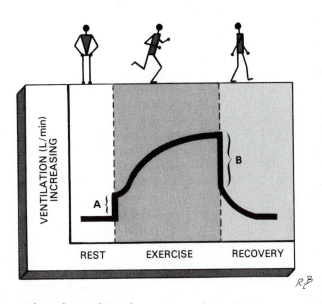

FIGURE 14–2. The relationship of exercise and ventilation. Note the abrupt increase in ventilation at the outset of exercise (*A*) and the even larger, abrupt decrease in ventilation at the end of exercise (*B*).

During very heavy exercise, the steady-state third stage may not be seen. In fact, when approximately 60 to 70 percent of the maximal exercise level is reached during the linear second stage, alveolar ventilation increases proportionately more than the oxygen uptake. The additional stimulation is thought to be caused primarily by the accumulation of lactic acid in the blood after the anaerobic threshold has been reached. It is suggested that the H^+ ions generated by the lactic acid stimulate the carotid chemoreceptors, which, in turn, send neural impulses to the medulla to increase alveolar ventilation (see Figure 10–3).

The maximum alveolar ventilation generated during heavy exercise under normal conditions is only about 50 to 65 percent of the maximum voluntary ventilation (also called maximum breathing capacity). This provides the athlete with an important reserve of alveolar ventilation, which may be required in such conditions as short bursts of increased exercise, exercise at high altitudes, or exercise during very hot and humid conditions. Because there is normally a large alveolar ventilatory reserve during exercise, it is not the limiting factor in the delivery of oxygen to the muscles during maximal muscular aerobic metabolism. As discussed later, the inability of the heart to pump sufficient blood to the working muscles is the major limiting factor.

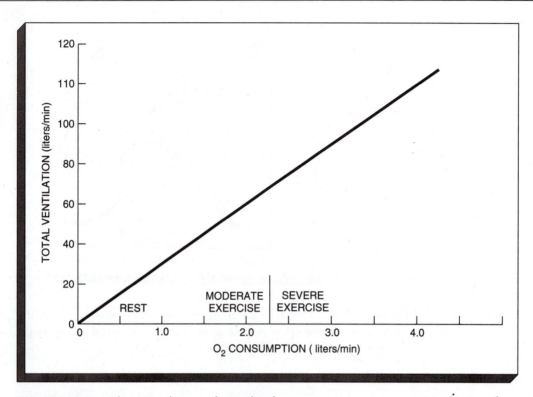

FIGURE 14–3.   There is a linear relationship between oxygen consumption ($\dot{V}_{O_2}$) and alveolar ventilation as the intensity of exercise increases.

Oxygen Consumption

At rest, normal oxygen consumption ($\dot{V}_{O_2}$) is about 250 ml per minute. The skeletal muscles account for approximately 35 to 40 percent of the total $\dot{V}_{O_2}$. During exercise, the skeletal muscles may account for more than 95 percent of the $\dot{V}_{O_2}$. During heavy exercise, the $\dot{V}_{O_2}$ of an untrained person may be more than 3500 ml of O_2 per minute. The $\dot{V}_{O_2}$ of a well-trained athlete while running a marathon may be over 5000 ml O_2 per minute. Figure 14–3 shows the linear relationship between $\dot{V}_{O_2}$ and alveolar ventilation as the intensity of exercises increases.

Arterial Blood Gases during Exercise

No significant Pa_{O_2}, Pa_{CO_2}, or pH changes are seen between rest and approximately 60 to 70% of maximal $\dot{V}_{O_2}$. During very heavy exercise, however, when lactic acidosis is present, both the pH and Pa_{CO_2} decline. Although

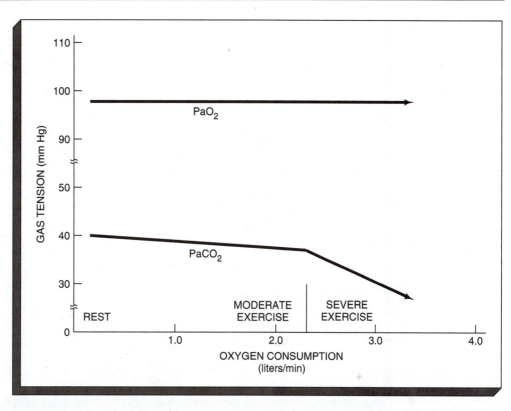

FIGURE 14–4. The effect of oxygen consumption on Pa_{O_2} and Pa_{CO_2} as the intensity of exercise increases.

controversial, it is believed that arterial acidosis stimulates the carotid chemoreceptors, causing increased alveolar ventilation and promoting respiratory acid-base compensation. The Pa_{O_2} remains constant during mild, moderate, and heavy exercise (Figure 14–4).

Oxygen Diffusion Capacity

The oxygen diffusion capacity increases linearly in response to the increased oxygen consumption ($\dot{V}_{O_2}$), during exercise (Figure 14–5). The oxygen diffusion capacity may increase as much as 3-fold during the state of maximum exercise. It has been shown that the increased oxygen diffusion capacity results from the increased cardiac output during exercise. The increased cardiac output causes the intravascular pressure in the pulmonary artery and left atrium to increase, which in turn serves to (1) distend the pulmonary capillaries that are not fully dilated, and (2) open, or recruit, closed pulmonary capillaries (see Figure 5–21). As more

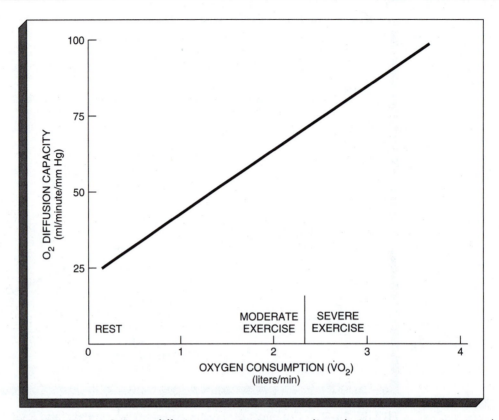

FIGURE 14–5. Oxygen diffusion capacity increases linearly in response to increased oxygen consumption, as the intensity of exercise increases.

blood flows through the lungs, more alveolar-capillary units become available for gas exchange. This provides a greater surface area through which oxygen can diffuse into the pulmonary capillary blood.

Alveolar-arterial PO_2 Difference

Normally, there is a mean alveolar-arterial oxygen tension difference $P_{(A-a)O_2}$ of about 10 mm Hg because of (1) mismatching of ventilation and perfusion, and (2) right-to-left pulmonary shunting of blood. In spite of increases in oxygen consumption ($\dot{V}_{O_2}$), alveolar ventilation, and cardiac output, the $P_{(A-a)O_2}$ remains essentially constant until 40% of the maximal $\dot{V}_{O_2}$ is reached. The $P_{(A-a)O_2}$ begins to increase when 40% of the maximal $\dot{V}_{O_2}$ is exceeded (Figure 14–6). An average $P_{(A-a)O_2}$ of 33 mm Hg has been reported for endurance runners who were exercising at their maximal $\dot{V}_{O_2}$.

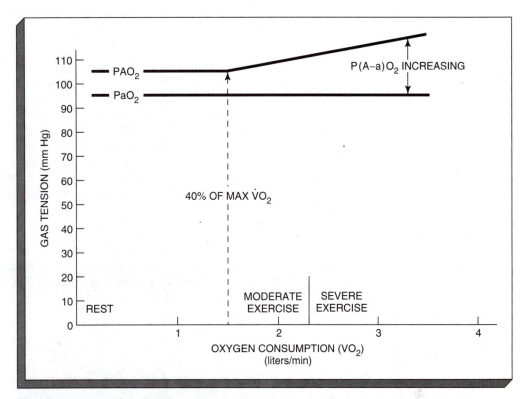

FIGURE 14–6. The alveolar-arterial oxygen tension difference $P_{(A - a)O_2}$ begins to increase when approximately 40% of the maximal $\dot{V}_{O_2}$ is exceeded.

CIRCULATION

Heavy exercise is one of the most stressful conditions the circulatory system encounters. Blood flow to the working muscles may increase as much as 25-fold, and the total cardiac output may increase as much as 6-fold.

The ability of an individual to increase cardiac output to the muscles is the major factor that determines how long and to what intensity the exercise can be sustained. In fact, the speed of a marathon runner or swimmer is almost directly proportional to the athletes' ability to increase their cardiac output. Thus, the circulatory system is as important as the muscles themselves in setting the limits for exercise.

During exercise, three essential physiologic responses must occur in order for the circulatory system to supply the working muscles with an adequate amount of blood. These are: (1) sympathetic discharge, (2) increase in cardiac output, and (3) increase in arterial blood pressure.

Sympathetic Discharge

At the onset of exercise, the brain transmits signals to the vasomotor center in the medulla oblongata to trigger a sympathetic discharge. This sympathetic discharge has two circulatory effects: (1) the heart is stimulated to increase its rate and strength of contraction, and (2) the blood vessels of the peripheral vascular system constrict, except for the blood vessels of the working muscles, which strongly dilate in response to local vasodilators in the muscles themselves. The net result is an increased blood supply to the working muscles while the blood flow to non-working muscles is reduced. It should be noted that vasoconstriction in the heart and brain does not occur during exercise, since both the heart and the brain are as important to exercise as the working muscles themselves.

Increased Cardiac Output

The increased oxygen demands during exercise are met almost entirely by an increased cardiac output. Figure 14–7 shows that there is a linear relationship between the cardiac output and the intensity of exercise. The increased cardiac output during exercise results from (1) increased stroke volume, (2) increased heart rate, or (3) a combination of both.

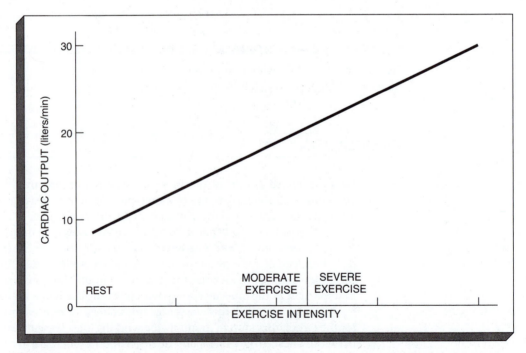

FIGURE 14–7. There is a linear relationship between cardiac output and the intensity of exercise.

Increased Stroke Volume. The increased stroke volume during exercise is primarily due to vasodilation in the working muscles. That is, the vasodilation in the working muscles increases the venous return to the heart. The heart, in turn, pumps more oxygenated blood back to the working muscles. Thus, the degree of vasodilation in the working muscles directly influences the stroke volume and, therefore, the greater the vasodilation in the working muscles, the greater the stroke volume and cardiac output. Another factor that facilitates an increased venous return during exercise is the sympathetic discharge. This causes a constriction of all venous blood reservoirs and forces more blood out of the veins and toward the heart.

As discussed in Chapter 5, the ability of the heart to accommodate the increased venous return and, subsequently, increase the cardiac output is due to the Frank-Starling mechanism (see Figure 5–19). When more venous blood returns to the heart, the heart chambers increase in size to accommodate the increased volume. As the heart chambers increase in size, the force of the heart muscle contractions increase, which in turn increases the stroke volume.

In addition to the Frank-Starling mechanism, the heart is also strongly stimulated by the sympathetic discharge. Increased sympathetic stimulation causes (1) increased heart rate (as high as 200 beats per minute), and (2) increased strength of contraction. The combined effect of these two mechanisms greatly increases the heart's ability to pump blood beyond what could be accomplished by the Frank-Starling mechanism alone.

Increased Heart Rate. An individual's maximum heart rate is estimated by the following formula:

maximum heart rate = 220 − age

Thus, the maximum heart rate for a 45-year-old is about 175 (220 − 45 = 175).

Although the heart rate increases linearly with oxygen consumption, the magnitude of the change is influenced by the size of the stroke volume. That is, when the stroke volume decreases, the heart rate increases, and when the stroke volume increases, the heart rate decreases. The stroke volume, in turn, is influenced by (1) the individual's physical condition, (2) the specific muscles that are working, and (3) the distribution of blood flow. The body's ability to increase the heart rate and stroke volume during exercise progressively declines with age.

Increased Arterial Blood Pressure

There is an increase in arterial blood pressure during exercise because of the (1) sympathetic discharge, (2) increased cardiac output, and (3) vasoconstriction of the blood vessels in the non-working muscle areas. Depending on the physical condition of the individual, as well as the intensity and duration of the exercise, the systolic arterial blood pressure may increase as little as 20 mm Hg or as much as 80 mm Hg.

Pulmonary Vascular Pressures

As oxygen consumption and cardiac output increase during exercise, the systolic, diastolic, and mean pulmonary arterial and wedge pressures also increase linearly (Figure 14–8). As discussed earlier, this mechanism enhances oxygen uptake by (1) distending the pulmonary capillaries, and (2) opening closed pulmonary capillaries.

Opening of Muscle Capillaries

At rest, approximately only 20 to 25 percent of the muscle capillaries are open. During heavy exercise, all these capillaries open up to facilitate the distribution of blood. This reduces the distance that oxygen and other nutrients must travel from the capillaries to the muscle fiber. At the same time, the blood vessels of the viscera and non-working muscles constrict.

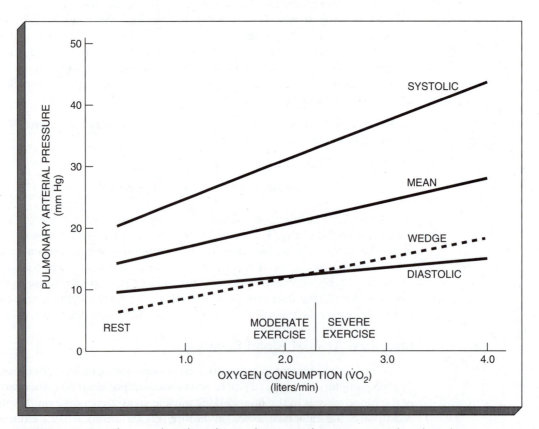

FIGURE 14–8.   The systolic, diastolic, and mean pulmonary arterial and wedge pressures increase linearly as oxygen consumption and cardiac output increase.

The dilation of the blood vessels in the working muscles is caused primarily by local vasodilators acting directly on the arterioles. The most important local vasodilator effect is the reduction of oxygen in the working muscles. It is suggested that a diminished oxygen concentration in the muscles causes vasodilation because either (1) the vessels are unable to maintain contraction at low oxygen levels, or (2) low oxygen levels cause the release of vasodilator substances. The most likely vasodilator substance is *adenosine*. Other vasodilator substances include potassium ions, acetylcholine, adenosine triphosphate, lactic acid, and carbon dioxide. The precise role of each of these substances in increasing blood flow to working muscles is not known.

Finally, because the vasodilation of the major working muscle groups is greater than the vasoconstriction of the non-working muscle groups, the overall peripheral vascular resistance decreases. This is why highly trained athletes can increase their cardiac output substantially with only a slight increase in their mean systemic arterial blood pressure. Untrained individuals have a high peripheral vascular resistance and, therefore, high arterial blood pressure in response to modest increases in cardiac output during exercise.

INTERRELATIONSHIPS BETWEEN MUSCLE WORK, OXYGEN CONSUMPTION, AND CARDIAC OUTPUT

Figure 14–9 shows that muscle work, oxygen consumption, and cardiac output are all related to each other. Increased muscle work increases oxygen consumption and the increased oxygen consumption, in turn, dilates the intramuscular blood vessels. As the intramuscular blood vessels dilate, venous return increases, causing the cardiac output to rise. Marathon runners can have a cardiac output as great as 40 L per minute. The maximum cardiac output of a young, untrained individual is less than 25 L per minute.

THE INFLUENCE OF TRAINING ON THE HEART AND ON CARDIAC OUTPUT

The increased cardiac output seen in marathon runners results mainly from the fact that the heart chambers and heart mass increase as much as 40 percent. Cardiac enlargement and increased pumping ability occur only in the endurance type of athletic training and not in the sprint type of activity. The "athlete's heart" is an effective and physiologically sound heart. It should not be considered a pathologic heart. At rest, the cardiac output of the well-trained athletic is almost the same as that of the average untrained individual. The well-trained individual, however, has a greater stroke volume and a reduced heart rate.

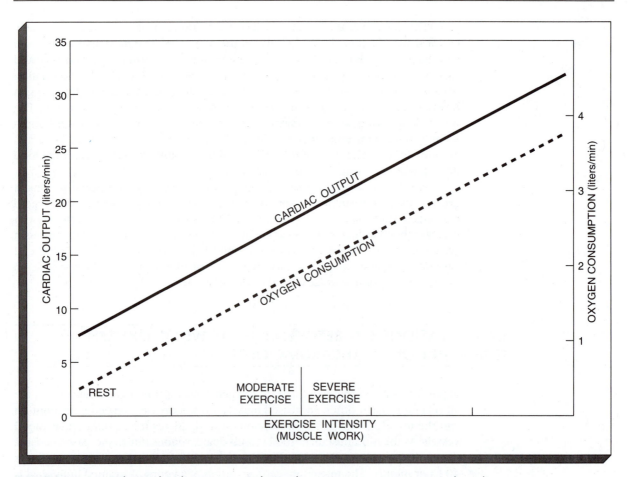

FIGURE 14–9. Relationship between muscle work, oxygen consumption, and cardiac output.

STROKE VOLUME VS. HEART RATE IN INCREASING THE CARDIAC OUTPUT

Figure 14–10 shows the approximate changes that occur in stroke volume and heart rate as the cardiac output increases from about 5 L per minute to 30 L per minute in a marathon runner. The stroke volume increases from about 100 ml to about 150 ml, an increase of about 50 percent. The heart rate increases from 50 to 180 beats per minute, an increase of 260 percent. Thus, during very heavy exercise the increase in heart rate accounts for a much greater proportion of the increased cardiac output than the increase in stroke volume. In fact, the stroke volume reaches its maximum when the maximum cardiac output is only at approximately

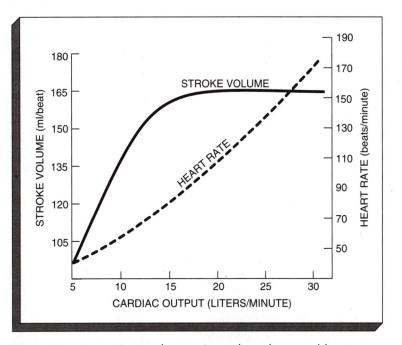

FIGURE 14–10. Approximate changes in stroke volume and heart rate that occur when the cardiac output increases from about 5 liters per minute to 30 liters per minute in a marathon runner.

50 percent. Thus, any further increase in cardiac output beyond the midway point is due solely to the increased heart rate.

At maximum exercise, cardiac output reaches about 90 percent of the maximum that can be achieved. Since maximum exercise taxes the respiratory system only about 65 percent of maximum, it can be seen that normally the cardiovascular system is a greater limiting factor on maximal exercise than the respiratory system. Thus, the maximum performance that a marathon runner can achieve is directly related to the condition of the cardiovascular system. Any type of heart disease that reduces the heart's ability to pump blood will also decrease an individual's muscle power. This partly explains why a patient in congestive heart failure may have difficulty in generating enough muscle power to climb out of bed, or to walk short distances.

BODY TEMPERATURE/CUTANEOUS BLOOD FLOW RELATIONSHIP

During exercise, the body generates a tremendous amount of heat and heat production may increase as much as 20-fold. Although some of the heat is stored in the body during exercise, most of the heat is dissipated through the skin. This requires a substantial increase in blood flow to the body surface. Nevertheless, even during normal temperature and humidity conditions the body temperature may rise from its normal 98.6°F to 102° to 103°F (37°C to 40°C) during endurance athletics.

When exercise is performed during very hot and humid conditions, or without adequately ventilated clothing, heat loss may be impaired and an unusually large amount of blood may be distributed to the skin. During these conditions the body temperature can easily rise to 106° to 108°F. As much as 5 to 10 lb of body fluid can be lost in one hour. When this happens, a number of symptoms may appear, which collectively are referred to as **heat stroke**. These symptoms include:

- Profuse sweating, followed by no sweating
- Extreme weakness
- Muscle cramping
- Exhaustion
- Nausea
- Headache
- Dizziness
- Confusion
- Staggering gait
- Unconsciousness
- Circulatory collapse

Heat stroke can be lethal if not treated immediately. Even when the individual stops exercising, the temperature does not readily return to normal. This is because of (1) the temperature-regulating mechanism often fails at a very high temperature, and (2) the intracellular metabolism is much faster at higher temperatures, which in turn generates still more heat.

The primary treatment of heat stroke is to reduce the victim's body temperature as fast as possible. This is done by (1) spraying cool water on the victim's body, (2) continually sponging the victim with cool water, (3) blowing air over the body with a strong fan, or (4) a combination of all three.

CARDIOVASCULAR REHABILITATION

Cardiovascular rehabilitation is now a well accepted, multidisciplinary health care service. It provides cardiac patients with a process of developing and maintaining a desirable level of physical, social, and psychologic well-being. The prominent components of a cardiovascular rehabilitation program are patient education, counseling, nutritional guidance, and graded exercise training. The rehabilitative process for the cardiac patient is commonly divided into the following four phases:

Phase I: Acute, In-Hospital

This phase consists of low-level exercise, patient and family education, group and individual counseling, and group discussion sessions.

Phase II: Outpatient, Immediately after Hospitalization

During this phase, the patient begins active range-of-motion exercises. Such exercises include work on the treadmill, air-dyne bike, arm ergometer, rowing machine, chest pulleys, and steps. The duration of phase II is between 2 and 4 months.

Phase III: Long-term Outpatient

This phase includes the long-term aspects of cardiac rehabilitation. The primary objective during this phase is the conditioning of the cardiovascular system (aerobic) and skeletal muscles. Long-term graded exercises are emphasized, such as walking, walking/jogging, stationary bicycling, and/or swimming. The duration of phase III is between 6 and 24 months.

Phase IV: Maintenance

Phase IV of rehabilitation is the maintenance of the patient's physical condition. Components of phase IV include efforts to modify risk factors (e.g., control of blood lipids, cigarette smoking, hypertension, and obesity) and a routine program of physical activity. This phase should continue indefinitely. The patient commonly goes through a yearly evaluation, which includes graded exercise testing. Some patients may require more frequent evaluations.

The benefits from cardiac rehabilitation include improved exercise capacity and decreased angina pectoris, dyspnea, and fatigue. Patients involved in exercise training after myocardial infarction demonstrate a 20 to 25 percent reduction in mortality and major cardiac mishaps. Cardiac rehabilitation may improve oxygen transport, reduce the myocardial oxygen requirements during work, and reduce myocardial ischemia during physical activity. Finally, the efforts to modify risk factors during cardiac rehabilitation has clearly shown a reduction in the progression of coronary artery disease, morbidity, and mortality.

SELF-ASSESSMENT QUESTIONS

1. During strenuous exercise, an adult's alveolar ventilation can increase as much as:

    a. 10-fold

    b. 20-fold

    c. 30-fold

    d. 40-fold

    e. 50-fold

2. The maximum alveolar ventilation generated during heavy exercise under normal conditions is about what percent of the maximum voluntary ventilation?

    a. 10 to 25 percent

    b. 20 to 35 percent

    c. 30 to 45 percent

    d. 40 to 55 percent

    e. 50 to 65 percent

3. During heavy exercise, the total cardiac output may increase as much as:

    a. 2-fold

    b. 4-fold

    c. 6-fold

    d. 8-fold

    e. 10-fold

4. At the onset of exercise, sympathetic discharge causes the:

    I. Heart rate to decrease

    II. Peripheral vascular system to constrict

    III. Heart to increase its strength of contraction

    IV. Blood vessels of the working muscles to dilate

    a. I only

    b. III only

    c. II and IV only

    d. I and II only

    e. II, III, and IV only

5. During exercise, the stroke volume reaches its peak when the cardiac output is at about what percent of its maximum:

    a. 30 percent

    b. 40 percent

    c. 50 percent

    d. 60 percent

    e. 70 percent

6. During exercise, heat production may increase as much as:

    a. 10-fold

    b. 20-fold

    c. 30-fold

    d. 40-fold

    e. 50-fold

7. During exercise, the oxygen consumption ($\dot{V}_{O_2}$) of the skeletal muscles may account for more than:

    a. 55 percent of the total $\dot{V}_{O_2}$

    b. 65 percent of the total $\dot{V}_{O_2}$

    c. 75 percent of the total $\dot{V}_{O_2}$

    d. 85 percent of the total $\dot{V}_{O_2}$

    e. 95 percent of the total $\dot{V}_{O_2}$

8. During very heavy exercise, the:

    I. pH increases

    II. Pa_{CO_2} decreases

    III. Pa_{O_2} remains constant

    IV. pH decreases

    V. Pa_{CO_2} increases

        a. I and II only

        b. IV and V only

        c. II and IV only

        d. II, III, and IV only

        e. III, IV, and V only

9. During maximum exercise, the oxygen diffusion capacity may increase as much as:

    a. 3-fold

    b. 6-fold

    c. 9-fold

    d. 12-fold

    e. 15-fold

10. During exercise, the $P_{(A-a)O_2}$ begins to increase when the oxygen consumption reaches about what percent of its maximum?

    a. 10 percent

    b. 20 percent

    c. 30 percent

    d. 40 percent

    e. 50 percent

Answers appear in Appendix VII.

CHAPTER 15

HIGH ALTITUDE AND ITS EFFECTS ON THE CARDIOPULMONARY SYSTEM

OBJECTIVES

By the end of this chapter, the student should be able to:

1. Describe the effects of high altitude on the following components of the cardiopulmonary system:
   —Ventilation
   —Red blood cell production
   —Acid-base status
   —Oxygen diffusion capacity
   —Alveolar-arterial oxygen tension difference
   —Ventilation-perfusion relationship
   —Cardiac output
   —Pulmonary vascular system
   —Myoglobin concentration
2. Describe other physiologic changes caused by high altitude, including:
   —Sleep
   —Acute mountain sickness
   —High-altitude pulmonary edema
   —High-altitude cerebral edema
   —Chronic mountain sickness
3. Complete the self-assessment questions at the end of this chapter.

HIGH ALTITUDE

The effects of high altitude on the cardiopulmonary system are of interest, since a better understanding of chronic oxygen deprivation can be applied to the treatment of chronic hypoxia caused by lung disease.

The barometric pressure progressively decreases with altitude (Figure 15–1). At an altitude of 18,000 to 19,000 ft, the barometric pressure is about half the sea level value of 760 mm Hg (380 mm Hg). The barometric pressure on the summit of Mount Everest (altitude: 29,028 ft) is about 250 mm Hg (the atmospheric P_{O_2} is about 43 mm Hg). At an altitude of about 65,000 ft, the barometric pressure falls below the pressure of water vapor and tissue fluids begin to "boil" or "vaporize."

When an individual who normally lives near sea level spends a period of time at high altitudes, a number of compensatory responses develop—a process known as **acclimatization**. For example, it is an interesting fact that after a period of acclimatization, an individual may reach the summit of Mount Everest without supplementary oxygen. However, when an individual is suddenly exposed to the oxygen tension found at the summit of Mount Everest, a loss of consciousness occurs within minutes.

The following are some of the major cardiopulmonary changes seen after a period of acclimatization at high altitude.

Ventilation

One of the most prominent features of acclimatization is increased alveolar ventilation. As already mentioned, when an individual ascends above the earth's surface, the barometric pressure progressively decreases and the atmospheric P_{O_2} declines. As the atmospheric P_{O_2} decreases, the individual's arterial oxygen pressure (Pa_{O_2}) also decreases. Eventually, the Pa_{O_2} will fall low enough (about 60 mm Hg) to stimulate the carotid and aortic bodies, known collectively as the **peripheral chemoreceptors** (see Figure 10–3). When the peripheral chemoreceptors are stimulated, they transmit signals to the medulla to increase ventilation (see Figure 10–4). Because the peripheral chemoreceptors do not acclimate to a decreased oxygen concentration, increased alveolar ventilation will continue for the entire time the individual remains at the high altitude.

Polycythemia

When an individual is subjected to a low concentration of oxygen for a prolonged period of time, the hormone *erythropoietin* from the kidneys stimulates the bone marrow to increase red blood cell (RBC) production. The increased hemoglobin available in polycythemia is an adaptive mechanism that increases the oxygen-carrying capacity of the blood. In fact, people who live at high altitudes

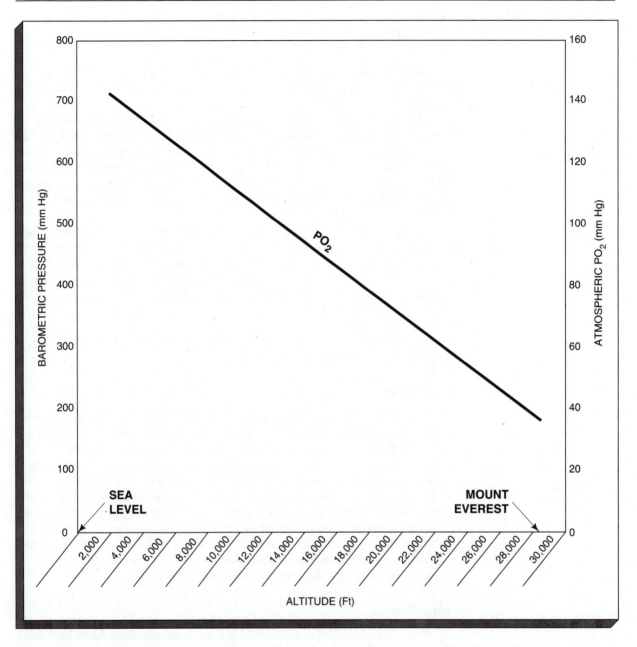

FIGURE 15–1. The barometric pressure and the atmospheric P_{O_2} decrease linearly as altitude increases.

often have a normal, or even above-normal, oxygen-carrying capacity, in spite of a chronically low Pa_{O_2} and oxygen saturation.

In lowlanders who ascend to high altitudes, the RBCs increase for about six weeks before the production rate levels off. As the level of RBCs increase the plasma volume decreases. Thus, there is no significant change in the total circulating blood volume. After six weeks, an average hemoglobin concentration of 20.5 g/dl has been observed in mountain climbers who were at altitudes greater than 18,000 ft.

Acid-base Status

Because of the increased ventilation generated by the peripheral chemoreceptors at high altitudes, the Pa_{CO_2} decreases, causing a secondary respiratory alkalosis. Over a 24 to 48 hour period, the renal system tries to offset the respiratory alkalosis by eliminating some of the excess bicarbonate. In spite of this mechanism, however, a mild respiratory alkalosis usually persists. In fact, even natives, who have been at high-altitudes for generations, commonly have a mild respiratory alkalosis.

It is assumed that respiratory alkalosis may be advantageous for the transfer of oxygen across the alveolar-capillary membrane, since alkalosis increases the affinity of hemoglobin for oxygen. In other words, the alkalosis enhances the loading of oxygen to the hemoglobin as desaturated blood passes through the alveolar-capillary system (see Figure 7–9). It is also argued, however, that the increased affinity interferes with the unloading of oxygen at the cells (see Figure 7–10).

There is both experimental and theoretical evidence that the increased oxygen affinity at high altitude is beneficial. This is further supported by the fact that a mild respiratory alkalosis usually persists in mountain climbers, high-altitude natives, and even in animals who live in low-oxygen environments. The alkalosis persists even after the kidneys should have had more than enough time to fully eliminate the excess bicarbonate.

Oxygen Diffusion Capacity

There is no significant change in the oxygen diffusion capacity of lowlanders who are acclimatized to high altitude. High-altitude natives, however, have been shown to have an oxygen diffusion capacity that is about 20 to 25% greater than predicted, both during rest and exercise. The increased oxygen diffusion may be explained by the larger lungs seen in the high-altitude natives. It is suggested that the larger lungs provide an increased alveolar surface area and a larger capillary blood volume.

This is further supported by studies that demonstrate that when animals are exposed to low-oxygen partial pressures during their active growth period, they develop larger lungs and greater diffusion capacity. On the other hand, animals exposed to a hyperoxic environment during their active growth period develop smaller lungs than expected.

Alveolar-arterial P_{O_2} Difference

At high altitude, oxygen diffusion across the alveolar-capillary membrane is limited and this results in an increased **alveolar-arterial oxygen tension difference** $P_{(A-a)O_2}$. Figure 15–2 shows that under normal circumstances there is ample time for oxygen to equilibrate between the alveoli and the end-capillary blood. In contrast, Figure 15–3 shows the estimated time necessary for oxygen to equilibrate for a climber at rest on the summit of Mount Everest. Note that the

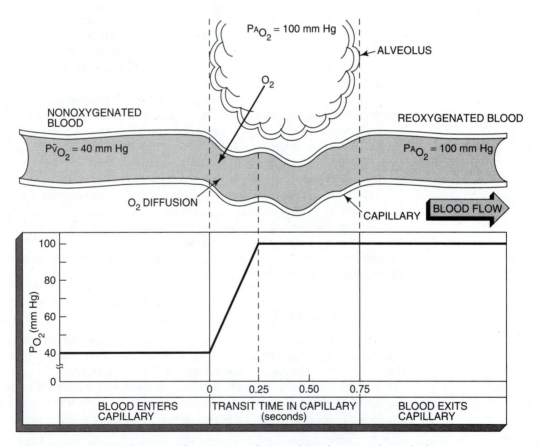

FIGURE 15–2. Under normal resting conditions, blood moves through the alveolar-capillary membrane in about 0.75 second. The oxygen pressure (P_{O_2}) reaches equilibrium in about 0.25 second—one-third of the time available.

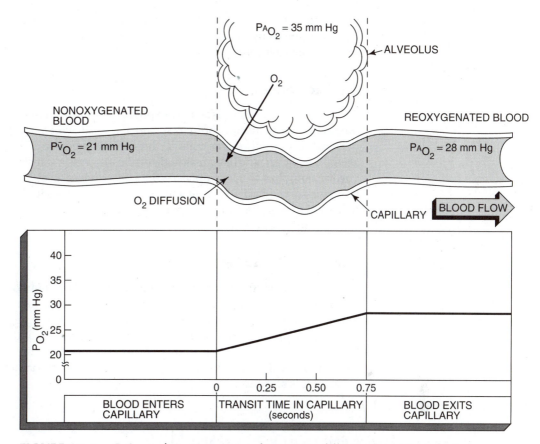

FIGURE 15–3. Estimated time necessary for oxygen diffusion for a climber at rest on the summit of Mount Everest. As the blood leaves the alveolar-capillary system, there is a large alveolar-arterial oxygen tension difference $P_{(A-a)O_2}$.

pulmonary blood enters the alveolar-capillary system with a P_{O_2} of about 21 mm Hg that slowly rises to about 28 mm Hg. As the blood leaves the alveolar-capillary system, there is thus a large $P_{(A-a)O_2}$ characteristic of oxygen diffusion-limitations. At high altitude, the $P_{(A-a)O_2}$ is further increased (1) during exercise (because of the increased cardiac output) and (2) in individuals with alveolar thickening caused by interstitial lung disease.

Ventilation-Perfusion Relationship

At high altitude, the overall ventilation-perfusion ratio improves as a result of the more uniform distribution of blood flow that develops in response to the increased pulmonary arterial blood pressure. Under normal circumstances the better gas exchange that results from the improved ventilation-perfusion ratio is relatively insignificant.

Cardiac Output

When an individual is acutely exposed to a hypoxic environment, the cardiac output increases during both rest and exercise which increases the oxygen delivery to the peripheral cells. In individuals who have acclimatized to high altitude, however, and in high-altitude natives, increased cardiac output is not seen. Cardiac output and oxygen uptake is the same as at sea level. The precise reason for the return of the cardiac output and oxygen uptake to sea level values is unknown. It has been suggested that the polycythemia that develops in well-acclimatized subjects may play a role.

Pulmonary Vascular System

As an individual ascends from the earth's surface, pulmonary hypertension progressively increases as a result of hypoxic pulmonary vasoconstriction. There is a linear relationship between the degree of ascent and the degree of pulmonary vasoconstriction and hypertension. The exact mechanism of this phenomenon is unclear (Figure 15–4). It is known, however, that it is the partial pressure of oxygen in the alveoli and not the partial pressure of arterial oxygen that chiefly controls this response.

OTHER PHYSIOLOGIC CHANGES

Sleep

During the first few days at high altitude, lowlanders frequently wake up during the night and complain that they do not feel refreshed when they awake in the morning. When sleeping, they commonly demonstrate breathing that waxes and wanes with apneic periods of 10 to 15 seconds duration (Cheyne-Stokes breathing). The arterial oxygen saturation fluctuates accordingly.

Myoglobin Concentration

The concentration of myoglobin in skeletal muscles is increased in high-altitude natives, and research in this group has shown a high concentration of myoglobin in the diaphragm, in the adductor muscles of the leg, in the pectoral

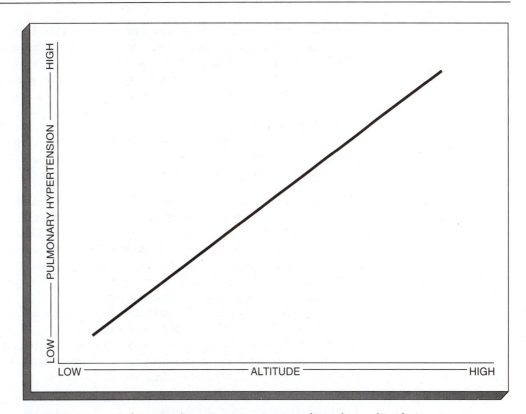

FIGURE 15–4. Pulmonary hypertension increases linearly as altitude increases.

muscles, and in the myocardium. Myoglobin enhances the transfer of oxygen between the capillary blood and peripheral cells, buffers regional P_{O_2} differences, and provides an oxygen storage compartment for short periods of very severe oxygen deprivation.

Acute Mountain Sickness

Newcomers to high altitude frequency experience what is known as **acute mountain sickness**. It is characterized by headache, fatigue, dizziness, palpitation, nausea, loss of appetite, and insomnia. Symptoms commonly do not occur until 6 to 12 hours after an individual ascends to a high altitude. The symptoms are generally most severe on the second or third day after ascent. Acclimatization is usually complete by the fourth or fifth day.

The precise cause of acute mountain sickness is not known. It is suggested that the primary cause is hypoxia, complicated by the hypocapnia and respiratory alkalosis associated with high altitude. It may also be linked to a fluid imbalance, since pulmonary edema, cerebral edema, and peripheral edema are commonly associated with acute and chronic mountain sickness.

Sensitivity to acute mountain sickness varies greatly among individuals. Being physical fit is no guarantee of immunity. Younger people appear to be more at risk. In some cases, descent may be the only way to reduce the symptoms.

High-altitude Pulmonary Edema

High-altitude pulmonary edema is sometimes seen in individuals with acute mountain sickness. A typical scenario is as follows: A lowlander rapidly ascends to a high altitude and is very active during the trip, or upon arrival. Initially, the lowlander demonstrates shortness of breath, fatigue, and a dry cough. Physical signs include tachypnea, tachycardia, and crackles at the lung bases. Orthopnea is commonly present at this time. In severe cases, the lowlander may cough up large amounts of pink frothy sputum. Death may occur.

The exact cause of high-altitude pulmonary edema is not fully understood. It may be associated with the pulmonary vasoconstriction that occurs in response to the alveolar hypoxia. It may also be associated with an increased permeability of the pulmonary capillaries. The best treatment of high-altitude pulmonary edema is rapid descent. Oxygen should be administered if available.

High-altitude Cerebral Edema

High-altitude cerebral edema is a serious complication of acute mountain sickness. It is characterized by photophobia, ataxia, hallucinations, clouding of consciousness, coma, and, possibly, death. The precise cause of high-altitude cerebral edema is unclear. It is suggested that it may be linked to the increased cerebral vasodilation and blood flow that results from hypoxia. Oxygen should be administered if available.

Chronic Mountain Sickness

Chronic mountain sickness (also known as Monge's disease) is sometimes seen in long-term residents at high altitude. It is characterized by fatigue, reduced exercise tolerance, headache, dizziness, somnolence, loss of mental acuity, marked polycythemia, and severe hypoxemia. The severe oxygen desaturation and polycythemia causes a cyanotic appearance. Hematocrit of 83% and hemoglobin concentrations as high as 28 g/dl have been reported. As a result of the high hematocrit, the viscosity of the blood is significantly increased. Right ventricular hypertrophy is common.

SELF-ASSESSMENT QUESTIONS

1. The barometric pressure is about half the sea level value of 760 mm Hg at an altitude of:
   a. 4,000–5,000 ft
   b. 9,000–10,000 ft
   c. 14,000–15,000 ft
   d. 18,000–19,000 ft
   e. 24,000–25,000 ft

2. The oxygen diffusion capacity of high-altitude natives is about
   a. 5–10% greater than predicted
   b. 10–15% greater than predicted
   c. 15–20% greater than predicted
   d. 20–25% greater than predicted
   e. 25–30% greater than predicted

3. Acute mountain sickness is characterized by:
   I. Insomnia
   II. Headache
   III. Dizziness
   IV. Palpitation
   V. Loss of appetite
       a. I and III only
       b. II and IV only
       c. III, IV, and V only
       d. II, III, and IV only
       e. I, II, III, IV, and V

4. The symptoms of acute mountain sickness are generally most severe on the:
   a. First or second day after ascent
   b. Second or third day after ascent
   c. Third or fourth day after ascent
   d. Fourth of fifth day after ascent
   e. Fifth or sixth day after ascent

5. When an individual is subjected to a high altitude for a prolonged period of time, which of the following is/are seen?
   I. An increased red blood cell production
   II. A decreased Pa_{CO_2}
   III. An increased $P_{(A-a)O_2}$
   IV. A decreased alveolar ventilation
       a. I and III only
       b. II and IV only
       c. III and IV only

    d. I, II, and III only
    e. I, III, and IV only

TRUE OR FALSE

1. At high altitude, the overall ventilation-perfusion   True _____   False _____
   ratio decreases.
2. In individuals who have acclimatized to a high   True _____   False _____
   altitude, an increased cardiac output is seen.
3. There is a linear relationship between the   True _____   False _____
   degree of ascent and the degree of pulmonary
   vasoconstriction and hypertension.
4. Natives who have been at high altitudes for   True _____   False _____
   generations commonly demonstrate a mild
   respiratory alkalosis.
5. The concentration of myoglobin in skeletal   True _____   False _____
   muscles is decreased in high-altitude natives.

Answers appear in Appendix VII.

CHAPTER 16

HIGH-PRESSURE ENVIRONMENTS AND THEIR EFFECTS ON THE CARDIOPULMONARY SYSTEM

OBJECTIVES

By the end of this chapter, the student should be able to:

1. Describe how the following relate to the effects of high-pressure environments on the cardiopulmonary system:
   —Breath-hold diving
   —The CO_2–O_2 paradox
   —The dive response
   —Decompression sickness
   —Hyperbaric medicine
2. Complete the self-assessment questions at the end of this chapter.

High-pressure environments have a profound effect on the cardiopulmonary system. In general, high-pressure environments include recreational scuba diving, deep sea diving, and hyperbaric medicine. The effects of high-pressure environments on the cardiopulmonary system are typically studied in (1) actual dives in the sea, (2) hyperbaric chambers where the subject is exposed to mixtures of compressed gases (known as "simulated dry dives"), and (3) a water-filled hyperbaric chamber that can simulate any depth by adjusting the gas pressure above the water (known as "simulated wet dives").

DIVING

Because water is incompressible, the pressure increases linearly with depth. For every 33 feet (10 m) below the surface, the pressure increases 1.0 atmosphere (760 mm Hg). Thus, the total pressure at a depth of 33 feet is 2 atmospheres (1520 mm Hg)—1.0 atmosphere is due to the water column and 1.0 atmosphere pressure is due to the gaseous atmosphere above the water. At 66 feet (20 m), the pressure is 3.0 atmospheres (2280 mm Hg) (Figure 16–1).

As an individual descends into water, the lung is compressed according to Boyle's law:

$$P_1 \times V_1 = P_2 \times V_2$$

where P_1 = the pressure prior to the dive, V_1 = the lung volume prior to the dive, P_2 = the pressure generated at a specific water depth, and V_2 = the lung volume at that water depth.

Thus, if an individual fully inhales to a total lung capacity of 6 liters at sea level, and dives to a depth of 33 feet, the lungs will be compressed to about 3 liters:

$$V_2 = \frac{P_1 \times V_1}{P_2}$$

$$= \frac{1 \times 6}{2}$$

$$= 3 \text{ liters}$$

At 66 feet, the lungs would be compressed to about 2 liters. At 99 feet, the lungs would be compressed to about 1.5 liters.

Boyle's law can also be used to calculate the pressure within a diver's lungs at a specific depth. For example, when the above diver descends from sea level (760 mm Hg) to a depth of 33 feet (compressing the lung volume from 6 to 3 liters), the pressure within the diver's lungs will increase to about 1520 mm Hg:

$$P_2 = \frac{P_1 \times V_1}{V_2}$$

$$= \frac{760 \times 6}{3}$$

$$= 1520 \text{ mm Hg}$$

At 66 feet, the pressure within a diver's lungs will be about 2,280 mm Hg. At 99 feet, the pressure will be about 3,040 mm Hg.

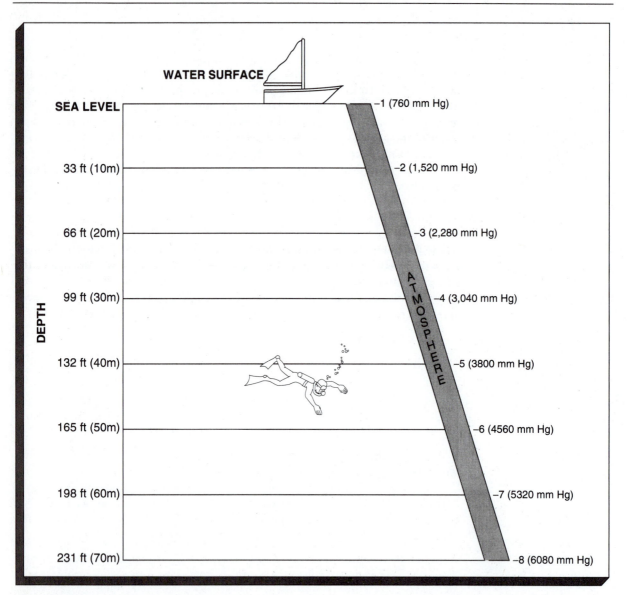

FIGURE 16–1. Pressure increases linearly with depth. For every 33 feet (10 m) below sea level, the pressure increases 1.0 atmosphere.

Breath-hold Diving

Breath-hold diving is the simplest and most popular form of diving. The maximum time of a breath-hold dive is a function of (1) the diver's metabolic rate, and (2) the diver's ability to store and transport O_2 and CO_2. A delicate balance exists between the diver's O_2 and CO_2 levels during a breath-hold dive. For example, the P_{CO_2} must not rise too rapidly and reach the so-called respiratory drive "**breaking point**" (generally about 55 mm Hg) before the diver returns to the surface. On the other hand, the diver's P_{CO_2} must rise fast enough (relative to the decrease in O_2) to alert the diver of the need to return to the surface before loss of consciousness develops from hypoxia.

Voluntary hyperventilation can prolong the duration of a breath-hold dive. Hyperventilation reduces the diver's CO_2 stores and, therefore, increases the time before the CO_2 stores are replenished and the "breaking point" is reached. It should be noted, however, that hyperventilation prior to a breath-hold dive can be dangerous. The diver's oxygen stores may fall to a critically low level before the CO_2 "breaking point" is reached. Should this happen, the diver could lose consciousness before reaching the surface, and drown.

The CO_2–O_2 Paradox

When an individual breath-hold dives to a great depth, there is a so-called paradoxical reversal in the flow of CO_2 and O_2 between the alveoli and the pulmonary capillary blood. This **CO_2–O_2 paradox** is caused by the pressure changes that develop around the diver's body during the dive. The CO_2 paradox occurs as the diver descends, and the O_2 paradox occurs as the diver ascends.

The reason for the CO_2 paradox is as follows: As the diver descends, the lungs are compressed and the pressure in the lungs increases. In fact, the gas pressure in the lungs is about doubled when the diver reaches a depth of 33 feet (2 atm). Thus, assuming a normal $P_{A_{O_2}}$ of about 100 mm Hg and $P_{A_{CO_2}}$ of about 40 mm Hg, at a depth of 33 feet the $P_{A_{O_2}}$ will be about 200 mm Hg and the $P_{A_{CO_2}}$ will be about 80 mm Hg.

In view of these pressure increases, it can be seen that as a diver progressively descends, a CO_2 paradox will occur when the $P_{A_{CO_2}}$ becomes greater than the $P_{\bar{v}_{CO_2}}$ of the pulmonary capillary blood (normally about 46 mm Hg). In other words, the CO_2 in the alveoli will move into the pulmonary capillary blood. As the diver returns to the surface, the alveolar air expands causing the $P_{A_{CO_2}}$ to decrease. When this happens, the CO_2 from the pulmonary capillary blood will again move into the alveoli. It is suggested that this mechanism might work to relieve the respiratory CO_2 drive (breaking point) as the diver moves toward the surface.

The reason for the O_2 paradox is as follows: Like the $P_{A_{CO_2}}$, the $P_{A_{O_2}}$ increases as the diver descends, causing more O_2 to move from the alveoli into the pulmonary capillary blood. This mechanism provides more dissolved O_2 for tissue metabolism. However, this physiologic advantage is lost as the diver returns to the surface and the lungs expand and the $P_{A_{O_2}}$ decreases. If a good portion of the O_2 is taken up from the lungs during descent, the $P_{A_{O_2}}$ decline during ascent may be significant. In fact, the $P_{A_{O_2}}$ can fall below the $P_{\bar{v}_{O_2}}$ of the pulmonary capillary blood. When this happens, the O_2 paradox occurs. That is, the O_2 in the pulmonary capillary blood moves into the alveoli. The fall in $P_{A_{O_2}}$ as a diver returns to the surface is also known as the **hypoxia of ascent**.

The Dive Response

The **dive response** consists of bradycardia, decreased cardiac output, and peripheral vasoconstriction elicited during a breath-hold dive. The dive response may partially explain the survival of numerous near-drowning cases in cold water after submersion lasting over 40 minutes. It is suggested that the peripheral vasoconstriction elicited during the dive response conserves oxygen for the heart and central nervous system by shunting blood away from less vital tissues.

Decompression Sickness

During a deep dive, the dissolved gases in the diver's blood will also move into body tissues. The amount of dissolved gas that enters the tissues is a function of (1) the solubility of the gas in the tissues, (2) the partial pressure of the gas, and (3) the hydrostatic pressure in the tissue.

During ascent (decompression) the pressure around the diver's body falls. This reduces the hydrostatic pressure in the tissues and, therefore, the ability of the tissues to hold inert gases. When the decompression is performed at an appropriately slow rate, the gases leaving the tissues will be transported (in their dissolved state) by the venous blood to the lungs and exhaled. When the decompression is conducted too rapidly, the gases will be released from the tissue as bubbles. Depending on the size, number, and location of the bubbles, they can cause a number of signs and symptoms, collectively referred to as **decompression sickness**. Decompression sickness includes, but is not limited to, joint pains (the bends), chest pain and coughing (the chokes), paresthesia and paralysis (spinal cord involvement), circulatory failure, and, in severe cases, death.

HYPERBARIC MEDICINE

The administration of oxygen at increased ambient pressures is now being used routinely to treat a variety of pathologic conditions. Clinically, this therapy is referred to as **hyperbaric medicine** and is accomplished by means of a compression chamber (also called a hyperbaric chamber). Most of the therapeutic benefits of hyperbaric oxygenation are associated with the increased oxygen delivery to the tissues.

As discussed in Chapter Seven, hemoglobin is about 97% saturated with oxygen at a normal arterial P_{O_2} of 80 to 100 mm Hg. Very little additional O_2 can combine with hemoglobin once this saturation level is reached. However, the quantity of dissolved O_2 will continue to rise linearly as the Pa_{O_2} increases. Approximately .3 ml of O_2 physically dissolves in each 100 ml of blood for every Pa_{O_2} increase of 100 mm Hg (Figure 16–2).

Indications for Hyperbaric Oxygenation

As shown in Table 16–1, the administration of hyperbaric oxygen is now indicated for a number of clinical conditions. Hyperbaric oxygen has long been

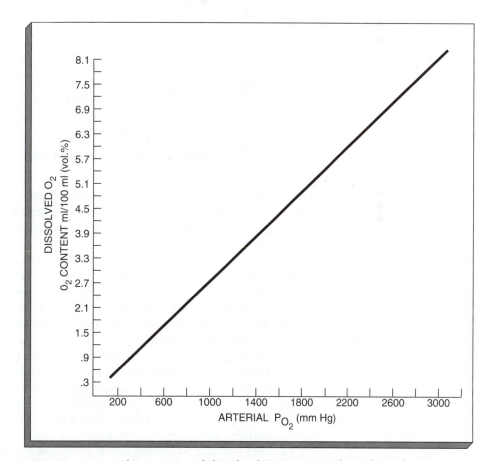

FIGURE 16–2. The quantity of dissolved O_2 increases linearly as the Pa_{O_2} increases. About 0.3 ml of O_2 physically dissolves in each 100 ml of blood for every 100 mm Hg increase in Pa_{O_2}.

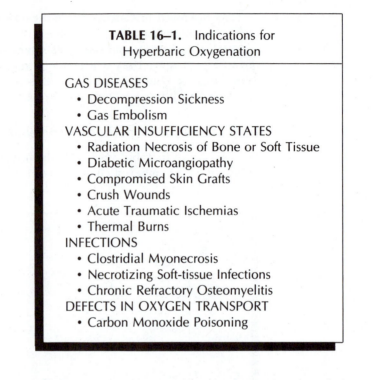

TABLE 16–1. Indications for Hyperbaric Oxygenation

GAS DISEASES
- Decompression Sickness
- Gas Embolism

VASCULAR INSUFFICIENCY STATES
- Radiation Necrosis of Bone or Soft Tissue
- Diabetic Microangiopathy
- Compromised Skin Grafts
- Crush Wounds
- Acute Traumatic Ischemias
- Thermal Burns

INFECTIONS
- Clostridial Myonecrosis
- Necrotizing Soft-tissue Infections
- Chronic Refractory Osteomyelitis

DEFECTS IN OXYGEN TRANSPORT
- Carbon Monoxide Poisoning

useful in the treatment of diseases, such as decompression sickness and gas embolism. Regardless of the cause of the bubbles, hyperbaric oxygen is effective in reducing bubble size, accelerating bubble resolution, and maintaining tissue oxygenation.

Hyperbaric oxygen is used empirically to enhance wound healing in conditions associated with ischemic hypoxia. Clinically, such conditions include radiation necrosis of bone or soft tissue, diabetic microangiopathy, compromised skin grafts, crush wounds, acute traumatic ischemias, and thermal burns. It appears that hyperbaric oxygen not only increases tissue oxygenation in these conditions, but increases capillary density as well.

Clinical evidence supports the use of hyperbaric oxygen for the treatment of anaerobic infections, including clostridial myonecrosis (gas gangrene), a variety of necrotizing soft tissue infections, and chronic refractory osteomyelitis. Hyperbaric oxygen added to surgery and antibiotics in the treatment of clostridial myonecrosis increases tissue salvage and decreases mortality.

Hyperbaric oxygen is effective in the treatment of carbon monoxide poisoning. Carbon monoxide poisoning, which is commonly caused by defective indoor heaters, automobile exhaust systems, or smoke inhalation, is the leading cause of death by poisoning in the United States. The severity of intoxication is a function of both the level and duration of carbon monoxide exposure. The administration of hyperbaric oxygen (1) increases the physically dissolved O_2 in the arterial blood, (2) increases the pressure gradient for driving oxygen into ischemic tissues, and (3) reduces the half-life of **carboxyhemoglobin** (COHb). The COHb half-life when a victim is breathing room air at one atmosphere is approximately 5 hours. That is, a 20% COHb will decrease to about 10% in 5 hours and 5% in another 5 hours. Breathing 100% oxygen at one atmosphere reduces the COHb half-life to less than 1 hour.

SELF-ASSESSMENT QUESTIONS

1. At what depth below the water surface does the pressure increase to 3.0 atmospheres?
   a. 13 feet
   b. 33 feet
   c. 66 feet
   d. 99 feet
   e. 132 feet

2. If an individual fully inhales to a total lung capacity of 5 liters at sea level (760 mm Hg), and dives to a depth of 66 feet, the lungs will be compressed to about:
   a. 0.5 liters
   b. 1.0 liters
   c. 1.5 liters
   d. 2.0 liters
   e. 2.5 liters

3. At sea level, a diver has:
   • Lung volume: 6 liters
   • Pressure within the lungs: 710 mm Hg

   If the above individual dives to a depth of 99 feet and compresses the lung volume to 2 liters, what will be the pressure within the diver's lungs?
   a. 960 mm Hg
   b. 1420 mm Hg
   c. 1765 mm Hg
   d. 2186 mm Hg
   e. 2615 mm Hg

4. The dive response consists of:
   I. Tachycardia
   II. Decreased cardiac output
   III. Bradycardia
   IV. Peripheral vasoconstriction
      a. I only

       b. II only

       c. III and IV only

       d. I and III only

       e. II, III, and IV only

5. The half-life of carboxyhemoglobin (COHb) when a victim is breathing room air at one atmosphere is approximately:

       a. 1 hour

       b. 2 hours

       c. 3 hours

       d. 4 hours

       e. 5 hours

TRUE OR FALSE

1. Hyperventilation prior to a breath-hold dive can be dangerous.   True _____   False _____

2. The fall in $P_{A_{O_2}}$ as a diver returns to the surface is known as the hypoxia of ascent.   True _____   False _____

3. Chest pain and coughing caused by decompression sickness is known as the bends.   True _____   False _____

4. The so-called P_{CO_2} respiratory drive "breaking point" during a dive is about 55 mm Hg.   True _____   False _____

5. Approximately 0.3 ml of O_2 is physically dissolved in each 100 ml of blood for every $P_{a_{O_2}}$ increase of 100 mm Hg.   True _____   False _____

Answers appear in Appendix VII

GLOSSARY

Abduct To draw away from the median plane of the body or from one of its parts.

Acclimatation Physiological or psychological adjustment to a new environment.

Acetylcholine A chemical found in most organs and tissues. Acetylcholine plays an important role in the transmission of parasympathetic nerve impulses at the synapses.

Acidemia Decreased pH and increased hydrogen ion concentration of the blood.

Acidosis Pathologic condition resulting from the accumulation of acid in, or loss of base from, the body.

Acinus (*pl.: acini*) The smallest division of a gland; a group of secretory cells surrounding a cavity. The functional part of an organ. The respiratory acinus includes the respiratory bronchioles, alveolar ducts, alveoli, and all other structures within the acinus.

Acromion process Lateral portion of the spine of the scapula that forms the point of the shoulder. It articulates with the clavicle and gives attachment to the deltoid and trapezius muscles.

Acute Sharp, severe; of rapid onset and characterized by severe symptoms and a short course; not chronic.

Adrenergic Nerve fibers that, when stimulated, release epinephrine at their endings. Adrenergic fibers include nearly all sympathetic postganglionic fibers except those innervating sweat glands.

Afferent Carrying impulses toward a center.

Afferent nerves Nerves that carry impulses from the periphery to the central nervous system.

Affinity Attraction between two substances that, when united, form new substances (i.e., oxygen and hemoglobin form oxyhemoglobin).

Air trapping The prevention of gas from leaving the alveoli during exhalation. This is usually caused by airway closure during exhalation.

Alkalemia Increased pH and decreased hydrogen ion concentration of the blood.

Allergen Any substance that causes an allergic reaction. It may or may not be a protein.

Allergy Acquired hypersensitivity to a substance (allergen) that normally does not cause a reaction.

Alpha receptor Site in the autonomic nerve pathways where excitatory responses occur when adrenergic agents such as norepinephrine and epinephrine are released.

Amniotic fluid Liquid produced by the fetal membranes and the fetus that surrounds the fetus throughout pregnancy, usually totaling about 1000 ml at term.

Analogous   Similar in function but having a different origin or structure.

Anastomosis   Joining of vessels, either naturally or surgically, to allow flow to other structures.

Anemia   Disorder characterized by a decrease in hemoglobin in the blood to levels below the normal range.

Anoxia   Deficiency of oxygen.

Anterior   Indicating the front of a structure or body surface relative to other body parts.

Antibody   Protein substance that develops in response to and interacts with an antigen. The antigen-antibody reaction forms the basis of immunity.

Antigen   Substance that induces the formation of antibodies that interact specifically with it. The antigen-antibody reaction forms the basis for immunity.

Antitrypsin   Inhibitor of trypsin; may be deficient in persons with emphysema.

Aperture   Opening or orifice.

Apex   Top end or tip of a structure.

Arrhythmia   Irregularity or loss of rhythm, especially of the heartbeat.

Arterial   Pertaining to one artery or a network of arteries.

Arteriole   A very small artery, especially one that, at its distal end, leads into a capillary.

Arteriosclerosis   A common arterial disorder characterized by thickening, loss of elasticity, and calcification of arterial walls, resulting in a decreased blood supply.

Asphyxia   Condition caused by an insufficient uptake of oxygen.

Aspiration   The act of inhaling. Pathologic aspiration of vomitus or other foreign substances into the respiratory tract.

Aspiration pneumonia   An inflammatory condition of the lungs and bronchi caused by the inhalation of foreign material or vomitus containing acid gastric contents.

Ataxia   An abnormal condition characterized by impaired ability to coordinate movement.

Atelectasis   Collapse of the lung. May be caused by obstruction.

Atherosclerosis   A common arterial disorder characterized by yellowish plaques of cholesterol, lipids, and cellular debris in the medial layer of the walls of the large and medium-sized arteries.

Atmospheric pressure   Pressure of the air on the earth at mean sea level; approximately 760 mm Hg (14.7 pounds per square inch).

Augment   To enlarge or increase in size, amount, or degree; make bigger.

Bacteriuria   The presence of bacteria in the urine.

Baroreceptor   A pressure sensor.

Basal   At the bottom, alkaline.

Basophil   A type of white blood cell that has a granular nucleus stained with basic dyes. These cells represent 1 percent or less of the total white blood cell count.

Beta receptor   Site in autonomic nerve pathways where inhibitory responses occur when adrenergic agents, such as norepinephrine and epinephrine, are released.

Bicarbonate   The HCO_3^- anion or any salt containing the HCO_3^- anion.

Bifurcation   A separation into two branches; the point of forking.

Blood-brain barrier   Membrane between the circulating blood and the brain that prevents certain substances from reaching brain tissue and cerebrospinal fluid.

Bradykinin   A nonapeptide produced by activation of the kinin system in a variety of inflammatory conditions. It is an extremely potent vasodilator; it also increases vascular permeability, stimulates pain receptors, and causes contraction of a variety of extravascular smooth muscles.

Bronchoconstriction   Narrowing of the pulmonary air passages.

Bronchodilation   Widening of pulmonary air passages.

Bronchospasm   Involuntary sudden movement or convulsive contraction of the muscular coats of the bronchus.

Calcification   Process in which organic tissue becomes hardened by the deposition of lime salts in the tissue.

Calculus   A pathologic stone formed of mineral salts. Calculi are usually found within hollow organs or ducts.

Caliber   The inside diameter of a tube, commonly given in millimeters and fractions of an inch.

Canalicular   Pertaining to a small channel or canal.

Capillary stasis   Stagnation of normal flow of fluids or blood in capillaries.

Carbon dioxide (CO_2)   Colorless, odorless, incombustible gas formed during respiration and combustion.

Cartilage   Dense, firm, compact connective tissue capable of withstanding considerable pressure and tension. Located in the tracheobronchial tree, all true joints, the outer ear, and the movable sections of the ribs.

Catecholamines   Biologically active amines that behave as epinephrine and norepinephrine.

Central venous pressure (CVP)   Pressure within the superior vena cava, which reflects the pressure under which the blood is returned to the right atrium.

Cerebrospinal fluid (CSF)   Fluid cushion that protects the brain and spinal cord from shock.

Chemoreceptor   Sense organ or sensory nerve ending, located outside the central nervous system, which is stimulated by and reacts to chemical stimuli.

Chronic   Denoting a process that shows little change and slow progression and is of long duration.

Cilia   Small, hairlike projections on the surface of epithelial cells. In the bronchi they propel mucus and foreign particles in a whiplike movement toward the throat.

Clinical manifestations   Symptoms or signs demonstrated by a patient.

Colloid   A state of matter composed of single large molecules or aggregations of smaller molecules of solids, liquids, or gases, in a continuous medium (dispersal medium), which also may·be a solid, liquid, or gas.

Composition   Makeup; what something is made of.

Compromise   A blending of the qualities of two different things; an unfavorable change.

Concave   A hollow surface, like the inside of a bowl.

Conception   The union of sperm and ovum.

Congenital   Existing at and usually before birth; referring to conditions that are present at birth, regardless of their cause.

Congestion   Excessive amount of blood or tissue fluid in an organ or tissue.

Congestive heart failure   Myocardial insufficiency of the left ventricle that results in pulmonary congestion.

Consolidation   The process of becoming solid; a mass that has solidified.

Constrict   Tighten or squeeze; making a part narrow.

Contiguous   Being in actual contact; touching along a boundary or at a point.

Contusion   Injury in which the skin is not broken; a bruise.

Convex   Having a rounded, somewhat elevated surface, resembling a segment of the external surface of a sphere.

Cor pulmonale   Failure of the right ventricle resulting from disorders of the lungs or pulmonary vessels.

Corpuscle   Any small, rounded body; an encapsulated sensory nerve ending.

Cortex   The outer layer of an organ.

Crackles   Abnormal, fine or medium crackling wet sounds typically heard during inspiration.

Creatinine   A substance formed from the metabolism of creatine, commonly found in blood, urine, and muscle tissue.

Density   Mass of a substance per unit of volume [g/cm^3].

Deoxyribonucleic acid (DNA)   A nucleic acid containing deoxyribose as the sugar component and found principally in the nuclei of animal and vegetable cells, usually loosely bound to protein (hence termed dioxyribonucleoprotein). Considered to be the autoreproducing component of chromosomes and of many viruses, and the repository of hereditary characteristics.

Depolarize   To reduce to a nonpolarized condition; to reduce the amount of electrical charge between oppositely charged particles (*ions*).

Desquamation   The process in which the cornified layer of the epidermis is sloughed in fine scales.

Determinant   An element that identifies or determines the nature of something or that fixes or conditions an outcome.

Diabetes   A general term referring to a variety of disorders characterized by excessive urination (polyuria), as in diabetes mellitus and diabetes insipidus.

Diagnostic Pertaining to the use of scientific and skillful methods to establish the cause and nature of a sick person's disease.

Diastole Normal period in the heart cycle during which the muscle fibers lengthen, the heart dilates, and the chambers fill with blood.

Differentiate To separate according to differences.

Digitation A fingerlike projection.

Distal Away from or being the farthest from any point of reference.

Dorsal Pertaining to the back or to the posterior portion of a body.

Driving pressure Pressure difference between two areas in any vessel or airway.

Ductus arteriosus Vessel between the left pulmonary artery and the aorta that bypasses the lungs in the fetus.

Edema A local or generalized condition in which the body tissues contain an excessive amount of extracellular fluid.

Efferent Carrying away from a central organ or section.

Efferent nerves Nerves that carry impulses from the brain or spinal cord to the periphery.

Electrocardiogram (ECG) Record of the electrical activity of the heart.

Electrolyte An element or compound that, when melted or dissolved in water or other solvent, dissociates into ions and is able to conduct an electric current.

Elongation The condition or process of being extended.

Embryonic Pertaining to the early stages (i.e., first three months) of fetal development.

Endothelium The layer of epithelial cells originating from the mesoderm, that lines the cavities of the heart, the blood and lymph vessels, and the serous cavities of the body.

Endotracheal Within the trachea.

Eosinophil A cell or cellular structure that stains readily with the acid stain eosin; specifically, a granular leukocyte.

Epinephrine One of two active hormones (the other is norepinephrine) secreted by the adrenal medulla.

Epistaxis Bleeding from the nose, also called *nosebleed*.

Equilibrium Condition in which one or more forces are evenly balanced by opposite forces.

Erythrocyte Red blood cell (RBC).

Etiology Cause of disease.

Excretion Elimination of waste products.

Excursion The extent of movement from a central position or axis.

Expectoration Clearing the lungs by coughing up and spitting out matter.

Extra-alveolar Pertaining to the area outside of the alveoli.

Extracellular Outside a cell or in the cavities or spaces between cell layers or groups of cells.

Extravascular   Outside a vessel.

Fascia   Fibrous membrane that covers, supports, and separates muscles.

Fertilization   The union of sperm and ovum.

Fetus   The developing human *in utero* from the third month to birth.

Fibrin   Whitish, filamentous protein formed by the action of thrombin on fibrinogen.

Fibroelastic   Composed of fibrous and elastic tissue.

Fibrosis   Formation of scar tissue.

Fissure   Cleft or groove on the surface of an organ, often marking the division of the organ into parts, such as the lobes of the lung.

Fistula   Abnormal passage or communication, usually between two internal organs or leading from an internal organ to the surface of the body.

Flex   To bend upon itself, as a muscle.

Foramen ovale   Opening between the atria of the heart in the fetus. This opening normally closes shortly after birth.

Functionally   According to its proper use or action; working as it should.

Gastrointestinal tract   The route taken by food from the stomach to the rectum.

Generation   The process of forming a new organism or part of an organism.

Gestation   The period of time from the fertilization of the ovum until birth.

Glomerulonephritis   Inflammation of the glomerulus in the nephron of the kidney.

Glomerulus   A tuft or cluster; a structure composed of blood vessels or nerve fibers, such as a *renal glomerulus*.

Glossopharyngeal nerve   The 9th cranial nerve.

Glycoprotein   Any of a class of conjugated proteins consisting of a compound of a protein with a carbohydrate group.

Goblet cell   A type of secretory cell found in the intestinal and respiratory tracts.

Gradient   A slope or grade; a difference in values between two points.

Hematocrit   Volume of erythrocytes packed by centrifugation in a given volume of blood, is expressed as the percentage of total blood volume that consists of erythrocytes.

Hemoglobin   Pigment of red blood cells containing iron.

Hemolysis   The breakdown of red blood cells and the release of hemoglobin.

Heparin   A polysaccharide produced by the mast cells of the liver and by basophil leukocytes that inhibits coagulation by preventing conversion of prothrombin to thrombin. It also inhibits coagulation by preventing liberation of thromboplastin from blood platelets.

Histamine   A substance that is normally present in the body and exerts a pharmacologic action when released from injured cells. It is produced from the amino acid *histidine*.

Hormone   A substance originating in an organ or gland that is conveyed through the body to another part of the body, which it stimulates by chemical action to increased functional activity and/or increased secretion.

Hydrostatic   Pertaining to the pressure of liquids in equilibrium.

Hydrous   Containing water, usually chemically combined.

Hypercapnia   Greater than normal amount of carbon dioxide in the blood; also called *hypercarbia*.

Hyperchloremia   Increased chloride level in the blood.

Hyperinflation   Distention by air, gas, or liquid, as in the hyperinflation of the alveoli.

Hyperkalemia   Increased amount of potassium in the blood.

Hypersecretion   Substance or fluid produced by cells or glands in an excessive amount or more than normal.

Hypersensitivity   Abnormal sensitivity to a stimulus of any kind.

Hypertension   Higher than normal blood pressure.

Hyperthermia   Higher than normal body temperature.

Hyperventilation   An increased alveolar ventilation.

Hypochloremia   A decreased amount of chloride in the blood.

Hypokalemia   A decreased amount of potassium in the blood.

Hypoperfusion   Deficiency of blood coursing through the vessels of the circulatory system.

Hypothalamus   Portion of the brain that controls certain metabolic activities.

Hypoventilation   A decreased alveolar ventilation.

Hypoxemia   Below-normal oxygen content in blood.

Hypoxia   Tissue oxygen deficiency.

Iliac crest   Long curved upper margin of the hip bone.

Immaturity   The state of being not fully developed or ripened.

Immunoglobulin   One of a family of closely related but not identical proteins that are capable of acting as antibodies.

Immunologic mechanism   Reaction of the body to substances that are foreign or are interpreted by the body as foreign.

Impede   To slow down; to stand in the way of; to fight against.

Inferior vena cava (IVC)   Venous trunk for the lower extremities and the pelvic and abdominal viscera.

Inflammation   Localized heat, redness, swelling, and pain as a result of irritation, injury, or infection.

Inguinal ligament   A fibrous band formed by the inferior border of the aponeurosis of the external oblique that extends from the anterior superior iliac spine to the pubic tubercle.

Inhibitory   Repressive; tending to restrain a function.

Innervation   Function of the nervous system that gives stimulation to a part of the body.

Interstitial Placed or lying between; pertaining to the interstices or spaces within an organ or tissue.

Intra- Prefix meaning within.

Intra-alveolar Within the alveoli.

Intrapleural Within the pleura.

Intrapulmonary Within the lungs.

Intrarenal Within the kidneys.

Intratubular Within a tube.

Intubation Passage of a tube into a body aperture; specifically, the insertion of a breathing tube through the mouth or nose or into the trachea.

Inverse Opposite in order, nature, or effect; being an inverse function.

Ion Atom, group of atoms, or molecule that has acquired a net electrical charge by gaining or losing electrons.

Ischemia Decreased blood supply to a body organ or part.

Isobar A line on a map, chart, or nomogram connecting areas of equal pressure.

Lactic acid Acid formed in muscles during activity by the breakdown of sugar without oxygen.

Ligamentum nuchae Upward continuation of the supraspinous ligament, extending from the 7th cervical vertebra to the occipital bone.

Linea alba "White line" of connective tissue in the middle of the abdomen from sternum to pubis.

Linear response Having or being a response or output that is directly proportional to the input.

Lipid Any of numerous fats generally insoluble in water that constitute one of the principal structural materials of cells.

Lobar Pertaining to a lobe, such as the lobes of the lung.

Lumen Inner open space of a tubular organ, such as a blood vessel or intestine.

Magnitude Pertaining to size.

Malar Pertaining to the cheek or cheekbones.

Malformation Deformity; abnormal shape or structure, especially congenital.

Mastoid process Projection of the posterior portion of the temporal bone; gives attachment to the sternocleidomastoid, splenius capitis, and longissimus capitis muscles.

Mean Occupying a middle position; being near the average.

Mechanical Relating to physical properties.

Mechanoreceptor Receptor that receives mechanical stimuli such as pressure from sound or touch.

Medial Pertaining to the middle.

Mediated Between two parts or sides.

Medulla oblongata Vital part of the brain; contains the cardiac, vasomotor, and respiratory centers of the brain.

Mesoderm   The middle of the three cell layers of the developing embryo, which lies between the ectoderm and endoderm.

Metabolism   Sum of all physical and chemical changes that take place within an organism; all energy and material transformations that occur within living cells.

Microvilli   Minute cylindrical processes on the free surface of a cell (especially cells of the proximal convoluted renal tubule and those of the intestinal epithelium), which increase the surface area of the cell.

Molecular weight   Weight of a molecule attained by adding the atomic weight of its constituent atoms.

Monocyte   A large, mononuclear leukocyte normally found in lymph nodes, spleen, bone marrow, and loose connective tissue.

Motor nerve   A nerve consisting of efferent fibers that conduct impulses from the brain or the spinal cord to one of the muscles or organs.

Mucous   Pertaining to or resembling mucus; secreting mucus.

Mucus   The gel-like substance of the mucous membranes, composed of mucin (secreted by the mucus glands), along with various inorganic salts, desquamated cells, and leukocytes.

Myelin   The substance that constitutes the sheaths of various nerve fibers throughout the body. It is largely composed of fat, giving the fibers a white, creamy color.

Myoepithelial cells   Spindle-shaped cells found around sweat, mammary and salivary glands. The myoepithelial cells are contractile and resemble smooth muscle cells.

Myoglobin   A ferrous globin complex consisting of one heme group and one globin polypeptide chain. It is responsible for the red pigment seen in skeletal muscle.

Necrosis   Localized tissue death that occurs in groups of cells in response to disease or injury.

Neoplasms   A new and abnormal formation of tissue.

Neuropathy   Any abnormal condition characterized by inflammation and degeneration of the peripheral nerves.

Nomogram   A graph consisting of several lines or curves (usually parallel) graduated for different variables in such a way that a straight line cutting the three lines gives the related values of the three variables.

Nonlinear   Having or being a response or output that is not directly proportional to the input.

Norepinephrine   One of two active hormones (the other is epinephrine) secreted by the adrenal medulla. It is chiefly a vasoconstrictor and has little effect on cardiac output.

Occipital   Referring to the back part or bone of the head.

Occlude   To close, obstruct, or join together.

Olfactory   Pertaining to the sense of smell.

Oncotic pressure   Osmotic pressure due to the presence of colloids in a solution.

Osmotic pressure   Pressure that develops when two solutions with different concentrations of solutes are separated by a semipermeable membrane.

Oxygen content   Total amount of oxygen in the blood.

Papillitis   An abnormal condition characterized by the inflammation of a papilla.

Paradoxical   Occurring at variance with the normal rule.

Parasympathetic nervous system   A division of the autonomic nervous system that is mediated by the release of acetylcholine and primarily involves the protection, conservation, and restoration of body resources.

Parenchyma   Essential parts of an organ that are concerned with its function.

Paroxysmal   Concerning the sudden, periodic attack or recurrence of symptoms of a disease.

Parturition   The action or process of giving birth to offspring.

Pathogen   Any agent causing disease, especially a microorganism.

Perfusion   Passing of blood or fluid through a vascular bed.

Peribronchial   Located around the bronchi.

Pericardium   A fibroserous sac that surrounds the heart and the roots of the great vessels.

Peripheral airways   Small bronchioles on the outer sections of the lung.

Peristalsis   A progressive wave movement that occurs involuntarily in hollow tubes of the body, especially the intestines.

Perivascular   Located around a vessel, especially a blood vessel.

Permeable   Capable of allowing the passage of fluids or substances in solution.

pH   Symbol for the logarithm of the reciprocal of the hydrogen ion concentration.

Phalanges   The bones of the fingers and toes.

Phosphate   A compound of phosphoric acid.

Photophobia   Abnormal sensitivity to light, especially by the eyes.

Pituitary gland   A small, gray, rounded body attached to the base of the brain.

Posterior   Back part of something; toward the back.

Prerenal   Located in front of the kidneys.

Pressure   In physics, the quotient obtained by dividing a force by the area of the surface on which it acts.

Prognosis   Prediction of outcome.

Proliferate   Increasing or spreading at a rapid rate; the process or result of rapid reproduction.

Prostaglandins   A group of fatty acid derivatives present in many organs that affect the cardiovascular system and smooth muscle and stimulate the uterus to contract.

Prostate   A gland in males that surrounds the neck of the bladder and the urethra and elaborates a secretion that liquefies coagulated semen.

Prostatic hypertrophy   Enlargement of the prostate gland.

Proximal   Nearest the point of attachment, center of the body, or point of reference.

Pubic symphysis   Junction of the pubic bones, is composed of fibrocartilage.

Pulmonary   Concerning or involving the lungs.

Pulmonary congestion   An abnormally large amount of fluid in the pulmonary system.

Pulmonary vascular resistance (PVR)   Pressure loss, per unit of blood flow, from pulmonary artery to the left ventricle.

Pyelonephritis   A diffuse pyogenic infection of the pelvis and parenchyma of the kidney.

Reflex   An involuntary response to a stimulus.

Renal   Pertaining to the kidneys.

Renal dysplasia   Abnormal development of tissue in the kidneys.

Resonance   Quality of the sound heard on percussion of a hollow structure such as the chest or abdomen.

Semipermeable   Permitting diffusion or flow of some liquids or solutes but preventing the transmission of others, usually in reference to a membrane.

Septic   Pertaining to infection or contamination.

Septicemia   Systemic infection in which pathogens and their toxins are present in the circulating blood stream, having spread from an infection in any part of the body.

Septum   Wall dividing two cavities.

Serotonin   A potent vasoconstrictor that is present in platelets, gastrointestinal mucosa, mast cells, and carcinoid tumors.

Serum   Clear watery fluid, especially that moistening surfaces of serous membranes or exuded inflammation of any of those membranes; the fluid portion of the blood obtained after removal of the fibrin clot and blood cells, sometimes used as a synonym for antiserum.

Shunt   To turn away from; to divert; an abnormal passage to divert flow from one route to another.

Sign   Any objective evidence or manifestation of an illness or disordered function of the body.

Smooth muscle   Muscle tissue that lacks cross-striations on its fibers, is involuntary in action, and is found principally in visceral organs.

Somatic nerve   Nerve that innervates somatic structures, i.e., those constituting the body wall and extremities.

Somnolence   The condition of being sleepy or drowsy.

Spasm   Involuntary sudden movement or convulsive muscular contraction.

Sputum   Substance expelled by coughing or clearing the throat that may contain a variety of materials from the respiratory tract, including one or more of the following: cellular debris, mucus, blood, pus, caseous material, and microorganisms.

Stasis   Stagnation of normal flow of fluids, as of the blood, urine, or intestinal mechanism.

Stroke volume   Amount of blood ejected by the ventricle at each beat.

Subcutaneous   Under the skin.

Sulfonamide   One of a large group of synthetic, bacteriostatic drugs that are effective in treating infections caused by many gram-negative and gram-positive microorganisms.

Superior vena cava   Venous trunk draining blood from the head, neck, upper extremities, and chest.

Surfactant   A substance important in controlling the surface tension of the air–liquid emulsion in the lungs; an agent that lowers surface tension.

Sympathetic nervous system   A division of the autonomic nervous system that accelerates the heart rate, constricts blood vessels, and raises blood pressure.

Sympathomimetic   Producing effects resembling those resulting from stimulation of the sympathetic nervous system.

Symptom   Any perceptible change in the body or its functions that indicates disease or the type or phases of disease. Symptoms may be classified as objective, subjective, cardinal, and sometimes constitutional.

Systemic   Pertaining to the whole body rather than to one of its parts.

Systemic reaction   Whole body response to a stimulus.

Systole   That part of the heart cycle in which the heart is in contraction.

Systolic pressure   Maximum blood pressure; occurs during contraction of the ventricle.

Tachycardia   An abnormal circulatory condition in which the myocardium contracts regularly but at a rate of greater than 100 beats per minute.

Thoracolumbar   Relating to the thoracic and lumbar portions of the vertebral column.

Tone   That state of a body or any of its organs or parts in which the functions are healthy and normal.

Transient   Passing especially quickly into and out of existence; passing through or by a place with only a brief stay.

Trimester   One of the three periods of approximately three months into which pregnancy is divided.

Unilateral renal agenesis   Failure of development of one of the kidneys.

Vagus   The 10th cranial nerve. It is a mixed nerve, having motor and sensory functions and a wider distribution than any of the other cranial nerves.

Vascular   Relating to or containing blood vessels.

Vasoconstriction   Decrease in the caliber of blood vessels.

Vasodilation   Widening of blood vessels, especially the small arteries and arterioles.

Venous   Pertaining to a vein or veins.

Venous return   The amount of blood returning to the atria of the heart.

Ventilation   Mechanical movement of air into and out of the lungs in a cyclic fashion.

Ventral   Pertaining to the anterior portion or front of the body.

Ventricle   Either of two lower chambers of the heart.

Viscosity   Stickiness or gumminess; internal friction resistance offered by a fluid to change of form or relative position of its particles due to attraction of molecules to each other.

Viscous   Sticky; gummy; gelatinous.

Viscus   Any organ enclosed within a cavity, such as the thorax or abdomen.

Volume percent (Vol%)   The number of milliliters (ml) of a substance contained in 100 ml of another substance.

SYMBOLS AND ABBREVIATIONS COMMONLY USED IN RESPIRATORY PHYSIOLOGY

Primary Symbols			
GAS SYMBOLS		**BLOOD SYMBOLS**	
P	Pressure	Q	Blood volume
V	Gas volume	$\dot{Q}$	Blood flow
$\dot{V}$	Gas volume per unit of time, or flow	C	Content in blood
F	Fractional concentration of gas	S	Saturation

Secondary Symbols			
GAS SYMBOLS		**BLOOD SYMBOLS**	
I	Inspired	a	Arterial
E	Expired	c	Capillary
A	Alveolar	v	Venous
T	Tidal	$\bar{v}$	Mixed venous
D	Deadspace		

Abbreviations	
LUNG VOLUME	
VC	Vital capacity
IC	Inspiratory capacity

LUNG VOLUME (cont'd.)	
IRV	Inspiratory reserve volume
ERV	Expiratory reserve volume
FRC	Functional residual capacity
RV	Residual volume
TLC	Total lung capacity
RV/TLC(%)	Residual volume to total lung capacity ratio, expressed as a percentage
V_T	Tidal volume
V_A	Alveolar ventilation
V_D	Deadspace ventilation
V_L	Actual lung volume

SPIROMETRY	
FVC	Forced vital capacity with maximally forced expiratory effort
FEV_T	Forced expiratory volume timed
$FEF_{200-1200}$	Average rate of airflow between 200–1200 ml of the FVC
$FEF_{25\%-75\%}$	Forced expiratory flow during the middle half of the FVC (formerly called the maximal midexpiratory flow MMF)
PEFR	Maximum flowrate that can be achieved
$\dot{V}_{max\ x}$	Forced expiratory flow related to the actual volume of the lungs as denoted by subscript x, which refers to the amount of lung volume remaining when measurement is made
MVV	Maximal voluntary ventilation as the volume of air expired in a specified interval

MECHANICS	
C_L	Lung compliance; volume change per unit of pressure change
R_{aw}	Airway resistance; pressure per unit of flow

DIFFUSION	
$D_{L_{CO}}$	Diffusing capacity of carbon monoxide

BLOOD GASES	
$P_{A_{O_2}}$	Alveolar oxygen tension
$P_{C_{O_2}}$	Pulmonary capillary oxygen tension
$P_{a_{O_2}}$	Arterial oxygen tension

Continued

BLOOD GASES (cont'd.)	
Pv_{O_2}	Mixed venous oxygen tension
PA_{CO_2}	Alveolar carbon dioxide tension
Pc_{CO_2}	Pulmonary capillary carbon dioxide tension
Pa_{CO_2}	Arterial carbon dioxide tension
Sa_{O_2}	Arterial oxygen saturation
Sv_{O_2}	Mixed venous oxygen saturation
pH	Negative logarithm of the H^+ concentration used as a positive number
HCO_3^-	Plasma bicarbonate concentration
mEq/L	The number of grams of solute dissolved in a normal solution
Ca_{O_2}	Oxygen content of arterial blood
Cc_{O_2}	Oxygen content of capillary blood
Cv_{O_2}	Oxygen content of mixed venous blood
$\dot{V}/\dot{Q}$	Ventilation-perfusion Ratio
Qs/Qt	Shunt
QT	Total cardiac output
OXYGEN TRANSPORT STUDIES	
$C(a - v)_{O_2}$	Arterial-venous oxygen content difference
$\dot{V}_{O_2}$	Oxygen consumption (oxygen uptake)
O_2ER	Oxygen extraction ratio
D_{O_2}	Total oxygen delivery

Hemodynamic Measurement Abbreviations	
DIRECT MEASUREMENTS	
CVP	Central venous pressure
RAP	Right atrial pressure
PA	Mean pulmonary artery pressure
PCWP	Pulmonary capillary wedge pressure

DIRECT MEASUREMENTS (cont'd.)	
PAW	Pulmonary artery wedge
PAO	Pulmonary artery occlusion
CO	Cardiac output

INDIRECT MEASUREMENTS	
SV	Stroke volume
SVI	Stroke volume index
CI	Cardiac index
RVSWI	Right ventricular stroke work index
LVSWI	Left ventricular stroke work index
PVR	Pulmonary vascular resistance
SVR	Systemic vascular resistance

Metric Measurement Abbreviations	
VOLUME MEASUREMENTS	
L	Liter
dl	deciliter (1×10^{-1})
ml	milliliter (1×10^{-3})
μl	microliter (1×10^{-6})
nl	nanoliter (1×10^{-9})

LINEAR MEASUREMENTS

m	meter
cm	centimeter ($m \times 10^{-2}$)
mm	millimeter ($m \times 10^{-3}$)
μ or μm	micrometer ($m \times 10^{-6}$)

WEIGHT MEASUREMENTS

g	gram
mg	milligram ($g \times 10^{-3}$)
μg	microgram ($g \times 10^{-6}$)
ng	nanogram ($g \times 10^{-9}$)

UNITS OF MEASUREMENT

Metric Weight				
GRAMS	**CENTIGRAMS**	**MILLIGRAMS**	**MICROGRAMS**	**NANOGRAMS**
1	100	1000	1,000,000	1,000,000,000
.01	1	10	10,000	10,000,000
.001	.1	1	1000	1,000,000
.000001	.0001	.001	1	1000
.000000001	.0000001	.000001	.001	1

Metric Liquid				
LITER	**CENTILITER**	**MILLILITER**	**MICROLITER**	**NANOLITER**
1	100	1000	1,000,000	1,000,000,000
.01	1	10	10,000	10,000,000
.001	.1	1	1000	1,000,000
.000001	.0001	.001	1	1000
.000000001	.0000001	.000001	.001	1

Metric Length				
METER	**CENTIMETER**	**MILLIMETER**	**MICROMETER**	**NANOMETER**
1	100	1000	1,000,000	1,000,000,000
.01	1	10	10,000	10,000,000
.001	.1	1	1000	1,000,000
.000001	.0001	.001	1	1000
.000000001	.0000001	.000001	.001	1

Weight Conversions (Metric and Avoirdupois)			
GRAMS	**KILOGRAMS**	**OUNCES**	**POUNDS**
1	.001	.0353	.0022
1000	1	35.3	2.2
28.35	.02835	1	$\frac{1}{16}$
454.5	.4545	16	1

Weight Conversions (Metric and Apothecary)					
GRAMS	**MILLIGRAMS**	**GRAINS**	**DRAMS**	**OUNCES**	**POUNDS**
1	1000	15.4	.2577	.0322	.00268
.001	1	.0154	.00026	.0000322	.00000268
.0648	64.8	1	$\frac{1}{60}$	$\frac{1}{480}$	$\frac{1}{5760}$
3.888	3888	60	1	$\frac{1}{8}$	$\frac{1}{96}$
31.1	31104	480	8	1	$\frac{1}{12}$
373.25	373248	5760	96	12	1

Approximate Household Measurement Equivalents (Volume)
1 tsp = 5 ml
1 tbsp = 3 tsp = 15 ml
1 fl oz = 2 tbsp = 6 tsp = 30 ml
1 cup = 8 fl oz = 240 ml
1 pt = 2 cups = 16 fl oz = 480 ml
1 qt = 2 pt = 4 cups = 32 fl oz = 960 ml
1 gal = 4 qt = 8 pt = 16 cups = 128 fl oz = 3840 ml

Courtesy of Des Jardins, *Clinical Manifestations of Respiratory Disease,* 2nd ed.
© 1990 by Mosby Year Book Medical Publishers, Inc., Chicago

Weight	
METRIC	**APPROXIMATE APOTHECARY EQUIVALENTS**
Grams	*Grains*
.0002	$1/300$
.0003	$1/200$
.0004	$1/150$
.0005	$1/120$
.0006	$1/100$
.001	$1/60$
.002	$1/30$
.005	$1/12$
.010	$1/6$
.015	$1/4$
.025	$3/8$
.030	$1/2$
.050	$3/4$
.060	1
.100	$1\frac{1}{2}$
.120	2
.200	3
.300	5
.500	$7\frac{1}{2}$
.600	10
1	15
2	30
4	60

Liquid Measure	
METRIC	**APPROXIMATE APOTHECARY EQUIVALENTS**
Milliliters	
1,000	1 quart
750	$1\frac{1}{2}$ pints
500	1 pint
250	8 fluid ounces *Continued*

Liquid Measure (cont'd.)	
200	7 fluid ounces
100	3½ fluid ounces
50	1¾ fluid ounces
30	1 fluid ounce
15	4 fluid drams
10	2½ fluid drams
8	2 fluid drams
5	1¼ fluid drams
4	1 fluid dram
3	45 minims
2	30 minims
1	15 minims
0.75	12 minims
0.6	10 minims
0.5	8 minims
0.3	5 minims
0.25	4 minims
0.2	3 minims
0.1	1½ minims
0.06	1 minim
0.05	¾ minim
0.03	½ minim

Volume Conversions (Metric and Apothecary)

MILLILITERS	MINIMS	FLUID DRAMS	FLUID OUNCES	PINTS	LITERS	GALLONS	QUARTS	FLUID OUNCES	PINTS
1	16.2	.27	.0333	.0021	1	.2642	1.057	33.824	2.114
.0616	1	$\frac{1}{60}$	$\frac{1}{480}$	$\frac{1}{7680}$	3.785	1	4	128	8
3.697	60	1	$\frac{1}{8}$	$\frac{1}{128}$	.946	$\frac{1}{4}$	1	32	2
29.58	480	8	1	$\frac{1}{16}$	.473	$\frac{1}{8}$	$\frac{1}{2}$	16	1
473.2	7680	128	16	1	.0296	$\frac{1}{128}$	$\frac{1}{32}$	1	$\frac{1}{16}$

Length Conversions (Metric and English System)

	MILLIMETERS	CENTIMETERS	INCHES	FEET	YARDS	METERS
1 A° =	$\frac{1}{10,000,000}$	$\frac{1}{100,000,000}$	$\frac{1}{254,000,000}$	$\frac{1}{3,050,000,000}$	$\frac{1}{9,140,000,000}$	$\frac{1}{10,000,000,000}$
1 nm =	$\frac{1}{1,000,000}$	$\frac{1}{10,000,000}$	$\frac{1}{25,400,000}$	$\frac{1}{305,000,000}$	$\frac{1}{914,000,000}$	$\frac{1}{1,000,000,000}$
1 μ =	$\frac{1}{1,000}$	$\frac{1}{10,000}$	$\frac{1}{25,400}$	$\frac{1}{305,000}$	$\frac{1}{914,000}$	$\frac{1}{1,000,000}$
1 mm =	1.0	0.1	0.03937	0.00328	0.0011	0.001
1 cm =	10.0	1.0	0.3937	0.03281	0.0109	0.01
1 in =	25.4	2.54	1.0	0.0833	0.0278	0.0254
1 ft =	304.8	30.48	12.0	1.0	0.333	0.3048
1 yd =	914.40	91.44	36.0	3.0	1.0	0.9144
1 m =	1000.0	100.0	39.37	3.2808	1.0936	1.0

POISEUILLE'S LAW

POISEUILLE'S LAW FOR FLOW REARRANGED
TO A SIMPLE PROPORTIONALITY

$$\dot{V} \simeq \Delta P r^4, \text{ or rewritten as } \frac{\dot{V}}{r^4} \simeq \Delta P.$$

When ΔP remains constant, then

$$\frac{\dot{V}_1}{r_1{}^4} \simeq \frac{\dot{V}_2}{r_2{}^4}$$

Example 1:
　　If the radius (r_1) is decreased to one-half its previous radius ($r_2 = \frac{1}{2} r_1$), then

$$\frac{\dot{V}_1}{r_1{}^4} \simeq \frac{\dot{V}_2}{(\frac{1}{2} r_1)^4}$$

$$\frac{\dot{V}_1}{r_1{}^4} \simeq \frac{\dot{V}_2}{(\frac{1}{16} r_1)^4}$$

$$(r_1{}^4) \frac{\dot{V}_1}{r_1{}^4} \simeq (r_1{}^4) \frac{\dot{V}_2}{(\frac{1}{16}) r_1{}^4}$$

$$\dot{V}_1 \simeq \frac{\dot{V}_2}{\frac{1}{16}}$$

$$(\frac{1}{16}) \dot{V}_1 \simeq (\frac{1}{16}) \frac{\dot{V}_2}{\frac{1}{16}}$$

$$(\frac{1}{16}) \dot{V}_1 \simeq \dot{V}_2$$

then gas flow ($\dot{V}_1$) is reduced to $\frac{1}{16}$ its original flow rate [$\dot{V}_2 \simeq (\frac{1}{16}) \dot{V}_1$].
Example 2:
　　If the radius (r_1) is decreased by 16% ($r_2 = r_1 - 0.16 r_1 = 0.84 r_1$), then

$$\frac{\dot{V}_1}{r_1{}^4} \simeq \frac{\dot{V}_2}{r_2{}^4}$$

$$\frac{\dot{V}_1}{r_1{}^4} \simeq \frac{\dot{V}_2}{(0.84r_1)^4}$$

$$\dot{V}_2 \simeq \frac{(0.84r_1)^4 \, \dot{V}_1}{r_1{}^4}$$

$$\dot{V}_2 \simeq \frac{0.4979 \, r_1{}^4 \, \dot{V}_1}{r_1{}^4}$$

$$\dot{V}_2 \simeq \tfrac{1}{2} \, \dot{V}_1$$

then the flow rate ($\dot{V}_1$) would decrease to one-half the original flow rate ($\dot{V}_2 \simeq \tfrac{1}{2}$ $\dot{V}_1$).

Courtesy of Des Jardins, *Clinical Manifestations of Respiratory Disease,* 2nd ed. © 1990 by Mosby Year Book Medical Publishers, Inc., Chicago.

POISEUILLE'S LAW FOR PRESSURE REARRANGED TO A SIMPLE PROPORTIONALITY

$$P \simeq \frac{\dot{V}}{r^4}, \text{ or rewritten as } P \cdot r^4 \simeq \dot{V}$$

when $\dot{V}$ remains constant, then

$$P_1 \cdot r_1{}^4 \simeq P_2 \cdot r_2{}^4$$

Example 1:

If the radius (r_1) is reduced to one-half its original radius [$r_2 = (\tfrac{1}{2})r_1$], then

$$P_1 \cdot r_1{}^4 \simeq P_2 \cdot r_2{}^4$$

$$P_1 \cdot r_1{}^4 \simeq P_2[(\tfrac{1}{2})r_1]^4$$

$$P_1 \cdot r_1{}^4 \simeq P_2 \cdot (\tfrac{1}{16})r_1{}^4$$

$$\frac{P_1 \cdot r_1{}^4}{r_1{}^4} \simeq \frac{P_2 \cdot (\tfrac{1}{16}) \, r_1{}^4}{r_1{}^4}$$

$$P_1 \simeq P_2 \cdot (\tfrac{1}{16})$$

$$16 \, P_1 \simeq 16 \cdot P_2 \cdot (\tfrac{1}{16})$$

$$16 \, P_1 \simeq P_2$$

then the pressure (P_1) will increase to 16 times its original level ($P_2 \simeq 16 \cdot P_1$).

Example 2:

If the radius (r_1) is decreased by 16% ($r_2 = r_1 - .16\,r_1 = 0.84r_1$), then

$$P_1 \cdot r_1{}^4 \simeq P_2 \cdot r_2{}^4$$

$$P_1 \cdot r_1{}^4 \simeq P_2\,(0.4979)r_1{}^4$$

$$\frac{P_1 r_1{}^4}{(0.4979 r_1)^4} = P_2$$

$$2\,P_1 = P_2$$

then the pressure (P_1) would increase to twice its original pressure ($P_2 \simeq 2 \cdot P_1$).

Courtesy of Des Jardins, *Clinical Manifestations of Respiratory Disease,* 2nd ed. © 1990 by Mosby Year Book Medical Publishers, Inc., Chicago

DUBOIS BODY SURFACE CHART

DIRECTIONS

To find body surface of a patient, locate the height in inches (or centimeters) on Scale I and the weight in pounds (or kilograms) on Scale II and place a straight edge (ruler) between these two points which will intersect Scale III at the patient's surface area.

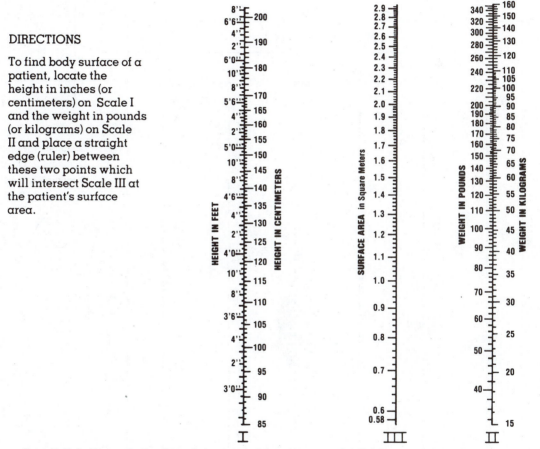

From DuBois, Eugene F.: *Basal Metabolism in Health and Disease*. Philadelphia: Lea and Febiger, 1924.

From DuBois, Eugene F.: *Basal Metabolism in Health and Disease*. Philadelphia: Lea and Febiger, 1924.

CARDIOPULMONARY PROFILE

A representative example of a cardiopulmonary profile sheet used to monitor the critically ill patient. See Chapters 5, 6, and 7 for explanations of the various components presented in this sample cardiopulmonary profile.

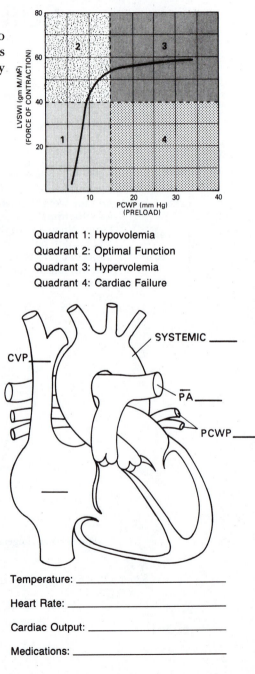

Quadrant 1: Hypovolemia
Quadrant 2: Optimal Function
Quadrant 3: Hypervolemia
Quadrant 4: Cardiac Failure

HEMODYNAMIC STATUS

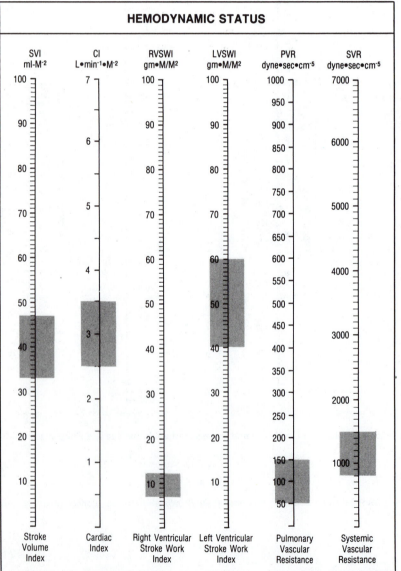

Temperature: _____

Heart Rate: _____

Cardiac Output: _____

Medications: _____

_____

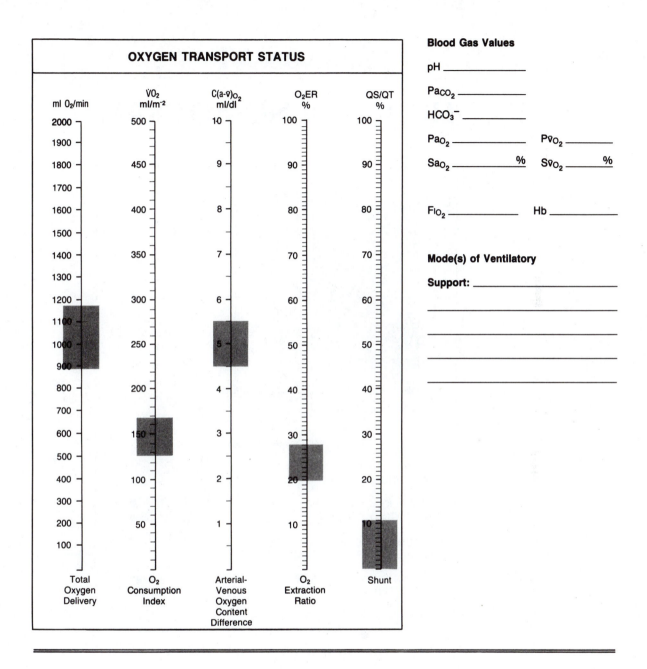

OXYGEN TRANSPORT STATUS

ml O₂/min	V̇O₂ ml/m⁻²	C(a-v̄)O₂ ml/dl	O₂ER %	QS/QT %

Total Oxygen Delivery | O₂ Consumption Index | Arterial-Venous Oxygen Content Difference | O₂ Extraction Ratio | Shunt

Blood Gas Values

pH _____

Paco₂ _____

HCO₃⁻ _____

Pao₂ _____   Pv̄o₂ _____

Sao₂ _____ %   Sv̄o₂ _____ %

Fio₂ _____   Hb _____

Mode(s) of Ventilatory

Support: _____

_____

_____

_____

_____

Patient's Name _____

Date _____

Time _____

APPENDIX VI

$P_{CO_2}/HCO_3^-/pH$ NOMOGRAM

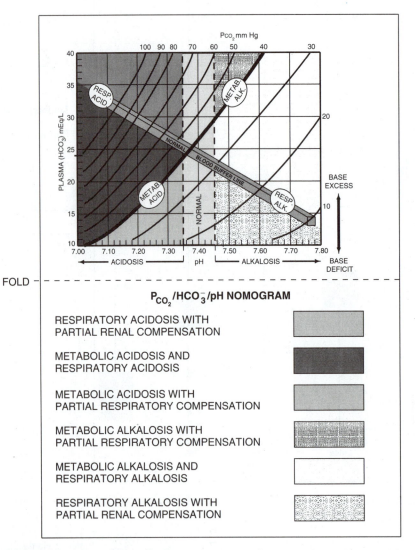

Copy the above $P_{CO_2}/HCO_3^-/pH$ nomogram, color it in if you like, and have it laminated for use as a handy, pocket-size reference tool.

See Chapter 8 on how to use the $P_{CO_2}/HCO_3^-/pH$ nomogram in the clinical setting.

ANSWERS TO SELF-ASSESSMENT QUESTIONS

CHAPTER 1

1. a	11. c
2. e	12. d
3. a	13. c
4. b	14. a
5. a	15. e
6. e	16. a
7. a	17. b
8. e	18. d
9. d	19. b
10. b	20. a

CHAPTER 2

1. a	12. d
2. b	13. d
3. d	14. 6,375 ml
4. d	15. Part I: 79 ml/cm H_2O
5. c	Part II: 70 ml/cm H_2O
6. c	Part III: decreasing
7. b	16. d
8. b	17. e
9. d	18. a
10. b	19. d
11. a	20. a

CHAPTER 3

1. c	7. c
2. b	8. e
3. a	9. a
4. e	10. b
5. b	11. a
6. c	

CHAPTER 4

1. d	6. b
2. b	7. d
3. e	8. b
4. e	9. b
5. c	10. b

CHAPTER 5

1. e	9. b
2. c	10. a
3. c	11. b
4. c	12. e
5. a	13. e
6. d	14. d
7. b	15. a
8. b	

CHAPTER 6

1. f	6. g
2. e	7. j
3. a	8. b
4. k	9. d
5. d	10. i

Multiple Choice

1. d
2. e
3. d
4. e
5. a

CHAPTER 7

1. a	6. e
2. c	7. e
3. c	8. c
4. b	9. d
5. b	10. e

Case Study: Automobile Accident Victim

Based on the questions asked and the information provided, the patient's $P_{A_{O_2}}$, $C_{c_{O_2}}$, $C_{a_{O_2}}$, and $C_{v_{O_2}}$ should first be calculated.

$$
\begin{aligned}
P_{A_{O_2}} &= (BP - P_{H_2O})\, F_{I_{O_2}} - P_{a_{CO_2}}\,(1.25) \\
&= (745 - 47)\, .50 - 38\,(1.25) \\
&= (698)\, .50 - 47.5 \\
&= 349 - 47.5
\end{aligned}
$$
Answer = 301.5 mm Hg

$$
\begin{aligned}
C_{c_{O_2}} &= (Hb \times 1.34) + (P_{A_{O_2}} \times 0.003) \\
&= (11 \times 1.34) + (301.5 \times 0.003) \\
&= 14.74 + 0.904
\end{aligned}
$$
Answer = 15.644 vol% O_2

$$
\begin{aligned}
C_{a_{O_2}} &= (Hb \times 1.34 \times S_{a_{O_2}}) + (P_{a_{O_2}} \times 0.003) \\
&= (11 \times 1.34 \times .90) + (60 \times 0.003) \\
&= 13.266 + 0.18
\end{aligned}
$$
Answer = 13.446 vol% O_2

$$
\begin{aligned}
C_{v_{O_2}} &= (Hb \times 1.34 \times S_{v_{O_2}}) + (P_{v_{O_2}} \times 0.003) \\
&= (11 \times 1.34 \times .65) + (35 \times 0.003) \\
&= 9.581 + 0.105
\end{aligned}
$$
Answer = 9.686 vol% O_2

With the above information and the data provided in the question, the following can now be calculated:

a. Total Oxygen = $QT \times (Ca_{O_2} \times 10)$
   Delivery $= 6\,L \times 13.446\ vol\% \times 10$
   $= 806.76\ ml\ O_2/minute$
   Answer: 806.76 ml O_2/minute

b. Arterial-Venous Oxygen Content Difference $C(a - \bar{v})_{O_2}$
   $C(a - \bar{v})_{O_2} = Ca_{O_2} - C\bar{v}_{O_2}$
   $= 13.446 - 9.686$
   $= 3.760\ vol\%\ O_2$
   Answer: 3.76 vol% O_2

c. Intrapulmonary Shunting $(\dot{Q}s/\dot{Q}t)$

   $\dot{Q}s/\dot{Q}T = \dfrac{Cc_{O_2} - Ca_{O_2}}{Cc_{O_2} - C\bar{v}_{O_2}}$
   $= \dfrac{15.644 - 13.446}{15.644 - 9.686}$
   $= \dfrac{2.198}{5.958}$
   $= .368$
   Answer: 36.8%

d. Oxygen Consumption $(\dot{V}_{O_2})$
   $\dot{V}_{O_2} = QT\,[C(a - \bar{v})_{O_2} \times 10]$
   $= 6\,L \times 3.760 \times 10$
   $= 225.6\ ml\ O_2/minute$
   Answer: 225.6 ml O_2/minute

e. Oxygen Extraction Rate $= \dfrac{Ca_{O_2} - C\bar{v}_{O_2}}{Ca_{O_2}}$
   $= \dfrac{13.446 - 9.686}{13.446}$
   $= \dfrac{3.760}{13.446}$
   $= .279$
   Answer: 27.9%

CHAPTER 8

1. e	6. d
2. b	7. e
3. a	8. e
4. c	9. e
5. e	10. b

CHAPTER 9

1. d	4. d
2. c	5. b
3. e	

CHAPTER 10

1. c	6. e
2. b	7. d
3. e	8. c
4. a	9. e
5. d	10. b

CHAPTER 11

1. b	6. c
2. b	7. d
3. a	8. e
4. d	9. e
5. a	10. d

CHAPTER 12

1. e	6. e
2. b	7. e
3. b	8. b
4. d	9. b
5. c	10. e

CHAPTER 13

1. e	6. c
2. e	7. d
3. e	8. d
4. b	9. e
5. d	10. c

CHAPTER 14

1. b	6. b
2. e	7. e
3. c	8. d
4. e	9. a
5. c	10. d

CHAPTER 15

	True or False
1. d	1. false
2. d	2. false
3. e	3. true
4. b	4. true
5. d	5. false

CHAPTER 16

1. c
2. e
3. b
4. e
5. e

True or False

1. true
2. true
3. false
4. true
5. true

BIBLIOGRAPHY

GENERAL ANATOMY AND PHYSIOLOGY

Anthony, C.P. and Thibodeau, G.A. *Anthony's Textbook of Anatomy and Physiology*. 13th ed. St. Louis: C.V. Mosby Co., 1990.

Clemente, C.D. *Anatomy: A Regional Atlas of the Human Body*, 3rd ed. Philadelphia: Wilkins/Wilcox, 1987.

Crouch, J.E. *Functional Human Anatomy*, 4th ed. Philadelphia: Lea and Febiger, 1985.

Gray, H. *Anatomy of the Human Body*, 30th ed. Philadelphia: Lea and Febiger, 1985.

Guyton, A.C. *Anatomy and Physiology*. Philadelphia: W.B. Saunders Co., 1985.

——— . *Physiology of the Human Body*, 6th ed. Philadelphia: W.B. Saunders Co., 1984.

Hole, J.W. *Essentials of Human Anatomy and Physiology*, 4th ed. Dubuque, Iowa: Wm. C. Brown Co., 1992.

Jacob, S.W., Francone, A.F., and Lossow, W.J. *Structure and Function in Man*, 5th ed. Philadelphia: W.B. Saunders Co., 1982.

McClintic, J.R. *Physiology of the Human Body*, 3rd ed. New York: John Wiley and Sons, 1985.

McClintic, J.R. *Human Anatomy*. St. Louis: C.V. Mosby Co., 1983.

McMinn, R.M.H., and Hutchings, R.T. *Color Atlas of Human Anatomy*, 2nd ed. Chicago: Year Book Medical Publishers, 1988.

Montgomery, R.L. *Basic Anatomy for the Allied Health Professions*. Baltimore: Urban and Schwarzenberg, 1981.

O'Rahilly, R. *Basic Human Anatomy*. Philadelphia: W.B. Saunders Co., 1983.

Snell, R.S. *Clinical Anatomy for Medical Students*, 2d ed. Boston: Little, Brown and Co., 1981.

Tortora, G.J. and Anagnostakos, N.P. *Principles of Anatomy and Physiology*, 6th ed. New York: Harper Collins, 1990.

Tortora, G.J. and Ronald, E.L. *Principles of Human Physiology*, 2d ed. New York: Harper and Row, 1986.

VanDeGraaff, K.M. *Human Anatomy*, 3rd ed. Dubuque, Iowa: Wm. C. Brown Co., 1992.

Vander, A.J., Sherman J.H. and Luciano, D.S. *Human Physiology: The Mechanisms of Body Function*, 5th ed. New York: McGraw-Hill Book Co., 1990.

Woodburne, R.T. *Essentials of Human Anatomy*, 8th ed. Oxford, England: Oxford University Press, 1988.

CARDIOPULMONARY ANATOMY AND PHYSIOLOGY

Bouhuys, A. *The Physiology of Breathing*. New York: Grune and Stratton, 1977.

Braun, H.A., Cheney, F.W., Jr. and Loehnen, C.P. *Introduction to Respiratory Physiology*, 2d ed. Boston: Little, Brown and Co., 1980.

Campbell, E.J.M., Agostoni, E., and Newsom-Davis, J.N. *The Respiratory Muscles: Mechanics and Neural Control*. Philadelphia: W.B. Saunders Co., 1970.

Cherniack, R.M., and Cherniack, L.C. *Respiration in Health and Disease*, 3d ed. Philadelphia: W.B. Saunders Co., 1983.

Comroe, J.H. *Physiology of Respiration*, 2d ed. Chicago: Year Book Medical Publishers, 1974.

Daily, E.K., and Schroeder, J.S. *Techniques in Bedside Hemodynamic Monitoring*, 4th ed. St. Louis, C.V. Mosby Co., 1989.

Davenport, H.W. *ABC of Acid-Base Chemistry*, 7th ed. Chicago: University of Chicago Press, 1978.

Fraser, R.G. and Pare, J.A.P. *Organ Physiology: Structure and Function of the Lung*, 2d ed. Philadelphia: W.B. Saunders Co., 1977.

Green, J.F. *Fundamental Cardiovascular and Pulmonary Physiology*, 2d ed. Philadelphia: Lea and Febiger, 1987.

Huber, Gary L. *Arterial Blood Gas and Acid-Base Physiology*. A Scope Current Concepts Publication. Kalamazoo: Upjohn Company, 1978.

Jacques, J.A. *Respiratory Physiology*. New York: McGraw-Hill Book Co., 1979.

Jones, N.L. *Blood Gases and Acid-Base Physiology*, 2nd ed. New York: Thieme-Stratton, 1987.

Levitzky, M.G. *Pulmonary Physiology*, 3rd ed. New York: McGraw-Hill Book Co., 1991.

Mines, A.H. *Respiratory Physiology*, 2nd ed. New York: Raven Press, 1986.

Murray, J.F. *The Normal Lung*, 2d ed. Philadelphia: W.B. Saunders Co., 1986.

Netter, F.H. *The CIBA Collection of Medical Illustrations*, vol. 7, Respiratory System, pp. 3–43. Summit, N.J.: CIBA Pharmaceutical Products, 1979.

Rosendorff, C. *Clinical Cardiovascular and Pulmonary Physiology*. New York: Raven Press, 1983.

Schweiss, J.F. *Continuous Measurement of Blood Oxygen Saturation in the High Risk Patient*, vol. 1. San Diego: Beach International, 1983.

Shapiro, B.A., Harrison, R.A., Roy, C.D., and Rozanna, T. *Clinical Application of Blood Gases*, 4th ed. Chicago: Year Book Medical Publishers, 1989.

Slonim, N.B., and Hamilton, L.H. *Respiratory Physiology*, 5th ed. St. Louis: C.V. Mosby Co., 1987.

West, J.B. *Respiratory Physiology, The Essentials*, 4th ed. Baltimore: Williams and Wilkins Co., 1990.

West, J.B. "State of the Art: Ventilation-Perfusion Relationships." *Am. Rev. Respir. Dis.*, 116:919–943 (1977).

SUPPLEMENTARY ANATOMY AND PHYSIOLOGY OF THE CARDIOVASCULAR SYSTEM

Berne, R.M., and Levy, M.N. *Cardiovascular Physiology*, 6th ed. St. Louis: C.V. Mosby Co., 1992.

Braunwald, E. "Regulation of the Circulation." *N. Engl. J. Med.* 290:1124, 1420 (1974).

Conover, M.H., and Zalis, E.G. *Understanding Electrocardiography: Physiological and Interpretive Concept*, 6th ed. St. Louis: C.V. Mosby Co., 1992.

Honig, C.R. *Modern Cardiovascular Physiology*, 2nd ed. Boston: Little, Brown and Co., 1988.

Hurst, J.W., and Logue, R.B., eds. *The Heart*, 7th ed. New York: McGraw-Hill Book Co., 1987.

Mohrman, D.E. and Heller, L.J. *Cardiovascular Physiology*, 3rd ed. New York: McGraw-Hill Book Co., 1991.

Netter, F.H. *The CIBA Collection of Medical Illustrations*, vol. 5, "The Heart." Summit, N.J.: CIBA Pharmaceutical Products, 1969.

Smith, J.J., and Kampine, J.P. *Circulatory Physiology: The Essentials*, 3rd ed. Baltimore: Williams and Wilkins, 1990.

RENAL SYSTEM

Coltman, K. "Urinary Tract Infections: New Thoughts on an Old Subject." *Practitioner* 223:351 (1979).

Grob, P.R. "Urinary Tract Infections in General Practice." *Practitioner* 221 (8): 237–244 (1978).

Kunin, C. *Detection, Prevention and Management of Urinary Tract Infections*, 4th ed., pp. 41, 99, 157. Philadelphia: Lea and Febiger, 1987.

Leaf, A., and Cotran, R. *Renal Pathophysiology*, pp. 167, 204. New York: Oxford University Press, 1980.

Marsh, D.J. *Renal Physiology*. New York: Raven Press, 1983.

Porth, C. *Pathophysiology—Concepts of Altered Health States*, 3rd ed. Philadelphia: J.B. Lippincott, 1982.

Rose, B.D. *Clinical Physiology of Acid-Base and Electrolyte Disorders*, 3rd Ed. New York: McGraw-Hill Book Co., 1989.

Sullivan, L.P., and Grantham, J.J. *Physiology of the Kidney*, 2d ed. Philadelphia: Lea and Febiger, 1982.

Turek, M. "Urinary Tract Infections." *Hosp. Pract.* 15(1): 49–58 (1980).

Valtin, H. *Renal Function*, 2d ed. Boston: Little, Brown and Co., 1983.

Vander, A.J. *Renal Physiology*, 4th ed. New York: McGraw-Hill Book Co., 1991.

Zeluff, G.W., Eknoyan, G., and Jackson, D. "Pericarditis in Renal Failure." *Heart Lung* 8(6):1139 (1979).

AGING AND CARDIOPULMONARY SYSTEM

Cassel, C.K., and Walsh, J.R. *Geriatric Medicine.* New York: Springer-Verlag, 1984.

Ebersole, P., and Hess, P. *Toward Healthy Aging,* 3rd ed. St. Louis: C.V. Mosby Co., 1990.

Fitzgerald, P.L. "Exercise for the Elderly." *Medical Clinics of North America* 69(1):189–196 (1985).

Gioiella, E.C., and Bevil, C.W. *Nursing Care of the Aging Client—Promoting Healthy Adaptation.* Norwalk, CT: Appleton-Century-Crofts, 1985.

Holm, K., and Kirchoff, K.T. "Perspective on Exercise and Aging." *Heart and Lung* 13(5):519–524 (1984).

McBee, S. "Here Come the Baby-Boomers." *U.S. News and World Report.* Nov. 5, 1984, pp. 68–73.

Newton, K.D. *Making the Mid-Years the Prime of Life.* Chicago: Budlong Press Co., 1978.

Powell, S. "Measuring Impact of the 'Baby Bust' on U.S. Future." *U.S. News and World Report.* Dec. 16, 1985, pp. 66–67.

Riffer, J. "Elderly 21 Percent of Population by 2040." *Hospital,* March 1, 1985, pp. 41–44.

Shepard, R.J. *Physical Activity and Aging,* 2nd ed. Gaithersburg, M.D., Aspen Pub., 1987.

Sivy, M. "The Middle-Aged Shape of Things To Come." *Money,* November 1985, pp. 66–72.

Stengel, R. "Snapshot of a Changing America—The U.S. Population is Growing Older and Thinking Smaller." *Time,* September 2, 1985, pp. 16–18.

CARDIOPULMONARY ANATOMY AND PHYSIOLOGY OF THE FETUS AND THE NEWBORN

Aloan, C.A. *Respiratory Care of the Newborn—A Clinical Manual,* 2nd ed. Philadelphia: J.B. Lippincott Co., 1992.

Avery, M.E., Wang, N., and Taeusch, H.W. "The Lung of the Newborn Infant." *Scientific American* 228:74–85 (Apr. 1973).

Bodegard, G. "Control of Respiration in Newborn Babies." IV, *Acta Paediatr. Scand.* 65:257 (1976).

Charnock, E.L., and Doershuk, C.F. "Development Aspects of the Human Lung." *Pediatr. Clin. North Am.* 20:275 (1973).

Crelin, E.S. "Development of the Lower Respiratory System." *Clin. Symp.* 27(4):3 (1975).

James, L.S., and Adamsons, K., Jr. "Respiratory Physiology of the Fetus and Newborn Infant." *N. Engl. J. Med.* 271:1352–1409 (1964).

Klaus, M.H., and Fanaroff, A.A. *Care of the High-risk Neonate*, 3rd ed. Philadelphia: W.B. Saunders Co., 1986.

Korones, S.B. *High-Risk Newborn Infants*, 4th ed. St. Louis: C.V. Mosby Co., 1986.

Lough, M.D., Williams, T.J., and Rawson, J.E. *Newborn Respiratory Care*. Chicago: Year Book Medical Publishers, 1974.

Lubchenco, L.O. *The High Risk Infant*. Philadelphia: W.B. Saunders Co., 1976.

Strang, L.B. "The Lungs at Birth." *Arch. Dis. Child.* 40:575 (1965).

Walsh, S.Z., Meyer, W.W., and Lind, J. *The Human Fetal and Neonatal Circulation*. Springfield, IL.: Charles C Thomas, 1974.

Wells, L.J., and Boyden, E.A. "The Development of the Bronchopulmonary Segments in Human Embryos of Horizons XVII to XIX." *Am. J. Anat.* 95:163 (1954).

EXERCISE AND ITS EFFECTS ON THE CARDIOPULMONARY SYSTEM

Appenzeller, O., and Atkinson, R. (eds.) *Health Aspects of Endurance Training*. New York, S. Karger, 1978.

Apple, D.F., Jr., and Cantwell, J.D. *Medicine for Sport*. Chicago, Year Book Medical Publishers, 1980.

Bevegard, GB.S., and Shepherd, J.T. Regulation of the circulation during exercise in man. *Physiol. Rev.* 47:178 (1967).

Clarke, D.H. *Exercise Physiology*. Englewood Cliffs, NJ., Prentice-Hall, 1975.

Fox, E.L. *Sports Physiology*, 2nd ed. Philadelphia, W.B. Saunders, 1984.

Rasch, P.J., and Burke, R.K. *Kinesiology and Applied Anatomy: The Science of Human Movement*, 7th ed. Philadelphia, Lea & Febiger, 1989.

Strauss, R.H. (ed.) *Sports and Medicine and Physiology*, 2nd ed. Philadelphia, W.B. Saunders, 1991.

Wyndham, C.H. The physiology of exercise under heat stress. *Annu. Rev. Physiol.*, 35:193 (1973).

HIGH ALTITUDE AND ITS EFFECTS ON THE CARDIOPULMONARY SYSTEM

Cassin, S.R., Gilbert, D., Bunnell, C.F., and Johnson, E.M. Capillary development during exposure to chronic hypoxia. *Am J Physiol* 220:448–451 (1971).

DeGraff, A.C., Grover, R.F., Johnson, R.L., Hammond, J.W., and Miller, J.M., Diffusing capacity of the lung in Caucasians native to 3100 m. *J Appl Physiol* 29:71–76 (1970).

Frisancho, A.R. Functional adaptation to high altitude hypoxia. *Science* 187:313 (1975).

Groves, B.M., Reeves, J.T., Sutton, J.R., Wagner, P.D., Cymerman, A., Malconian, M.K., Rock, P.B., Young, P.M., and Houston, C.S. Operation Everest II: elevated high-altitude pulmonary resistance unresponsive to oxygen. *J Appl Physiol* 63:521–530 (1987).

Guleria, J.S., Pande, J.N., Sethi, P.K., and Roy, S.B. Pulmonary diffusing capacity at high altitude. *J Appl Physiol* 31:536–543 (1971).

Kreuzer F. Van Lookeren, and Champagne, P. Resting pulmonary diffusing capacity for CO and O_2 at high altitude. *J Appl Physiol* 20:519–524 (1965).

Lahiri, S. Physiological responses and adaptations to high altitude. *Int. Rev. Physiol.* 15:217 (1977).

Oelz, O., Howald, H., di Prampero, P.E., Hoppeler, H., Claassen, A.H., Jenni, R., Biihlmann, A., Ferretti, G., Bruckner, J.C., Veicsteinas, A., Gussoni, M., and Certetelli, P. Physiological profile of world-class high-altitude climbers. *J Appl Physiol* 60:1734–1742 (1986).

Reite, M., Jackson, D., Cahoon, R.L., and Weil, J.V. Sleep physiology at high altitude. *Electroencephalogr Clin Neurophysiol* 38:463–471 (1975).

Reynafarje, B. Myoglobin content and enzymatic activity of muscle and altitude adaptation. *J Appl Physiol* 17:301–305 (1962).

Schoene, R.B., Lahiri, S., Hackett, P.H., Peters, R.M., Jr., Milledge, J.S. Pizzo, C.J., Sarnquist, F.H., Boyer, S.J., Graber, D.J., Maret, K.H., and West, J.B. Relationship of hypoxic ventilatory response to exercise performance on Mount Everest. *J Appl Physiol: Respir Environ Exercise Physiol* 56:1478–1483 (1984).

Singh, I., Khanna, P.K., Srivastava, M.C., Lah, M., Roy, S.B., and Subramanyam, C.S.V. Acute mountain sickness. *N Engl J Med* 280:175–184 (1969).

Vogel, J.A., and Harris, C.W. Cardiopulmonary responses of resting man during early exposure to high altitude. *J Appl Physiol* 22:1124–1128 (1967).

Vogel, J.A., Hartley, L.H., and Cruz, J.C. Cardiac output during exercise in altitude natives at sea level and high altitude. *J Appl Physiol* 36:173–176 (1974).

Wagner, P.D., Saltzman, H.A., and West, J.B. Measurement of continuous distributions of ventilation-perfusion ratios: theory. *J Appl Physiol* 36:588–599 (1974).

Ward, M.P., Milledge, J.S., and West, J.B. *High Altitude Medicine and Physiology*. London: Chapman & Hall Medical, 1989.

Weil, J.V., Kryger, M.H., and Scoggin, C.H. Sleep and breathing at high altitude. In: Guilleminault C., Dement W., eds. *Sleep Apnea Syndromes*. New York: Alan R. Liss, 1978, pp. 119–136.

West, J.B. Climbing Mt. Everest without supplementary oxygen: an analysis of maximal exercise during extreme hypoxia. *Respir Physiol* 52:265–279 (1983).

West, J.B. Diffusing capacity of the lung for carbon monoxide at high altitude. *J Appl Physiol* 17:421–426 (1962).

West, J.B., Boyer, S.J., Graber, D.J., Hackett, P.H., Maret, K.H., Milledge, J.S., Peters, R.M. Jr., Pizzo, C.J., Samaja, M., Sarnquist, F.H., Schoene, R.B., and Winslow, R.M. Maximal exercise at extreme altitudes on Mount Everest. *J Appl Physiol: Respir Environ Exercise Physiol* 55:688–698 (1983).

West, J.B., Lahiri, S., Maret, K.H., Peters, R.M. Jr., and Pizzo, C.J. Barometric pressures at extreme altitudes on Mt. Everest: physiological significance. *J Appl Physiol: Respir Environ Exercise Physiol* 54:1188–1194 (1983).

West, J.B., Peters, R.M. Jr., Aksnes, G., Maret, K.H., Milledge, J.S., and Schoene, R.B. Noctural periodic breathing at altitudes of 6300 meters and 8050 meters. *J Appl Physiol* 61:280–287 (1986).

Winslow, R.M., and Monge, C.C. *Hypoxia, Polycythemia, and Chronic Mountain Sickness.* Washington, DC: Johns Hopkins University Press, 1987, pp. 184–196.

HIGH-PRESSURE ENVIRONMENTS AND THEIR EFFECT ON THE CARDIOPULMONARY SYSTEM

Bakker, D.J. Clostridial myonecrosis. In: Davis, J.C., Hunt, T.K., eds. *Problem Wounds. The Role of Oxygen.* New York: Elsevier, 1988, pp. 153–172.

Craig, A.B. Jr. Depth limits of breath-hold diving (an example of Fennology). *Respir Physiol* 5:14–22 (1968).

Davis, J.C., Dunn, J.M., and Heimbach, R.D. Hyperbaric medicine: patient selection, treatment procedures, and side-effects. In: Davis, J.C., Hunt, T.K., eds. *Problem Wounds. The Role of Oxygen.* New York: Elsevier, 1988, pp. 225–235.

Davis, J.C., Hunt, T.K., eds. *Problem Wounds. The Role of Oxygen.* New York: Elsevier, 1988.

Gamarra, J.A. *Decompression Sickness.* Hagerstown, MD: Harper & Row, 1974.

Hempelman, H.V., and Lockwood, A.P.M. *The Physiology of Diving in Man and Other Animals.* London, Edward Arnold, 1978.

Lundgren, C.E.G., Farhi, L.E. Pulmonary circulation in diving and hyperbaric environment. In: Weir, E.K., Reeves, J.T., eds. *Pulmonary Vascular Physiology and Pathophysiology, Lung Biology in Health and Disease.* New York: Marcel Dekker, 1989, pp. 199–240.

Mader, J.T., ed. *Hyperbaric Oxygen Therapy Committee Report.* Bethesda, MD: Undersea and Hyperbaric Medical Society, 1989.

Marx, R.E., and Johnson, R.P. Problem wounds in oral and maxillofacial surgery: the role of hyperbaric oxygen. In: Davis, J.C., Hunt, T.K., eds. *Problem Wounds. The Role of Oxygen.* New York: Elsevier. 1988, pp. 65–123.

Nemiroff, M.J., Saltz, G.R., and Weg, J.G. Survival after cold-water near-drowning: the protective effect of the diving reflex. *Am Rev Respir Dis* 115:145 (1977).

Olszowka, A.J., and Rahn, H. Breath hold diving. In: Sutton, J.R., Houston, C.S., Coates, G., eds. *Hypoxia and Cold.* New York: Praeger, 1987, pp. 417–428.

Physiological and human engineering aspects of underwater breathing apparatus.

In: Lundgren, C., Warkander, D., eds. *Proceedings of an Undersea and Hyperbaric Medical Society Workshop*. Bethesda, MD: Undersea and Hyperbaric Medical Society, 1989; 270.

Schaefer, K.E., Allison, R.D., Dougherty, J.H. Jr., Carey, C.R., Walker, R., Yost, F., and Parker, D. Pulmonary and circulatory adjustments determining the limits of depths in breathhold diving. *Science* 162:1020–1023 (1968).

Shilling, C.W., and Beckett, M.W. (eds.) *Underwater Physiology IV*, Bethesda, MD: Federation of American Societies for Experimental Biology, 1978.

The physiological basis of decompression. In: Vann, R.D., ed. *Thirty-eighth Undersea and Hyperbaric Medical Society Workshop*. Bethesda, MD: Undersea and Hyperbaric Medical Society, 1989, 437 pp.

Thom, S.R. Hyperbaric oxygen therapy. *J Intensive Care Med* 4:58–74 (1989).

CARDIOVASCULAR REHABILITATION

American Association of Cardiovascular and Pulmonary Rehabilitation. Scientific evidence of the value of cardiac rehabilitation services with emphasis on patients following myocardial infarction. Section I. Exercise conditioning component (position paper). *J Cardiopulm Rehabil* 10:79–87 (1990).

Burgess, A.W., Lerner, D.J., D'Agostino, R.B., Vokonas, P.S., Hartman, C.R., Gaccione, P. A randomized control trial of cardiac rehabilitation. *Soc Sci Med* 24:359–370 (1987).

DeBusk, R.F., Haskell, W.L., Miller, N.H., Berra, K., Taylor, C.B., Berger, W.E. III, and Lew, H. Medically directed at home rehabilitation soon after clinically uncomplicated acute myocardial infarction: a new model for patient care. *Am J Cardiol* 55:251–257 (1985).

Ehsani, A.A., Martin, W.H. III, Health, G.W., and Coyle, E.F. Cardiac effects of prolonged and intense exercise training in paients with coronary artery disease. *Am J Cardiol* 50:246–254 (1982).

Froelicher, V., Jensen, D., Genter, F., Sullivan, M., McKirnan, M.D., Witztum, K., Scharf, J., Strong, M.L., and Ashburn, W. A randomized trial of exercise training in patients with coronary heart disease. *JAMA* 252:1291–1297 (1984).

Health and Public Policy Committee, American College of Physicians: Cardiac rehabilitation services (position paper). *Ann Intern Med* 109:671–673 (1988).

O'Connor, G.T., Buring, J.E., Yusuf, S., Goldhaber, S.Z., Olmstead, E.M., Paffenbarger, R.S. Jr., and Hennekens, C.H. An overview of randomized trials of rehabilitation with exercise after myocardial infarction. *Circulation* 80:234–244 (1989).

Paffenbarger, R.S. Jr., and Hyde, R.T. Exercise in the prevention of coronary heart disease. *Prev Med* 13:3–22 (1984).

Rehabilitation: Status, 1990. *May Clin Proc* 65:731–755 (1990).

Squires, R.W., Gau, G.T., Miller, T.D., Allison, T.G., and Lavie, C.J. Cardiovascular.

Squires, R.W., Gau, G.T., and Orszulak, T.A. Cardiac rehabilitation: benefits of a structured, brief inpatient program after coronary bypass surgery (abstract). *Med Sci Sports Exerc* 19(Suppl):S20 (1987).

Squires, R.W., and Lavie, C.J. New trends in cardiac rehabilitation exercise. *Cardio* 5:85–87; 91–92; 112 (July 1988).

Sullivan, M.J., Higginbotham, M.B., Cobb, F.R. Exercise training in patients with severe left ventricular dysfunction: hemodynamic and metabolic effects. *Circulation* 78:506–515 (1988).

Thompson, P.D. The benefits and risks of exercise training in patients with chronic coronary artery disease. *JAMA* 259:1537–1540 (1988).

Williams, R.S. Exercise training of patients with ventricular dysfunction and heart failure. *Cardiovasc Clin* 15(2):219–231 (1985).

SUPPLEMENTARY RESPIRATORY CARE

Burton, G.G., Hodgkin, J.E.K., and Ward, J.J. *Respiratory Care: A Guide to Clinical Practice*, 3rd ed. Philadelphia: J.B. Lippincott Co., 1991.

Rau, J.L. *Respiratory Therapy Pharmacology*, 3rd ed. Chicago: Year Book Medical Publishers, 1989.

Ruppel, G. *Manual of Pulmonary Function*, 5th ed. Mosby-Year Book, Inc. 1991.

Shapiro, B.A., Kacmark, R.M., Cane, R.D., and Hauptman, D. *Clinical Application of Respiratory Care*, 4th ed. Chicago: Mosby-Year Book, Inc. 1991.

INDEX